CELL BIOLOGY RESEARCH PROGRESS

OXIDATIVE STRESS

CAUSES, ROLE IN DISEASES AND BIOLOGICAL EFFECTS

CELL BIOLOGY RESEARCH PROGRESS

CELL BIOLOGY RESEARCH PROGRESS

OXIDATIVE STRESS

CAUSES, ROLE IN DISEASES AND BIOLOGICAL EFFECTS

CASSIDY CROFT
EDITOR

NOVA BIOMEDICAL

New York

For permission to use material from this book please contact us:
Telephone 631-231-7269; Fax 631-231-8175
Web Site: http://www.novapublishers.com

Additional color graphics may be available in the e-book version of this book.

Library of Congress Cataloging-in-Publication Data

ISBN: 978-1-63117-578-7

Library of Congress Control Number: 2014934751

Published by Nova Science Publishers, Inc. † New York

Contents

Preface

Active oxygen species are produced as inescapable by-products of a normal aerobic metabolism, and their production is further enhanced by exposure to certain environmental conditions, or as a result of some diseases. Oxidative stress is defined as an imbalance between the production of free radicals (FR) and antioxidant defenses in favor of the former, which can result from an excess of prooxidant, antioxidant deficiency or both factors. There are many kinds of FR, but these can be grouped together under the name of reactive oxygen species (ROS) or reactive nitrogen species (RNS), determined by the ability of each species according to the four basic characteristics: reactivity, specificity, selectivity and diffusivity. This book aims to discuss the biological effects, role in diseases, and causes of oxidative stress. Some of the topics provided include oxidative stress in biofilms; age relation to oxidative stress; controlling of oxidative stress in non-alcoholic steatohepatitis; and the role of nitric oxide toxicity and oxidative stress in graft vs. host disease.

Chapter 1 – During recent years researchers have shown reactive oxygen species (ROS) to have an essential role in the origin of a large number of diseases. This has resulted in extensive research within the molecular mechanisms of ROS. Excessive amounts of ROS are known to damage mtDNA, proteins and lipids and to activate the cell death pathways. It has been known since the 70s that the main source of cellular superoxide is the mitochondrion, more specifically the mitochondrial electron transport chain (ETC). The mitochondrial ROS originates mainly from electrons leaking from complex I and III during oxidative phosphorylation (OXPHOS), and probably also from Electron Transfer Flavoprotein (ETF) and Electron Transfer Flavoprotein ubiquinone oxidoredutase (ETF-QO); the latter of which is also a part of the ETC within the mitochondria. At physiological low levels, ROS is known to have an essential function as beneficial redox signaling molecules in cellular signaling and gene regulation systems, maintaining cell homeostasis. However, when ROS generation overwhelms the cellular defense system, either by generation of excessive amounts of ROS, by decrease in the antioxidant defense system or when challenged by external or internal factors like starvation, infections or inherited gene defects, oxidative stress occurs. Upon additional increases in cellular ROS levels, the cellular systems can no longer manage with the increasing amount of ROS, resulting in reversible cell damage, activating cellular death pathways. Thus, the amounts of cellular ROS determine the consequences of cellular adaption to oxidative stress.

Mitochondrial defects and oxidative stress are central factors in human health and disease. Any disease could theoretically be related to mitochondria defect, and mitochondrial dysfunction has already been shown to be the core of a surprising range of both common and rare disorders as the mitochondria are responsible for energy production, are key sources of oxidative stress, regulate apoptosis and calcium homeostasis, and are central in many other aspects of well-being/survival of cells. There is evidence that oxidative stress plays a prominent role in neuromuscular disorders such as: amyotrophic lateral sclerosis (ALS), mitochondrial/metabolic disease and Friedreich's ataxia. It's not clear, however, whether oxidative stress is the main cause of symptoms or merely a symptom itself. Oxidative stress is without doubt a common factor in the pathophysiological mechanism of neuromuscular disorders, like many other diseases. However, despite this association between disease and oxidative stress, knowledge about how oxidative stress is produced and the types of reactive oxygen species (ROS) that are involved in neuromuscular diseases is lacking.

Chapter 2 – Active oxygen species are produced as inescapable by-products of a normal aerobic metabolism, and their production is further enhanced by exposure to certain environmental conditions, or as a result of some diseases. Oxidative stress is defined as an imbalance between the production of free radicals (FR) and antioxidant defenses in favor of the former, which can result from an excess of prooxidant, antioxidant deficiency or both factors. There are many kinds of FR, but these can be grouped together under the name of reactive oxygen species (ROS) or reactive nitrogen species (RNS), determined by the ability of each species according to the four basic characteristics: reactivity, specificity, selectivity and diffusivity.

The defense mechanisms of living organisms have developed antioxidant physiological defenses that prevent the formation of FR, recognize oxidative damage and repair. Antioxidant defenses can be classified according to their nature as enzymatic or non-enzymatic antioxidants, and depending on their origin, as endogenous or exogenous antioxidants. The reactive species not neutralized by antioxidant defenses can damage the cellular membranes by oxidation lipids, critical enzymes of the intermediary metabolism or other proteins, and also break DNA chains.

Oxidative stress is involved in various disease processes such as cardiovascular and neurological disorders, diabetes, ischemia and cancer; it being one of the most important causative agents of mutagenesis, tumorigenesis and even aging. Furthermore, it has been also associated with the chronic inflammation caused by the biofilms of the FR that are generated during bactericidal attack of macrophages and neutrophils.

Biofilms are microbial communities containing sessile cells embedded in a self-produced extracellular polymeric matrix (containing polysaccharides, DNA and other components). In comparison with their planktonic (free-living) counterparts, sessile cells are often much more resistant to various stress conditions, with this increased resistance having a considerable impact on the treatment of biofilm-related infections.

In the first part of this review, the reactivates of active species of oxygen and the antioxidant system of the oxidative stress responses will be highlighted briefly, and their physiological role in biofilms discussed. Subsequently, the similarities and differences between oxidative stress responses in bacteria and eukaryotic microorganism biofilms will be reviewed, and finally the phenotypic adaptation of microbial biofilms is discussed in response to stress resulting from exposure to environmental pollutants, disinfectants and antibiotics is discussed Despite some progress, better understanding of the genotypic and phenotypic adaptation of sessile (biofilm-associated) microorganisms to various forms of stress is still required in order to develop more effective anti-biofilm strategies.

Chapter 3 – The oxidative stress may cause injury to the retinal pigment epithelium, the Bruch's membrane and the choroid, which are layers in the eye involved in the pathophysiology of age related degeneration macular (AMD). These oxidative processes are thought to contribute to the clinical manifestation of pigment dispersion, accumulation of intracellular lysosomal lipofuscin and extracellular drusen deposits.

The purpose of this chapter is to analyze the possible routes of oxidative stress in the AMD and the biomarkers of oxidative eye damage. The mitochondria may be especially important in this process because the reactive oxygen species (ROS) produced in their electron transport chain can damage cellular components. In several studies, the increase in mitochondrial DNA (mtDNA) damage and mutations (for example, production of oxidized derivatives of the DNA bases, 8-oxoguanine), and the decrease in the efficacy of DNA repair have been correlated with the occurrence and the stage of AMD. Also, lymphocytes from AMD patients displayed a higher amount of total endogenous basal and oxidative DNA damage, exhibited a higher sensitivity to hydrogen peroxide and UV radiation, and repaired the lesions. Furthermore, there is increasing evidence that constant oxidative stress impairs autophagy and heterophagy, as well as increases protein aggregation and causes inflammaome activation leading to the pathological phenotype of AMD. Other mechanism is the iron accumulation in AMD, that it is a toxic in the visual phototransduction cascade and catalyzes the conversion of hydrogen peroxide to hydroxyl radical, which is the most damaging of the ROS. This has therapeutic potential for diminishing iron-induced oxidative damage to prevent or treat AMD.

Finally, dietary factors play an important role in the control of oxidative stress. In a large clinical trial, dietary supplements of antioxidants including carotenoids, vitamin C, vitamin E and zinc, experienced reduced progression to advanced AMD. The effect of lutein was a significant reduction in malonyldialdehide (MDA) level and increase in the gene expression of antioxidant enzyme activities (SODs and catalase). In the chapter analyzed all antioxidant therapies and future lines of investigation in oxidative stress.

Chapter 4 – Myocardial infarction (MI) remains one of the leading causes of death and disability throughout the world. MI and related complications (e.g., heart failure) are great socio-economic burdens to society and healthcare systems. Blood flow restoration through the culprit coronary artery is necessary to save endangered myocardium after acute myocardial infarction. It is well established that early reperfusion limits infarct size and improves clinical outcome of patients with acute MI. The process of restoring blood flow to the ischemic myocardium, however, can induce injury, myocardial reperfusion injury, which can paradoxically reduce the beneficial effects of myocardial reperfusion and cause contractile dysfunction and cellular damage. Despite intensive research, therapeutic strategies are limited and there is as yet no routine effective, generally accepted and promising approach for myocardial ischemia/reperfusion (I/R) injury. In recent years, there is a growing interest in the treatment of myocardial I/R-induced cardiac dysfunction with plant-based therapy including traditional Chinese medicine, for which extensive experience has been accumulated over thousands of years. In this chapter the authors propose a systematic approach to the molecular basis of the cardioprotective effects of antioxidant traditional Chinese medicine that could offer a novel therapeutic opportunity against this oxidative tissue damage.

Chapter 5 – Non-alcoholic steatohepatitis (NASH) is a severe form of non-alcoholic fatty liver disease (NAFLD), in which most patients exhibit non-progressive non-alcoholic fatty liver (NAFL) representing simple steatosis of the liver. Multiple hits, including genetic differences, fat accumulation, insulin resistance and intestinal microbiota changes, account for the progression NASH. NAFLD is strongly associated with obesity, which induces adipokine secretion, endoplasmic reticulum (ER) and oxidative stress at the cellular level, and induces hepatic steatosis, inflammation and fibrosis. Among these factors, oxidative stress is considered a key contributor to the progression from NAFL to NASH. Although several clinical trials have shown that anti-oxidative therapy with vitamin E can effectively control the effects of hepatitis in the short term, the long-term effects remains obscure. Several trials of long-term anti-oxidant protocols aimed at treating cerebrovascular diseases or cancer development have failed to demonstrate benefits. This might be attributed to the non-selective anti-oxidant properties or excessive anti-oxidative effects of these drugs. Molecular hydrogen has recently been identified as an effective antioxidant that specifically reduces cytotoxic reactive oxygen species (ROS). Several diseases associated with oxidative stress, such as ischemia reperfusion injury of brain or heart, Parkinson's disease, post-chemotherapeutic renal injury, or transplant rejection, are responsive to hydrogen. The progress of NASH and transition of NASH to hepatocellular carcinoma can be controlled using hydrogen-rich water in mouse models. Long-term clinical intervention is required to control this complex lifestyle-related disease.

Chapter 6 – Multiple sclerosis (MS) is a heterogeneous disease with the different and unpredictable clinical courses. Investigations of MS are very wide due to its complex pathogenesis that involves several components: autoimmune, inflammatory, demyelinisation, neurodegeneration and oxidative stress. The development of effective antioxidative therapy for MS patients is intricated by the heterogenity of pathophysiological mechanisms involved. There is a strong need for further research in this field especially in progressive subtypes of MS that have no effective pharmacological treatment. In this chapter the authors try to focus on the oxidative stress not only as a specific biochemical process of this complex disease but also as a potential target of the therapies in MS, therefore some exogenous compounds have been proposed as such approach to MS treatment.

The redox therapeutic approach can target: degenerative, inflammatory/autoimmune and neurodegenerative components. Redox therapy should not be applied uniformly, and must be developed to target specific mechanisms. The results of redox studies could lead to new therapies in MS, as well as to knowledge about life style adjustments that would contribute to well being of the MS patients.

Chapter 7 – Allogeneic Hematopoietic Stem Cell Transplantation (HSCT) is widely used for treatment of malignant and non-malignant hematological diseases. Allogeneic transplantation is associated with the beneficial Graft vs. Leukemia/lymphoma (GVL) effect that prevents disease relapse. Often though, allogeneic HSCT leads to graft-versus-host disease (GVHD) which remains a major cause of morbidity and mortality in allogeneic HSCT patients. Clinically, GVHD manifestations present acute and/or chronic form. Acute GVHD is characterized by multi-organ damage targeting mainly skin, liver and gastrointestinal tract, while chronic GVHD can target many organ systems, including acute GVHD target organs as well as connective tissue and exocrine glands.

Monocytes/Macrophages are phagocytic cells that serve as a first-line defense against invading pathogens through the generation of reactive oxygen species (ROS), reactive nitrogen species (RNS, e.g., nitric oxide, NO•), and production of inflammatory cytokines. In pathological inflammatory conditions, overproduction of ROS/RNS coupled with deficiency in enzymatic and non-enzymatic antioxidants can be harmful. In allogeneic HSCT and GVHD, the ROS/RNS balance is disturbed.

Here the authors review the cumulative knowledge from the past two decades, on the effect of allogeneic HSCT on blood markers for free radicals' toxicity in patients. The role of RNS in the patho-etiology of GVHD, as it emerges from studies in experimental models is presented. In addition, the issue whether drug intervention in ROS/RNS pathways could improve the clinical results after allogeneic HSCT is addressed. The authors describe the PreImplantation Factor and its projected therapeutic role in reducing GVHD by modulating inflammation and reducing NO production. Evidence suggests that restored free radicals balance is an efficient way to improve clinical GVHD manifestations.

Chapter 8 – Inner ear hair cells are know to be highly energy demanding and oxygen consuming cells. The damage of the inner ear cells cell can occur as a result of local ROS (reactive oxygen species) production. The main source of these molecules within the cochlea appear to be the hair cells' mitochondria, or enzymes such as xanthine oxidase and NADPH oxidase.

Once generated, ROS are responsible for direct cellular damage to lipids, proteins and DNA, triggering apoptosis or necrosis and may also diffuse among the inner ear scalae. In animal models, several conditions of ROS production related to cochlear damage have been reported, including exposure to noise and drugs (amynoglycosides and cisplatin). In humans, ROS appear to be involved in hairs cell damage in some cases of genetic hearing loss (i.e., Pendred syndrome, presbycusis and Meniere's syndrome). Several animal or in vitro models have been proposed for treatment against ROS-mediated damage (interruption of the lipid peroxidation process and preservation of the cell membrane integrity; prevention of noise induced inner ear damage by cochlear ischemia/ re-perfusion; and prevention of cell apoptosis).

In otosclerosis (localized bone dysplasia of the human otic capsule) the ROS could be produced in the otosclerotic foci and diffuse to the inner ear compartment through the cochlear endosteum, causing cochlear damage and sensorineural hearing loss. Indeed, recent studies for the first time confirmed the presence of ROS secondary messengers (4-hydroxynonenal) in the otosclerotic specimens. Different distribution pattern of HNE antibodies has been observed in otosclerotic specimens compared to the control ones, suggesting its potential role in the pathophysiology of the disease. However, further studies (both experimental and clinical ones) are needed in order to better understand and clarify the role of ROS in the pathophysiology of otosclerosis and different hearing disorders.

Chapter 9 – Eales' Disease (ED) is an idiopathic, inflammatory, venous occlusive disease which primarily affects the peripheral retina of young adult males. The disease is more prevalent in the Indian subcontinent. ED was described by Henry Eales in 1880. Despite of the rigorous research effects, the etiopathogenesis of disease remains ambiguous. ED presents with inflammation, non-perfusion in peripheral veins, and retinal neovascularization. Loss of vision is due to repeated vitreous haemorrhage and its sequlae. Various research findings associate the disease with autoimmunity, oxidative stress and exposure to Mycobacterium *tuberculin* for the cause of the disease. There is no specific laboratory test available till date for its diagnosis. Therefore, the diagnosis of ED is arrived at by excluding other similar diseases. The scope of the present review is in highlighting the new findings on the strong association of oxidative stress with the disease.

There is strong evidence, for the involvement of oxidative stress and ED, both at the level of the local environment (i.e., vitreous humour and epiretinal membrane) and at systemic circulation. Elevated levels of thiobarbituric acid reactive substances (TBARS) were observed in serum, vitreous and monocytes samples of ED, as compared to controls. The authors have reported damage to DNA and proteins, from the accumulated 8-hydroxy-2'deoxyguanosine and 3-Nitrotyrosine in leucocytes respectively. Elevated levels of homocysteine (Hcy), and its metabolite thiolactone (HcyTL), are observed in the disease and are associated with the functional impairment of proteins due to homocysteinylation. Plasma Hcy and HcyTL levels are positively correlated with TBARS, while plasma glutathione (GSH) is negatively correlated with Hcy and HcyTL levels. Increased oxidative stress is also evidenced from the accumulation of advanced glycation and lipid oxidation end products in epiretinal membranes, observed in patients with ED who underwent vitrectomy. The antioxidant enzymes superoxide dismutase (SOD) and glutathione peroxidase (GPX) and GSH levels were found to be reduced in the vitreous and the erythrocytes of patients with ED. Most interestingly, significant increase in the levels of intra-cellular iron and copper in circulating monocytes was observed in the vitreous of patients afflicted with ED. A novel iron binding protein, 88 kDa in molecular weight and with a presumable antioxidant function has been characterized for its possible role in ED as a biomarker, and its involvement in its etiopathogenesis. Several iron binding proteins in circulation have been analyzed systematically and have been found to vary in ED, indicating a strong role for iron in the disease. A complete study into the significance of iron binding proteins in the mechanism of the disease is needed to decode their relevance in etiopathogenesis, and for subsequent application of this knowledge in therapeutics.

In: Oxidative Stress
Editor: Cassidy Croft
ISBN: 978-1-63117-578-7

Chapter 1

Oxidative Stress and Mitochondrial Defect in Neuromuscular Disorders: Source or Symptoms?

***Nanna Cornelius*[*1], *Niels Gregersen*[†2], *Zeynep Tümer*[‡1] *and Rikke K. J. Olsen*[§2]**

[1] Applied Human Molecular Genetics, Kennedy Center, Copenhagen University Hospital, Rigshospitalet, Glostrup, Denmark

[2]Research Unit for Molecular Medicine, Department of Clinical Medicine, Aarhus University and Aarhus University Hospital, Aarhus, Denmark

Abstract

During recent years researchers have shown reactive oxygen species (ROS) to have an essential role in the origin of a large number of diseases. This has resulted in extensive research within the molecular mechanisms of ROS. Excessive amounts of ROS are known to damage

[*] Correspondence to: Nanna Cornelius (e-mail: nanna.cornelius@regionh.dk), Applied Human Molecular Genetics, Kennedy Center, Copenhagen University Hospital, Rigshospitalet, Glostrup, Denmark.

[†] E-mail: NIG@ki.au.dk.

[‡] E-mail: Zeynep.Tumer@regionh.dk.

[§] email: Rikke.Olsen@ki.au.dk.

mtDNA, proteins and lipids and to activate the cell death pathways. It has been known since the 70s that the main source of cellular superoxide is the mitochondrion, more specifically the mitochondrial electron transport chain (ETC). The mitochondrial ROS originates mainly from electrons leaking from complex I and III during oxidative phosphorylation (OXPHOS), and probably also from Electron Transfer Flavoprotein (ETF) and Electron Transfer Flavoprotein ubiquinone oxidoredutase (ETF-QO); the latter of which is also a part of the ETC within the mitochondria. At physiological low levels, ROS is known to have an essential function as beneficial redox signaling molecules in cellular signaling and gene regulation systems, maintaining cell homeostasis. However, when ROS generation overwhelms the cellular defense system, either by generation of excessive amounts of ROS, by decrease in the antioxidant defense system or when challenged by external or internal factors like starvation, infections or inherited gene defects, oxidative stress occurs. Upon additional increases in cellular ROS levels, the cellular systems can no longer manage with the increasing amount of ROS, resulting in reversible cell damage, activating cellular death pathways. Thus, the amounts of cellular ROS determine the consequences of cellular adaption to oxidative stress.

Mitochondrial defects and oxidative stress are central factors in human health and disease. Any disease could theoretically be related to mitochondria defect, and mitochondrial dysfunction has already been shown to be the core of a surprising range of both common and rare disorders as the mitochondria are responsible for energy production, are key sources of oxidative stress, regulate apoptosis and calcium homeostasis, and are central in many other aspects of well-being/survival of cells. There is evidence that oxidative stress plays a prominent role in neuromuscular disorders such as: amyotrophic lateral sclerosis (ALS), mitochondrial/metabolic disease and Friedreich's ataxia. It's not clear, however, whether oxidative stress is the main cause of symptoms or merely a symptom itself. Oxidative stress is without doubt a common factor in the pathophysiological mechanism of neuromuscular disorders, like many other diseases. However, despite this association between disease and oxidative stress, knowledge about how oxidative stress is produced and the types of reactive oxygen species (ROS) that are involved in neuromuscular diseases is lacking.

Introduction

During recent years the role of reactive oxygen species (ROS), in the pathogenesis of a large number of diseases, has become more apparent. This has resulted in extensive research within the molecular mechanisms of ROS.

Excessive amounts of ROS are known to damage DNA, proteins and lipids and to activate cell death pathways [1-3]. Since the 70s, it has been known that the main source of cellular superoxide is the mitochondria, more specifically the mitochondrial electron transport chain (ETC). The mitochondrial ROS originates mainly from electrons leaking from complex I and III during oxidative phosphorylation (OXPHOS), and probably also from Electron Transfer Flavoprotein (ETF) and Electron Transfer Flavoprotein ubiquinone oxidoredutase (ETF-QO) [4-6]. At physiological low levels, ROS is known to have an essential function as beneficial redox signaling molecules in cellular signaling and gene regulation systems, maintaining cell homeostasis [7, 8]. However, when ROS generation overwhelms the cellular defense system, by generation of excessive amounts of ROS, by decrease in the antioxidant defense system or when challenged by external or internal factors like starvation, infections or inherited gene defects, oxidative stress occurs [3]. Upon additional increases in cellular ROS levels, the cellular systems can no longer manage with the increasing amount of ROS, resulting in reversible cell damage, activating cellular death pathways. Thus, the amounts of cellular ROS determine the consequences of cellular adaption to oxidative stress [9, 131, 132].

Mitochondrial defects and oxidative stress are central factors in human health and disease. Any disease could theoretically be related to mitochondria defect, and mitochondrial dysfunction has already been shown to be the core of a surprising range of both common and rare disorders as the mitochondria are responsible for energy production, are key sources of oxidative stress, regulate apoptosis and calcium homeostasis, and are central in many other aspects of well-being/survival of cells [1]. Neuromuscular disorders are a very broad and relatively undefined (pleiotropic) term that includes many different diseases and syndromes. Collectively neuromuscular disorders are disorders that affect the skeletal muscles, the muscles that move the limbs and trunk, and/or their direct nervous system control, by affecting the signaling from the nerves to the muscles [10, 11]. There is evidence that oxidative stress plays a prominent role in neuromuscular disorders, with primary mitochondrial defect, such as: inborn errors of metabolism (IEM) and Friedreich's ataxia (FA) [9-12]. It's not clear, however, whether oxidative stress is the main cause of symptoms or merely a symptom itself. Oxidative stress is without doubt a common factor in the pathology of neuromuscular disorders, like many other diseases. However, despite this association between disease and oxidative stress, knowledge about how oxidative stress is produced and the types of ROS that are involved in neuromuscular diseases is lacking.

Despite the fact that ROS and mitochondrial dysfunction is also becoming increasingly recognized in neuromuscular disorders, there are many unanswered questions: Is oxidative stress an epiphenomenon of dysfunctional mitochondria, or does oxidative stress itself cause the dysfunctionality of mitochondria? How does oxidative stress result in selective muscular neural vulnerability shown to be involved in many neuromuscular diseases? And if oxidative stress is truly fundamental to pathogenesis, then why has the use of natural antioxidant therapy been thus far largely unsuccessful in such diseases? The answer does not seem simple.

In this review, to address these questions above, we first will give a background definition of mitochondria, oxidative stress, and the cells own antioxidant defense. We then present a short introduction to oxidative stress involved in neuromuscular disease, we then in further detail describe the proof and mechanisms of oxidative stress in IEM and in the mitochondrial disease FA, trying to clarify the involvement of oxidative stress in these neuromuscular disorders. Finally we discuss the use of mitochondrial therapeutic targets, as treatment options to target mitochondrial dysfunction and oxidative stress.

1. Mitochondria, Oxidative Stress and the Antioxidant System

1.1. Mitochondria

Mitochondria are known as the power plant of the cells, referring to mitochondria's involvement in the adenosine triphosphate (ATP) production. Mitochondrial ATP production includes many different metabolic processes; in general it includes the fatty acid β-oxidation, the citric cycle, also known as the tricarboxyl acid cycle (TCA cycle), and ultimately the ETC, which is the greatest source of ATP. The ETC consist of a series of complexes that transfer electrons from electron donors to electron acceptors via redox reactions, and couples this electron transfer with the transfer of protons (H^+ ions) across the mitochondrial membrane. The transfer of protons creates an electrochemical proton gradient that drives the ATP synthesis. The most common source of proton transfer into the ETC arises from the conversion of Acetyl-CoA in the citric acid cycle. An alternative link to the electron transport chain is via ETF and ETF-QO, which transfers electrons from the mitochondrial fatty acid β-oxidation, amino acid metabolism, and the choline metabolism into the ETC [13]. In addition to supplying cellular energy, mitochondria are involved in other tasks such as signaling, cellular differentiation, cell death (autophagy, apoptosis and mitochondrial specific autophagy; mitophagy), as well as the control of the cell cycle and cell growth [14].

1.2. Reactive Oxygen Species (ROS)

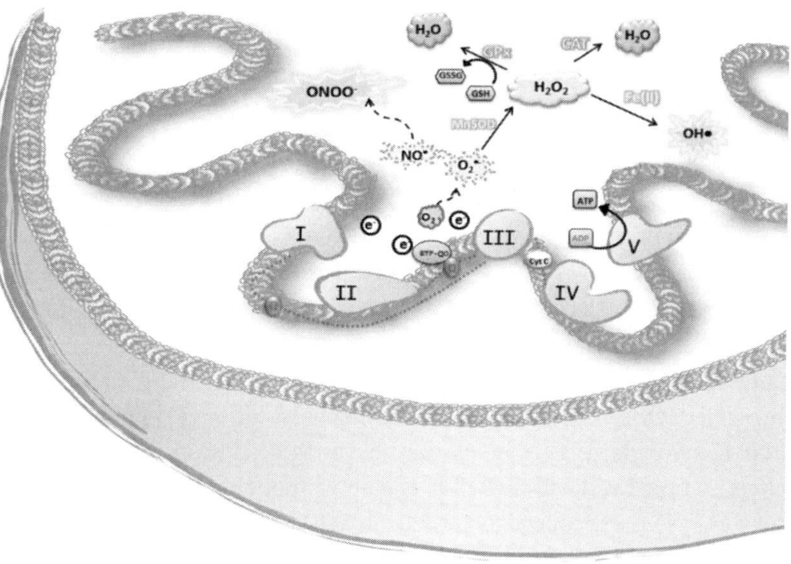

Figure 1. Reactive species and the counter acting antioxidants. The primary source of ROS production is the ETC, which resides in the inner mitochondrial membrane. Upon leakage of electrons these will quickly react with oxygen to create the reactive redical; Superoxide ($O_2^{\bullet-}$). MnSOD, is one of the main antioxidants of the mitochondria and catalyze the dismutation of $O_2^{\bullet-}$ to H_2O_2. While H_2O_2 can rapidly diffuse cross the cell membrane, its reactivity is restricted to proteins containing transition metals (such as Fe-S clusters) or low pKa thiols. Cells have numerous enzymatic mechanisms to detoxify H_2O_2, including catalase, glutathione peroxidase, and the peroxiredoxins, which reduce H_2O_2 to H_2O and O_2. Upon the Fenton reaction H_2O_2 is converted to OH•. This radical is highly reactive and oxidizes lipids, nucleic acids, and amino acids. OH• is primarily detoxifyed by small-molecule reductants, such as glutathione and ascorbate. When these detoxification mechanisms are insufficient to neutralize the ROS, cellular components may become oxidatively damaged, and oxidative stress occurs.

ROS and reactive nitrogen species (RNS) are produced continuously during normal cellular function. At physiological low levels the amount of reactive species and the counter acting antioxidants, exists in a healthy homodynamic balance, where these reactive species is known to have an essential function as beneficial redox signaling molecules in intracellular signaling and gene regulation systems [7, 8]. However, when this homodynamic balance is disturbed either by external or internal stressors like starvation, infections or inherited gene defects, the amount of ROS and/or RNS increases and oxidative stress occurs. This oxidative stress will shift the cells towards additional activation of the cell maintaining/survival systems resulting in a disturbed cell growth control and proliferation. If the cells cannot restore the homodynamic balance, cellular ROS levels will increase further resulting in damage to cellular molecules causing cellular dysfunction and activation of cell death pathways like the apoptosis/necrosis systems [3, 15-17]. It has been known since the 70's that one of the major intracellular sources of ROS is the mitochondria, more precisely the electron transport chain complexes I and III [5, 7]. ROS and RNS include substances like; hydroxyl radicals (OH•), superoxide anion ($O_2^{\bullet -}$), hydrogen peroxide (H_2O_2), nitric oxide (NO•) and peroxynitrite ($ONOO^-$) [18]. Superoxide anions are a product of a one electron reduction of oxygen, and it is the main precursor of most of the ROS produced in the cell. Dismutase of the $O_2^{\bullet -}$ radical produces hydrogen peroxide, H_2O_2, which may be further reduced to form the highly reactive hydroxyl radical, OH•, for examples though the Fenton reaction (see figure 1). RNS is produced when $O_2^{\bullet -}$ reacts with radicals like nitric oxide, NO•, to create peroxynitrite, $ONOO^-$, which is also classified as a powerful oxidant. These radicals are very reactive species due to their high chemical reactivity and can lead to damage to mtDNA, proteins, and lipids [2, 3, 19].

1.3. Producers of ROS

Although nine potential mitochondrial ROS generating enzymes have been identified until now, the ETC, as already mentioned, is still considered the major generator of intracellular ROS [20]. It is believed that electron leakage, causing superoxide, comes predominantly from the ETC complex I (NADH:ubiquinone oxidoreductase) and complex III (Ubiquinol:cytochrome C oxidoreductase; cytochrome bc) [5], however, other mitochondrial enzyme complexes have also been reported to produce ROS. Examples include the dihydrolipoamide dehydrogenase-containing FAD-linked pyruvate and αketoglutarate dehydrogenase complexes [21], as well as the flavoenzymes α-glycerophosphate dehydrogenase [22], and the ETF/ETF-QO proteins [4, 23, 24]. The production rate of superoxide in isolated mitochondria depends on specific local conditions, such as the $NADH/NAD^+$ ratio, the membrane protonmotive force, the QH_2/Q ratio, and the local O_2 concentration. The sites of electron leakage causing superoxide production in the ETC are considered to be a semiquinone radical, or a reduced flavin [5, 18].

1.4. The Cellular Defense Systems, the Antioxidant System

Direct ROS Scavenging

Antioxidants delay, inhibit or reverse the oxidation of cellular oxidizable substrates. The various antioxidants exert their effects by either directly scavenging superoxide, or the free radicals, or by activation of antioxidant defensive proteins. The antioxidant defense system consist of two major groups; i) Enzymes, including manganese superoxide dismutase (MnSOD), catalase and glutathione peroxidase. MnSOD is one of the first line defenses that catalyze the dismutation of $O_2^{\cdot-}$ to H_2O_2 and O_2. The second line of defense is the removal of H_2O_2, which is done by glutathione in association with glutathione peroxidase and glutathione reductase. The cytosol contains the catalase as an additional mechanism for removal of H_2O_2, and ii) low molecular weight antioxidants like ascorbate, glutathione, phenolic compounds, etc., which remove free radicals by a non-enzymatically mechanism [25]. In addition to the immediate accessible antioxidants, the cell induces the expression of various oxidative stress genes, one example is *HMOX1*, which encodes Heme Oxygenase 1 (HO1) that catabolises heme groups into the antioxidant biliverdin. Biliverdin is subsequently converted into bilirubin, a more powerful antioxidant [26]. Additionally, it has by now been shown that CoQ10, which resides in the inner mitochondrial membrane as a part of the electron transport system, has an antioxidative role and that a deficiency in CoQ10 may result in oxidative stress [27-29]. Also it is interesting, especially in relation to metabolic diseases, to notice that B2-vitamin, also known as riboflavin, has been found to exhibit anti-oxidant properties in the cell [30].

ROS Activation of Transcriptional Regulation and Metabolic Switching

Besides triggering the direct antioxidant defense of the cell, ROS can diffuse through the mitochondrial membranes to the cytosol and oxidize thiol residues in regulatory proteins like kinases/phosphatases, hereby controlling their activity. Here we will focus on two pathways (Nrf2 and HIF-1) in which evidence have indicated that ROS might have a regulative mechanism.

Transcriptional Regulation by Activation of Nrf2

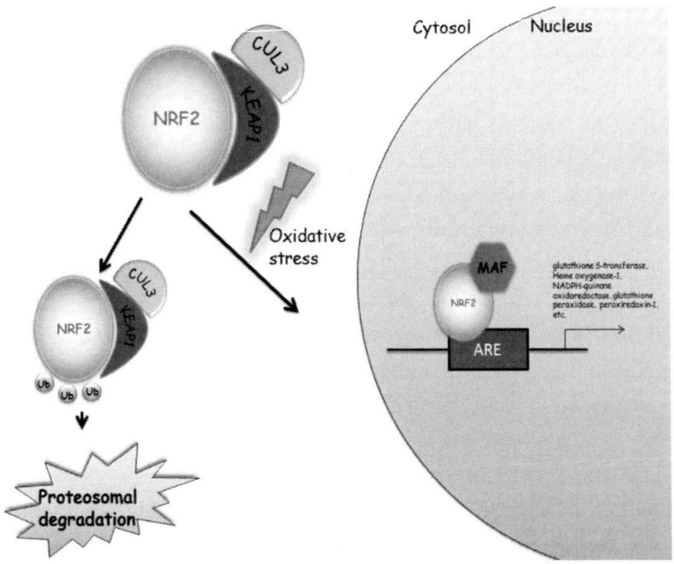

Figure 2. Model of the Nrf2 activation by oxidative stress. Under normal conditions, Nrf2 is located in the cytoplasm by binding of the Keap1-Cul3 complex, which rapidly degrades Nrf2, in the ubiquitin-proteasome dependent manner. Oxidative stress cause dissociation of Nrf2-Keap1-Cul3 complex, which culminates in ubiquitination of Keap1 and Cul3 and nuclear translocation of Nrf2. After nuclear relocation, Nrf2 associates with other transcription factors such as small Maf, and promotes transcriptional activation of antioxidant and detoxifying enzymes by binding to the antioxidant responsive elements (ARE) in the promoter regions of the target genes.

Under normal, unstressed conditions the nuclear factor erythroid 2-related factor 2 (Nrf2) is kept in the cytoplasm by Kelch like-ECH-associated protein 1 (Keap1) and Cullin 3 (Cul3), which quickly degrade Nrf2 by ubiquitination [31]. Keap1 is a substrate adaptor, which helps Cul3 ubiquitinate Nrf2. When Nrf2 is ubiquitinated, it is transported to the proteasome, where it is degraded and its components recycled [32]. However, there is evidence that ROS react with critical redox sensitive cysteine residues in Keap1, hereby disrupting the Keap1-Cul3 ubiquitination system. When Nrf2 is not ubiquitinated it instead translocates to the nucleus [33-35]. In the nucleus, it creates a heterodimer with a small Maf protein. The heterodimer binds to the Antioxidant Response Element (ARE), which is located in the upstream promoter region of many antioxidative genes such as glutathione S-transferase, Heme oxygenase-1, NADPH-quinone oxidoredoctase, glutathione peroxidase, peroxiredoxin-1, and many others, and initiates their transcription [35, 36] (Figure 2).

Transcriptional Regulation and Metabolic Switching Through HIF-1

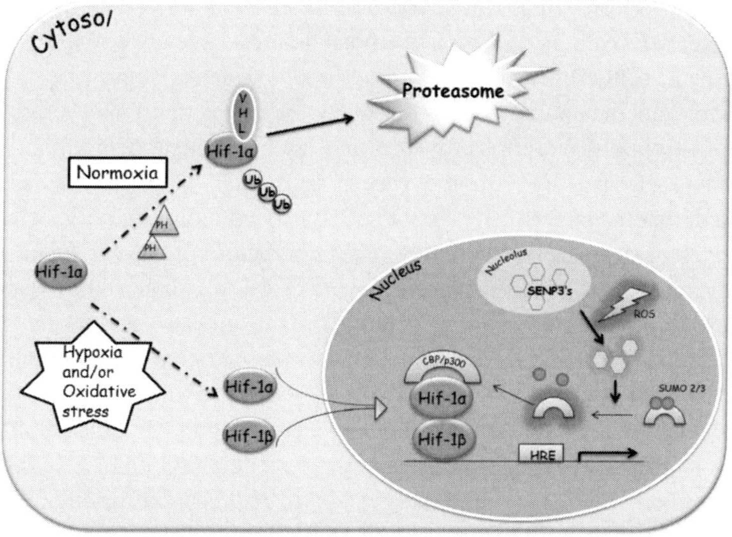

Figure 3. When oxygen is present (nomoxia), there is a continuous targeting of HIF-1α for degradation. The degradation targeting is controlled by the prolyl hydroxylase (PH), which hydroxylates HIF-1α, mediating recognition of the VHL–elongins complex and ubiquitination (Ub) of HIF-1α and hence targeting for proteasomal degradation. When oxygen is low (hypoxia) or the presence of oxidative stress, HIF-1α fails to be degraded by inhibition of the PH activity, stabilizing the HIF-1α which localizes to the nucleus and then associates with HIF-1β, which binds to cognate hypoxia-responsive elements (HREs) and initiate transcription. In addition oxidative stress in the form of H_2O_2 have been shown to oxidizes a SUMO-specific protease (SENP3), which also promotes the transcriptional activity of HIF-1α by de SUMOylation of a p300 co-activator of HIF-1α **transcription.**

Hypoxia-inducible factor-1 (HIF-1) is known to control the transcriptional response to hypoxia. However, more evidence recently suggests that HIF-1 can also be activated under normoxic conditions and in relation to various disease conditions, where oxidative stress is involved [37, 38], suggesting that HIF-1 activation might be an adaptive mechanism for cell survival, not only under hypoxia, but also under increased ROS production.

Besides activating genes responsible for increasing oxygen supply during hypoxia, under conditions of oxidative stress, HIF-1 also induces a metabolic reprogramming, where glycolytic genes are up-regulated and OXPHOS genes are down-regulated under aerobic conditions (also known as the Warburg switch/effect), allowing cells to use oxygen independent glycolysis instead of oxygen dependent OXPHOS [37, 39-41] (Figure 4).

The Warburg effect was originally found as a major hallmark of cancer cells. The Warburg effect was discovered more than 50 years ago [42], but only in recent years it has attracted great interest, because of the possible involvement, of this metabolic switching, upon oxidative stress [38, 42]. The reason for the metabolic switch in cancer cells has for many years been obscure. Originally Warburg proposed that the mechanism behind the switch was damage to the ETC in the cancer cells [42]. But later it has been suggested, that the cancer cells do not necessarily undergo Warburg switching, because of damage to the oxidative phosphorylation. Instead it might result from dysregulation of the expression of genes regulating the glycolytic enzymes. Recent results propose a more flexible mechanism, where cancer cells use gene regulation to suppress and activate oxidative phosphorylation to sustain their energy demand [43, 44]. More than 70% of cancers worldwide show overexpression of an enzyme in the transport or consumption of glycolysis [45], and several studies have shown that inhibition of glycolysis, or the biosynthetic pathways linked to glycolysis, reduced cell proliferation and tumor growth, supporting the hypothesis of Warburg switching involvement in cancers [46-48]. Despite the energetic disadvantage for the cancer cells in switching from oxidative phosphorylation to glycolysis, there are many other advantages for the cancer cells in the glycolysis. Glucose and its metabolites provide the backbone for the synthesis of nucleotides, lipids, and amino acids, which are all vital components for proliferation [49-51]. It was also suggested that the increased glycolysis in cancer cells may be an adaption to intermittent hypoxia/anoxia that develops in the early stages of tumor growth [52]. Glycolysis also increases lactate levels, creating an acidic environment which are toxic to normal cells, but which stimulates cancer growth and metastasis [53, 54]. Although not completely understood, the shift towards aerobic glycolysis appears to increase resistance toward apoptosis [39, 55]. Another advantage is the increased production of reducing equivalents, which are important regulators of the cellular redox potential [39]. In relation to oxidative stress, the major advantage of the Warburg shift would most properly be decrease in the transport of electron and therefore a decreased source for electron leakage.

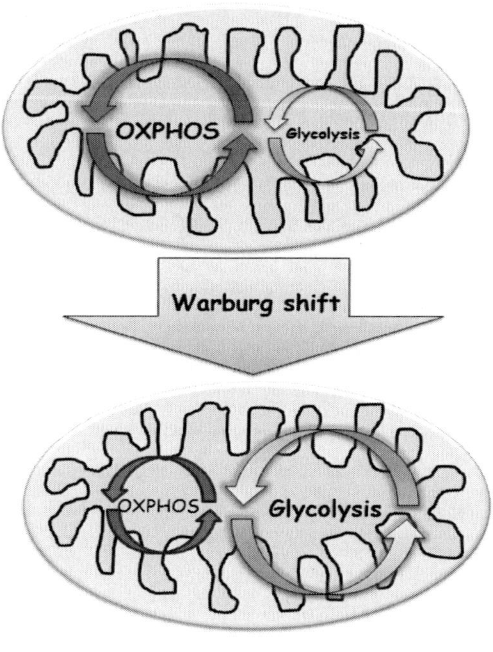

Figure 4. During Warburg shift cells undergo a shift from mitochondrial respiration to glycolytic and glutamine-addicted profile. The warburg shift is mainly known from cancer cells that use glucose and glutamine as the major sources of energy carbon precursors. The carbon flux through glycolysis and glutaminolysis is increased in cancer cells and provides abundant energy production and increase biosynthesis pathways such as nucleotide, lipid and amino acid synthesis that are used for making new cells. In relation to oxidative stress, it might be a defense mechanism to avaoid further electron transport leakage as a result of non-efficient electron transport in the ETC.

Several studies have now established that ROS is involved in the stabilization and activation of HIF-1 and thereby involvement in the same regulatory mechanisms as involved in the mechanism of Warburg [56-62]. HIF-1 is composed of two subunits; a constitutively expressed β-subunit (HIF-

1β) and a regulated α-subunit (HIF-1α). The stability of HIF-1α is tightly controlled by a family of oxygen dependent prolyl hydroxylase (PH) enzymes, which target HIF-1α for protesomal degradation, hereby inhibiting HIF-1 activation [38]. During hypoxia this reaction is inhibited, HIF-1α is stabilized and dimerize with HIF-1β. Upon dimerizing, the dimer binds HIF-response elements (HRE) and initiates gene transcription. Results have shown that PH enzymes may be inhibited by cellular factors like metabolites (succinate, fumarate and 2-OH glutarate). These results reveal that HIF-1 may play a broader role in sensing metabolic changes in relation to mitochondrial stress [63]. Although the role of ROS in HIF-1 activation is still controversial [64] studies have shown that H_2O_2 can inhibit the activity of the PH enzymes, probably by oxidizing cysteines or the essential non-heme bound iron [65, 66]. Other recent studies propose a mechanism by which the activity of stabilized HIF-1α can be further regulated directly by different levels of ROS [67, 68]. Supporting this it has been shown that low levels of H_2O_2 oxidizes a SUMO-specific protease (SENP3) at a specific cysteine residue (C243), which promotes the transcriptional activity of HIF-1α by de SUMOylation of a p300 co-activator of HIF-1α transcription. Additional oxidation of another cysteine residue (C532) at increased H_2O_2 levels inactivates SENP3 and consequently de-SUMOylation of p300 and co-activation of HIF-1α transcription. Another regulator of HIF1 is MnSOD. As already mentioned, MnSOD, is a major antioxidant enzyme in the mitochondria, where it has an important function in the first defense against ROS by converting superoxide anions to hydrogen peroxide. Several studies have shown MnSOD to have an important role in regulation of the HIF-1α subunit of HIF-1, both on the stabilization and the transcriptional activity [69-71] (Figure 3).

2. Oxidative Stress and Neuromuscular Disorders

2.1. The Role of Oxidative Stress in Neuromuscular Disorders

One of the major features of neuromuscular disease is the selective vulnerability of muscles and/or of different neuronal populations associated with muscle control, that are affected in a progressive and often stereotyped manner. Therefore, in addition to a global oxidative stress that affects all neurons, there must be additional factors that determine the selective cell death in each disease.

Cell specific features that may predispose for neuromuscular degeneration have earlier been reviewed [72, 73].

Certain neuronal groups have high intrinsic levels of oxidative stress and are therefore more vulnerable to additional disease-related oxidative stress. Neurons, like motor neurons which are the neuron type found in muscles, have long axons and multiple synapses and have high bioenergetic requirements for axonal transport or long-term plasticity. A high ATP demand combined with relative mitochondrial dysfunction will render these groups of neurons far more sensitive to degeneration than other neuronal groups. One interesting hypothesis for the vulnerability of specific neuronal groups comes from the discovery that in Parkinson's disease the dopaminergic neurons have an autonomous pacemaker mechanism that utilizes L-type calcium channels resulting in intracellular calcium oscillations. This creates a metabolic stress for such neurons as the repeated and persistent entry of calcium into cells needs to be counterbalanced by ATP demanding pumps to restore the calcium concentration. In fact it has been demonstrated that the opening of these L-type ion channels results in higher levels of oxidative stress in the mitochondria of such neurons. Moreover, other nondopaminergic groups of neurons that are also selectively affected in Parkinson's disease such as the dorsal motor nucleus of the vagus, the serotonergic neurons of the raphe nuclei, and neurons of the locus coeruleus all engage the same L-type calcium channel pacing mechanism. Therefore, this represents an example of a cell-specific factor that renders certain neuronal groups highly vulnerable to the disease process [74].

Proper mitochondrial functioning is very important to neurons. Neurons have high energy requirements. They are terminally differentiated cells which consume a lot of ATP to maintain ion gradients across membranes for proper neurotransmission. The high energy metabolisms because of the high energy demand, is a factor which will lead to an increase in metabolic biproducts hereby increasing the ROS. Additionally these neurons may also, because of their high energy demand, be especially vulnerable to energy depletion, which are seen in almost all neuromuscular diseases [75]. Combined with a decreased antioxidant defense this will potentially result in more oxidative injury to the motor neurons [76]. Efficient mitochondrial transport and positioning are also critical because different regions of the neuron have different energy requirements. Active growth cones and presynaptic terminals need more ATP than other parts of the cell. Calcium buffering by mitochondria is important to neurons. Presynaptic mitochondria are responsible for clearing calcium for proper neurotransmitter release and can affect the rate of recovery from synaptic depression after moderate synaptic activity [77]. Also, neurons have lipid membranes with high proportions of polyunsaturated fatty acids which are susceptible to oxidative damage by reactive oxygen species. Therefore, neuronal functioning relies heavily on the presence of healthy mitochondria, and consequently mitochondrial dysfunction is a fundamental part of neurodegeneration [75]. Furthermore, alternations in the axonal transport have been linked to several neuromuscular diseases like amytrophic lateral sclerosis [78, 79], Parkinson's disease [80-82] and Huntington disease [83] and it has been shown by live cell imaging that oxidative stress, in the form of hydrogen peroxide, inhibit axonal transport, especially mitochondrial transport is affected very early. In this study they also show that axons are more sensitive to ROS than the cell bodies and the dendrites [84]. Supporting this, a study in a *Drosophila* model of Friedreich's ataxia (FA) showed specific axonal transport deficits [85].

Below we will discuss two major neuromuscular disease types; inborn errors of metabolism (IEM) and FA, as examples of diseases for which oxidative stress has been shown to play a key role in disease pathogenesis.

2.2. Inborn Errors of Metabolism (IEM)

Inborn errors of metabolism (IEM) are a relatively rare cause of neuromuscular disease. They are, however important to discuss here as they are perhaps the most clearly defined and etiologically understood neuromuscular disorders. Traditionally they are considered monogenetic disorders and divided into so-called *metabolic myopathies* of intermediary metabolism (carbohydrates, fatty acids and proteins) and *mitochondrial myopathies* with primary defects in components of the ETC [86]. Common to these diseases are genetic defects in metabolic enzymes/transporters and a compromised ability to maintain adequate mitochondrial adenine triphosphate (ATP) and cellular energy level, with affections of tissues having a relatively high energy demand and content of mitochondria, like skeletal muscles, heart and brain. The precise cellular mechanisms, causing degeneration of especially neuro and/or muscular tissue in these disorders, are still not fully understood. However, it is increasingly being recognized that inadequate energy production, caused by impaired substrate oxidation, is not the sole and perhaps also not the most important factor. Rather, a general mitochondrial dysfunction with cellular oxidative stress, driven by retrograde signaling and activation of mitochondrial stress adaption and cell growth pathways, seems to play a key role. Such mitochondrial processes have been studied and documented in particular for inborn errors of ETC components (reviewed in [87-89]), fatty acid oxidation (FAO) enzymes (reviewed in [90-92]) and organic acidurias (OAs) (reviewed in [93-95]). Here we will summarize and discuss current knowledge on the mechanisms by which IEM can induce a state of chronic oxidative stress, with mitochondrial dysfunction and disturbed cell growth control, which is increasingly appreciated to be the driving force in their tissue degenerative phenotypes. The discussion will focus mainly on examples from own and others studies of inborn errors of FAO, but also knowledge from inborn errors of the ETC and OAs will be discussed when relevant. Before discussing oxidative stress in IEM, a brief overview of mitochondrial oxidative metabolism and the type of gene defects associated with its dysfunction will be given.

Energy Metabolism

Cells use ATP as the most important source of energy to drive biological activities. The energy required for ATP production comes from oxidation of carbohydrates, fats and proteins. Inside the cell, smaller units of these fuel molecules are metabolized, mainly to acetyl-CoA, which is then completely oxidized to CO_2 in the TCA cycle. Oxidation of fatty acids and amino acids occurs almost entirely in the mitochondrial matrix, where activated fatty acyl-CoAs are oxidized to acetyl-CoA in the β-oxidation spiral, and deaminated amino acids are metabolized to acetyl-CoA or an intermediate of the TCA cycle. Carbohydrates are initially oxidized through glycolysis to pyruvate in the cytosol. Pyruvate may further be converted into lactate, or taken up by mitochondria, where it is metabolized to acetyl-CoA. Electrons derived from the oxidation of fuel molecules during glycolysis, the TCA cycle and the β-oxidation spiral are transferred to the electron carriers nicotinamide adenine dinucleotide (NAD^+) and flavin adenine dinucleotide (FAD) to yield NADH and $FADH_2$, respectively. The NADH and $FADH_2$ electrons are transferred to oxygen through the four ETC enzyme complexes in the inner mitochondrial membrane yielding H_2O and a proton gradient, which is used by complex V to produce ATP. NADH is oxidized by complex I (NADH:ubiquinone oxidoreductase) whereas $FADH_2$ mainly is oxidized by complex II (succinate:ubiquinone oxidoreductase) or ETF-QO (electron transfer flavoprotein:ubiquinone oxidureductase), which in complex with ETF (electron transfer flavoprotein), transfers electrons gained from the first oxidation step in the β-oxidation of fatty acids to the ETC. The electrons gained from complex I, II or ETF-QO are transferred to complex III (ubiquinole:cytochrome c oxidoreductase) by coenzyme Q10 (CoQ10), and further to complex IV by cytochrome c, where they react with oxygen to form H_2O. Full oxidation of a molecule of glucose or palmitate by OXPHOS yields more than 30 ATPs. ATP can also be produced directly in the cytosol during glycolysis yielding only two molecules of ATP per oxidized molecule of glucose [87]. Therefore tissues having a high energy demand rely mainly on mitochondrial OXPHOS for ATP production. Only when oxygen supply is limited, as during impaired blood flow or intense physical activity, cells switch to glucose fermentation and cytosolic ATP production. Interestingly and relevant for the discussion below, this balance between cytosolic and mitochondrial ATP production is often disturbed in IEM, where impairment of OXPHOS capacity - induced directly by genetic defects in its components or over time by pathological levels of ROS or other molecular stressors - may force the cell to shift from mitochondrial to glycolytic ATP production, even under normoxic conditions (Warburg shift) as will be discussed below.

IEM and Their Association to Oxidative Stress

A number of IEM are known to give neuromuscular symptoms [86, 96, 97]. Here we will focus on some of the IEM, where oxidative stress have been studied and shown to play a role in disease progression. Because of the considerable heteogeneity in genetic, biochemical and clinical findings, a detailed description of each disorder is beyond the scope of this chapter, and only the most common clinical and molecular genetic findings will be summarized.

Most IEM are inherited in an autosomal recessive manner. ETC disorders can also be caused by variations in mitochondrial DNA, which are inherited almost entirely from the mother and results in a more complex heritability with copies of normal and mutated mitochondrial DNA in each cell (heteroplasmy). Clinical presentations vary with age with newborns and infants having mostly metabolic decompensation, with metabolic acidosis and hypotonia, often combined with severe multisystemic disease (encephalopathy, cardiomyopathy, endocrinopathy), whereas adults frequently have muscle weakness, cramps sometimes with rhabdomyolysis, or a more progressive peripheral or proximal neuropathy, the latter of which may cause respiratory arrest. CNS symptoms like seizures, strokes, and developmental delay are also seen. Sensorineural hearing loss and optic atrophy are more often observed in patients with mitochondrial DNA defects. Attacks are often precipitated with feverish infections or exercise during which cells rely mainly on mitochondrial respiration for ATP production [86, 87, 96, 97].

Two of the most common ETC disorders, associated with myopathies, are myoclonic epilepsy with ragged red fibers (MERRF) and mitochondrial encephalopathy, lactic acidosis, and stroke-like episodes (MELAS). They are most often caused by variations in mitochondrial DNA genes encoding transfer RNA [89], and both diseases have been associated with oxidative stress [89, 98, 99]. Oxidative stress and mitochondrial dysfunction have also been documented in isolated deficiencies of complex I, like Leigh Syndrome (LS) and Leber hereditary optic neuropathy (LHON) as reviewed in [87].

Like isolated complex 1 deficiencies, organic acidurias (OAs) mainly present with neurological symptoms sometimes accompanied by skeletal and cardiac symptoms. Several studies by Wajner's and Kolker's research groups have, in recent years, shown mitochondrial dysfunction with secondary ETC deficiency and oxidative stress induced by toxic metabolites that accumulate in patients suffering from different OAs; mainly inborn errors of amino acid metabolism [93-95].

A number of inborn errors of long-chain fatty acids are known to give neuromuscular symptoms and oxidative stress. These include deficiencies of 1) carnitine palmitoyltransferase 2 (CPT2), which is involved in the mitochondrial import of long-chain fatty acylcarnitines and catalyzes their transesterification back into fatty acyl-CoAs, which can then be oxidized in the mitochondrial β-oxidation spiral, 2) very-long-chain acyl-CoA dehydrogenase (VLCAD), which is involved in the initial and FAD-dependent step of the mitochondrial β-oxidation spiral, 3) mitochondrial trifunctional protein (MTP), a multi-enzyme complex catalyzing the remaining three steps in the β-oxidation of long-chain fatty acyl-CoAs and finally 4) the ETF/ETF-QO electron transfer enzyme complex, which transfers electrons gained in the FAD-dependent β-oxidation step to CoQ10 in the ETC [86. 96, 97]. For all these deficiencies a genotype-phenotype relationship has been documented, in which genetic variations, resulting in no or very low residual enzyme activity, cause severe neonatal and multisystemic disease, whereas genetic variations causing substitution or deletion of a single amino acid more often are associated with later-onset and myopathic forms [100-105]. In contrast to these deficiencies of long-chain fatty acid oxidation, genetic deficiencies of short-chain acyl-CoA dehydrogenase (SCAD), which oxidize short-chain fatty acyl-CoAs and which may cause neuromuscular symptoms in neonates and infants, do not show any relation between genotype and phenotype [91, 106].

ROS and cellular signs of oxidative stress in inborn errors of FAO have been documented in number of studies of patient cells, model cells and animals. We have recently summarized these studies and argued that ROS produced as a consequence of primary genetic FAO defects, by redox activation of mitochondrial stress adaption pathways, are the driving force in the creation of a state of chronic oxidative stress and disturbed growth control in these patient cells [90]. Mass spectrometric (MS) protein profile analysis of primary patient skin fibroblasts have to a great extent been the key to the creation of this hypothesis, which requires further experiments to be finally proven. Using such proteomic analyses, we have shown that fibroblasts, derived from patients with SCAD or ETF-QO deficiency, show adaptation to cellular stress by regulating antioxidant systems, protein quality control systems, cell death pathways and metabolic reprogramming [107-110]. Furthermore, we have shown that some of these disease-associated gene variants, when overexpressed in model cells or *in vitro*, produce mitochondrial and/or cellular ROS [111-113]. Mitochondrial ROS production was also demonstrated in cultured skin fibroblasts from patients with ETF-QO deficiency [114], and the same cells showed altered mitochondrial dynamic with decreased fusion and increased fission (Cornelius et al., unpublished results), as did astrocyte cells overexpressing a disease-causing variant SCAD protein [115]. Treatment with the natural antioxidant CoQ10 or its synthetic form MitoQ decreased ROS production and mitochondrial fractionation in both studies; reflecting that mitochondrial dynamic is controlled by ROS to inhibit healthy mitochondria in fusing with oxidatively damaged and fractionated mitochondria, which are then removed by mitophagy [116].

A number of studies have shown impaired function of ETC complexes, sometimes combined with CoQ10 deficiency or decreased expression of FAO enzymes in skin fibroblasts or skeletal muscle biopsies from patients with genetic deficiencies of ETF-QO [109, 114, 117-120], whereas other studies found normal ETC function in such samples [121, 122]. Impaired ETC function has also been documented in patients suffering from MTP deficiency [123] and moderate CoQ10 deficiency has recently been shown in patients suffering from genetic deficiencies of VLCAD or ETF [124]. Some of the FAO metabolites, which accumulate in FAO deficient patients, have been shown, by them self, to disrupt ETC function [125-127]. Thus, primary genetic deficiencies of FAO enzymes seem to cause secondary impairment of the ETC. In case of ETF and ETF-QO deficiencies, this impairment of the ETC has been shown to be compensated with increases in glycolytic enzymes indicating that a transcriptional metabolic reprogramming (Warburg switch) is taken place [109. 128]. In ETF and ETF-QO deficient Zebrafish this metabolic reprogramming was elegantly shown to be controlled by the mTORC1/PPARG-ERK signaling pathway [128, 129]. mTOR1 activates anabolic processes sustaining cell survival and proliferation by activating among others HIF-1 (shift from OXPHOS to glycolysis), PPARG-ERK (shift from FAO to lipogenesis) and PGC-1α (mitochondrial biosynthesis) [130] resulting in an apoptosis resistant proliferative phenotype with enlarged cell size, mitochondrial dysfunction and proliferation, fatty acid accumulation, and multi-organ failure [128, 129]. We speculate that this cell survival signaling pathway and metabolic reprogramming is activated by ROS to reduce further ROS production and leakage from an impaired ETC, which if uncontrolled directly will damage cellular DNA, proteins and lipids and cause further ROS and activation of cell death pathways [90]. Persistent activation of these signaling pathways keeps the cell in a state of chronic oxidative stress with oxidant/antioxidant imbalance combined with compromised mitochondrial respiration and an increased susceptibility to additional stressors like infections, fasting and exercise, which can increase the cellular ROS level further and shift the balance from cell survival to mostly cell death [90, 131, 132]. This innate predisposition to cell stress is illustrated in a study in which cultured fibroblasts, derived from patients with genetic deficiencies of SCAD, MTP or CPT2, as compared to control cells, suffered from early death when challenged with the ROS-inducing anticancer drug menadione [133]. Interestingly, in the same study, cell death was increased further by physiological stressors, such as high temperature or glucose fasting, whereas survival was increased when the cells were treated with antioxidants or the PPARα agonist bezafibrate. This suggests that also in these cells mitochondrial respiration and stress tolerance might be limited by ROS-induced signaling defects as shown in the ETF/ETF-QO deficient Zebrafish, where metabolic reprogramming and to some extent tissue degeneration could be alleviated by mTORC1 and PPARG antagonists. Like bezafibrate, resveratrol is known to increase mitochondrial function and respiration; although in a more direct manner by binding to and stimulating Complex I, thereby increasing the NAD+/NADH ratio and causing post-translational activation of mitochondrial respiration by the deacetylase activities of sirtuins like SIRT1 and SIRT3 [134]. Accordingly, not only bezafibrate [135-137], but also resveratrol [138] have been shown to boost FAO and sometimes ETC capacity in FAO patient cells, with or without clinical improvement [139, 140]. Likewise, resveratrol has been shown to reverse metabolic reprogramming in fibroblasts from patients with primary genetic deficiencies of complex I and complex IV [141], and nicotinic acid, another activator of sirtuins, was shown to improve ETC function and restore mTORC1 and AMPK signaling in fibroblasts and skeletal muscles from a diverse group of patients with primary ETC gene defects [142]. All together these data suggest that a common signaling network, that involves mTORC1, PPARs, HIF-1 and also AMPK and sirtuins, may sense and respond to mitochondrial stress induced by primary gene defects of FAO and ETC enzymes causing global alteration of downstream cellular pathways with impaired mitochondrial respiration and disturbed cellular growth control. It is important to mention here that not all studies have shown impaired mitochondrial respiration in inborn errors of FAO. Some studies have shown no or even compensatory increases in mitochondrial respiration in patients and animals with long-chain FAO deficiencies [121, 143-145]. Further studies are needed to clarify if these differences in cellular adaptation to stress relate to genetic differences between different cells or to experimental conditions.

ROS as Inducer and Mediator of Mitochondrial Dysfunction in IEM

In vitro and cellular studies have shown that certain gene variations of ETC enzymes, like complex I [146], complex II [147, 148] and ETF-QO [90, 113] but also the matrix located flavoenzyme ETF [112], may allow an increased flow of electrons out of the enzymes to oxygen, or they may increase access of oxygen to the partially reduced flavosemiquinones or ubisemiquinone and thereby give rise to ROS. Besides direct ROS generation, from mutated metabolic enzymes, it has also been suggested, and in some cases indicated, that aggregated or misfolded proteins and/or some of the metabolic substrates, that accumulate due to IEM, may interact and inhibit components of the ETC or cause disturbances in ETC or FAO supercomplex integration; thereby increasing electron leakage with lipid peroxidation and further ROS production [90, 92-94, 112, 149, 150]. For certain gene defects of ETC complexes and ETF-QO, the increased ROS has directly been tied to activation of survival signaling [98, 128, 129, 146, 151]. This interconnection between mitochondria ROS and metabolic reprogramming is most likely explained by ROS directly oxidazing thiol residues in stress regulatory proteins, such as enzymes or transcription factors, that control the signaling pathways and activates downstream targets to protect the cells from the harmful effects of pathological amounts of ROS. Metabolic reprogramming, to shuttle metabolites away from an impaired and electron leaky ETC, is increasingly recognized as one of these oxidative stress adaptive cell mechanisms. Alternatively or additionally, other signaling molecules like

AMP/ATP, NADH/NAD+ and acetyl-CoA, which may be dysregulated secondary to an IEM, may cause epigenetic/post-translational modification and activation of signaling pathways that lead to metabolic reprogramming with coordinated down-regulation of antioxidant mechanisms, making the cells more prone to accumulation of oxidative stress. Even though the exact molecular triggers of mitochondrial dysfunction still remains to be elucidated, it is clear from the above mentioned studies that similar stress adaption mechanisms, controlled by signaling pathways, exist in a number of IEM with different genetic etiologies. It is reasonable to suggest that ROS could be a key regulator of these cell processes, which should be investigated in future studies.

2.3. Friedreich's Ataxia (FA)

Clinics

The word Ataxia origins from the Greek "lack of order". Ataxia in general is a neurological condition consisting of lack of voluntary coordination of muscle movements. Ataxia is a non-specific clinical manifestation implying dysfunction of the parts of the nervous system, such as cerebellum, that coordinate movement. Both sporadic and hereditary forms of Ataxia exist. For the sporadic Ataxia no specific acquired or genetic cause can be found. The hereditary ataxias are categorized by the way of inheritance and causative gene or chromosomal locus. The hereditary ataxias can be inherited in an autosomal dominant, autosomal recessive or X-linked manner [152, 153]. In this chapter we will focus on the involvement of oxidative stress and mitochondrial defect in FA, even though some of the other ataxia forms like spinocerebellar ataxia and ataxia telangiectasia [154-158] have also recently shown indications of oxidative stress and therefore it is interesting to further investigate if more of the ataxia's have oxidative stress involved in the pathology of these disease. FA is the most common form of the autosomal recessive ataxias. The first indication of FA is generally difficulty in walking. The condition typically progresses to the arms and trunk. Muscles weaken and degrade over time, resulting in deformities, particularly in the feet, lower legs and hands. As the disease progress other signs and symptoms such as slow speech, fatigue, rapid, involuntary eye movements, spinal curvature and heart disease, including heart enlargement (cardiomyopathy) and heart failure may develop [159, 160].

Frataxin

The vast majority of autosomal recessive FA is caused by a homozygous expansion of the trinucleotide (GAA) repeat within the first intron of frataxin (FXN) located on chromosome 9q21. Normal individuals have 5-30 GAA repeat expansions, whereas affected individuals have more than 70 (up to 1000) GAA-triplets. This mutation causes a transcriptional defect and hereby lack of frataxin. In a small percentage of patients nonsense or frameshift mutations resulting in aberrant or premature termination of translation, and loss-of-function missense mutations have been reported [161, 162]. FXN encodes a small mitochondrial protein, frataxin, which is located in the mitochondrial matrix in association with the inner mitochondrial membrane. Frataxin is an iron-binding protein responsible for forming iron–sulphur clusters, making it essential to the activity of many proteins. It is by now widely accepted that the pathological mechanisms in FA is caused by frataxin deficiency [161, 163, 164]. Some of the initial understanding of the molecular mechanism to FA came from studies in yeast with deletion of the yeast frataxin homolog YFH1. These deletions resulted in a 10-fold increase of iron inside the mitochondria along with an increase in ROS [165-167]. This has later also been confirmed with results from other models like C. elegans [168], in FA patients [169] and in mice [170].

Iron Metabolic Pathway in FA

The Fe-S cluster biogenesis hypothesis is currently the most accepted regarding the biochemical function of frataxin. Some of the major consequence of frataxin deficiency is abnormal function of enzymatic activities and uncoupling of the electron transport chain [171-177]. Iron is vital for the cell to survive, and it is of outmost importance that the levels of iron are constantly regulated due to irons redox activity and involvement in ROS generation. It is by now known that mitochondria have an essential role in maintaining cellular iron homeostasis, however the in depth understanding of the regulatory mechanism are not yet clear [178]. However, the importance of iron in relation to Fe-S clusters (ISC) and heme groups, in the mitochondria, are well known [179] and will be discussed below. Iron is necessary for a variety of important cellular processes, such as oxygen transport, cellular respiration, and DNA synthesis, and there is also a tight link between the metabolism of iron and key metabolic processes such as cell growth, inflammatory pathways, and cell death [180]. Iron that is not tightly sequestered within a redox-inactive state has the potential to generate ROS, which can be disastrous in the environment of the cell. To minimize these reactions, cellular mechanisms exist to tightly regulate the metabolism of iron depending on intracellular iron levels and metabolic requirements. Within the cell, the regulation of iron metabolism is largely controlled by the iron regulatory proteins (IRP1 and 2), which regulate cellular iron uptake, utilization, export, and storage in a tightly controlled manner. However, at the systemic level, iron homeostasis is primarily regulated by the "hormone of iron metabolism," hepcidin, which acts through the modulation of eukaryotic Ferroportin1 expression [181].

There are three major iron metabolic pathways within the mitochondrion: (i) heme synthesis, (ii) ISC biogenesis, and (iii) mitochondrial iron storage. Heme synthesis occurs both in the mitochondria and in the cytoplasm of the cell. Research has shown that frataxin is involved in the heme biosynthesis [182]. Supporting this it was shown that knockdown of frataxin in mammalian cells decreases mitochondrial heme metabolite level and at the same time increases the heme biosynthesis, suggesting a role for frataxin in the biogenesis of heme-containing proteins [183, 184]. The mitochondrion is a major generator of ISCs that are essential for the electron transport ability of various ISC proteins that contain them [185, 186]. Finally, dysregulation of mitochondrial iron processing can have direct consequences for cellular iron homeostasis, as vital proteins such as IRP1 require ISCs for their proper function. Notably, a number of neurodegenerative diseases are associated with misregulated mitochondrial iron metabolism [187].

Metabolic Defect in FA

There is evidence for multiple metabolic disturbances in the pathogenesis of FA covering both the ETC, the TCA cycle, and the lipid metabolism. Here we will try to sum up some of the results. Several studies have shown a defect in the ETC in FA pathogenesis. In relation to the ISC defect found in FA this is not surprising, as many of the ETC components contain ISC's. In FA patient samples of cardiac muscle the oxidative phosphorylation was found to be impaired, with severe deficiency of the mitochondrial ETC I, II and III [188, 189].

Experiments has shown an interaction between frataxin and complex II subunits in yeast, human cells [190] and *Caenorhabditis elegans* [191], suggesting that there is a direct role of frataxin in the electron transport chain and mitochondrial respiration. Thus, frataxin deficiency could involve a disruption of the electron transport chain.

A regulatory mechanism resulting in aggravating the deficiency of the oxidative phosphorylation, as a defense mechanism to minimize further ROS development, have been shown recently, where a study demonstrated that the respiratory chain defects, accompanying frataxin deficiency, cause progressive hyperacetylation of cardiac mitochondrial proteins. In this study, the found hyperacetylation was shown to be due to the inhibition of one of the major positive regulator of oxidative metabolism, the NAD-Dependent Deacetylase Sirtuin-3 (SIRT3). These findings present a novel disease phenotype and reveal a negative feedback mechanism that may serve to coordinately suppress mitochondrial oxidative pathways, as a ROS defense mechanism [192]. SIRT3-mediated deacetylation has recently emerged as one of the major mechanism regulating the activity of mitochondrial oxidative and intermediary metabolism. SIRT3 is also found to respond to the flux of mitochondrial NAD+ and NADH, which is determined by the capacity of the respiratory chain to oxidize NADH, showing the sensitivity of SIRT3 to detect defects in the respiratory chain [193]. The capacity to oxidize NADH was found to be severely decreased in FA, leading to accumulation of NADH [192]. Analyzing these results together with the accumulating results showing respiratory chain deficiency in FA, it seems logical to hypothesis that the mitochondria in FA patients, would have a defense mechanism to decrease oxidative metabolism, hereby also the further generation of NADH, sparing the cell from damaging ROS that would be produced by forcing electrons through a dysfunctional respiratory chain. It has been known for several decades that a decrease in NAD+/NADH redox balance has a largely inhibitory effect on many enzymes of intermediary mitochondrial metabolism [194]. Summing up, the results indicate a key role for SIRT3 in the maintenance of oxidative metabolism which might be related to the found respiratory defects in FA. In relation to the pathology in FA, these results might be the link to the muscular defect found in FA, since as much as 90% of its ATP from oxidative phosphorylation is used by muscles, especially important to cardiac muscles, which is also severely affected in FA [195]. Further supporting this, SIRT3-deficient mice showed reduced cardiac ATP levels, were hypersensitive to cardiac stress and furthermore developed an early onset cardiac hypertrophy [195, 196]. In addition to its metabolic functions, SIRT3 is known to directly activate antioxidant defense mechanisms via deacetylation of mitochondrial manganese superoxide dismutase and isocitrate dehydrogenase of the glutathione system [197-200].

Deficiency of aconitase, an essential component of the tricarboxylic acid cycle (TCA), was also found [201]. Another recent study supporting this showed reduced aconitase activity, together with increased oxidative stress in a transgenic mouse model with the expanded GAA repeat [202]. The finding of reduced aconitase activity might suggest an induction of a vicious cycle of oxidative stress [201], as it has been shown to be, in contrast to other TCA cycle enzymes, selectively inactivated by oxidative stress [203]. The activity of aconitase was monitored in frataxin-RNAi flies, where frataxin was knocked out by RNAi [204]. Interestingly, when exposing these flies to hyperoxia, it led to a marked reduction of aconitase activity. This result indicates a role for frataxin in protecting aconitase activity against ROS-mediated inactivation, showing frataxin to have a function as an aconitase chaperone. Oxidative stress induced the release of the Fe-α aconitase Fe-S cluster leading to its inactivation. Thus, without the protection of frataxin, aconitase might not be reactivated at normal rates when oxidative stress reaches high levels, as happens in hyperoxia or during the aging process, resulting in its irreversible inactivation.

Finally, an indication of dysregulation/deficiency of the lipid metabolism in FA has been shown [205-207]. Very little is known about lipid homeostasis in FA. A typical symptom of FA is diabetes mellitus, and studies from patient autopsies or plasma samples showed decreased levels of phosphatidylethanolamine, phosphatidylserine and linoleic acid [208-211]. Also, electron microscopy analysis of cardiac muscle from frataxin-deficient mouse, revealed the presence of numerous lipid droplets, indicating a defective metabolism of lipids [212]. Very recently, lipid metabolism was associated with frataxin deficiency in fly [207]. Deregulated lipid metabolism and increased lipid peroxide levels are recurrent events in pathologies related to mitochondrial dysfunction [192]. Furthermore, lipid imbalance has been reported to have a pivotal effect in the pathophysiology of multiple neurological disorders, including bipolar disorders, schizophrenia, Alzheimer's, Parkinson's, and Huntington's diseases, connecting dysfunctional lipid metabolism with neuron damage [213]. Since SIRT3 is an important regulator of fatty acid β-oxidation, lipid metabolism regulations needs to be further investigated for involvement in the pathogenesis of FA.

FA and the Antioxidant System

Recent results have suggested a role for frataxin as an antioxidant, showing that overexpression of human frataxin in mice can increase the activation of glutathione peroxide together with elevated amount of reduced triols. [214]. Reduction in the level of free glutathionone levels together with an increase in the gluthathione bound to hemoglobin in erythrocytes have been found in blood samples from FA patients [215].

Further supporting these results it has been shown that MnSOD is not upregulated in FA fibroblasts when exposed to iron or H_2O_2 [159, 216]. In addition to the lacking activation of MnSOD, a lack in activation of the redox-sensitive nuclear factor; NFkB was found [217]. NFkB is activated by free radical species, especially hydroxyl radicals and is a primary upstream mediator of MnSOD activation [218-22]. Reasoning these results it has been proposed, that the reduced activity of NFkB and MnSOD is a defense mechanism, which results in a reduced amount of hydroxyl radicals, hereby preventing the reaction of these toxic radicals with the excess overload iron producing Fenton cofactor hydrogen peroxide. However the consequences are a high level of superoxide, resulting in damage to the cell. So in the end the defense mechanism just seems to give other ways of damage contributing to the disease mechanisms [217].

Oxidative Stress in the Pathology of FA

Oxidative stress may have a central role in the pathology of FA disease mechanism, as we have aldready presented some of the many indications. Deficiency in frataxin protein has already been associated with increased oxidative stress [191, 202, 221]. Increased levels of oxidative stress markers such as 8-hydroxy-2'-deoxyguanosine and lipid peroxidation have been found in both urine and blood from FA patients [222, 223]. In culturd cells with low frataxin free radical production is increased [224-227] and FA fibroblasts are more sensitive to oxidants than controls [228, 229]. Furthermore, the Fenton reaction may be enhanced in FA because of the excess mitochondrial iron and may contribute to pathogenesis.

FA and Mitochondrial Biogenesis

The peroxisome proliferation activator receptor Υ-coactivator 1 alpha (PGC-1α) is a transcriptional co-activator that has emerged as yet another master regulator in metabolic programming, often by stimulating mitochondrial biogenesis [230]. It has now also been identified as a target pathway in FA [231]. Superoxide anion levels and the expression of PGC-1α and the mitochondrial transcription factor TFAM were increased in the fibroblasts of two patients with late onset disease. Moreover, levels of the upstream signals p38 MAPK and AMPK kinases were also increased. These findings suggest a relationship between oxidative stress and mitochondrial biogenesis in FA. Interestingly, PGC-1α and TFAM expression was down-regulated by the presence of the antioxidant idebenone (the antioxidant function will be discussed later) in cell culture. On the contrary, such an increase in PGC-1α and TFAM expression was not observed in fibroblasts from an early onset patient [231]. The positive effect found with idebenone may prove two pathways in which it function: Idebenone may directly work as an antioxidant; reduce ROS levels into the cells, reducing p38 activation or, idebenone may improve the efficiency of the mitochondrial respiratory chain, and then decreasing the levels of activated AMPK. Furthermore these results just as other discussed results within the FA pathology suggest that oxidative stress is an early event in FA and early treatment with antioxidants are essential for an efficient effect against oxidative stress.

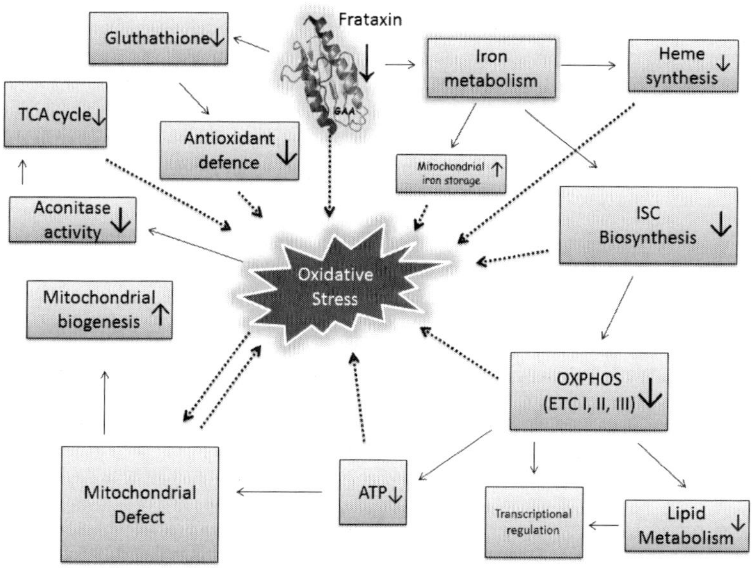

Figure 5. The involvement in the pathogenesis of FA. From the primary genetic defect in Frataxin leading to an overall defect in the iron metabolism, it seems that oxidative stress have a central role in all the defects/regulations involved in the pathogenesis of FA.

3. Oxidative Stress As a Target for Treatment in Neuromuscular Disorders

The realization that mitochondrial dysfunction and oxidative stress are involved in the pathogenesis of a wide specter of diseases has opened a path for new therapeutic strategies aimed at the mitochondrial function. It seems that nearly all cases where mitochondrial dysfunction contributes to disease, a major cause of damage is overproduction of ROS by mitochondria, either directly or as a secondary consequence of other dysfunctions [232, 233]. For many years trials with natural antioxidants, like vitamin E and CoQ10, have been ongoing, however with minor effects. One plausible explanation for the failure of natural antioxidants, to show beneficial effects, might possibly be that these antioxidants do not accumulate properly or in full amount, in the mitochondria, the major site of ROS generation or it might be that antioxidant treatment has to be initiated at a very early stage in the delevopment of the disease, maybe even before significant symptoms appear for the patients, and therefore too early for diagnosis and initiation of treatment, whereas the disease-models, in which many of these treatments are tested, the diagnosis are pre-knowledge and therefore the treatment can be tested earlier than realistically possible in the patients. Due to the very extensive amount of data on therapeutic targets for the mitochondria we will focus on reviewing the potential therapeutic efficiency of metabolic antioxidants, mitochondrial-directed antioxidants and mitochondria-targeting peptides (Szeto-Schiller peptides (SS peptides), for a more extensive review see Gruber et al. and Moreira P, et al. [234, 235]. Finally we will briefly discuss the targeting of transcriptional regulation as a mean of treatment, as the importance of these transcriptional mechanisms in oxidative stress-involved diseases are becoming more clear, as already mentioned.

3.1. Metabolic/Natural Antioxidants

Creatine

Creatine phosphokinase (CPK), is an enzyme expressed by various tissues and cell types. CPK catalyzes the conversion of creatine and consumes ATP to create phosphocreatine (PCr) and ADP. The reversible CPK enzyme reaction thus generates ATP from PCr and ADP [236].

In tissues and cells that consume ATP rapidly, like skeletal muscle, but also brain, and other tissues, PCr therefore serves as an important energy reservoir for a rapid buffering and regeneration of ATP when the energy demand increases [237, 238].

Use of the supplement Creatine has recently gained more attention. The guanidine compound creatine is endogenously produced in neurons, but can to some extent be obtained from the diet [239]. In relation to ROS, creatine has been shown to provide an antioxidant capacity and buffer intracellular energy reserves, stabilizing intracellular calcium, and inhibit activation of the mitochondrial pore transition [239]. Supplementation was found to be neuroprotective in several *in vitro* and *in vivo* studies. Chronic administration of creatine was shown to significantly increase survival, tyrosine hydroxylase, immunoreactive fiber density, and size of dopaminergic neurons in mesencephalic cultures by protecting against neurotoxic insults induced by serum and glucose deprivation, MPP+ and 6-hydroxydopamine [240-242]. Furthermore, it has been shown that creatine treatment can reduce serum 8-hydroxy-2'-deoxyguanosine levels [243]. However, while creatine has shown positive short-term improvements in patients with mitochondrial and neuromuscular diseases, there are documented side effects with creatine use. Specifically, side effects of creatine can include: diarrhea, dehydration, weight gain, kidney dysfunction, which should be seriously considered.

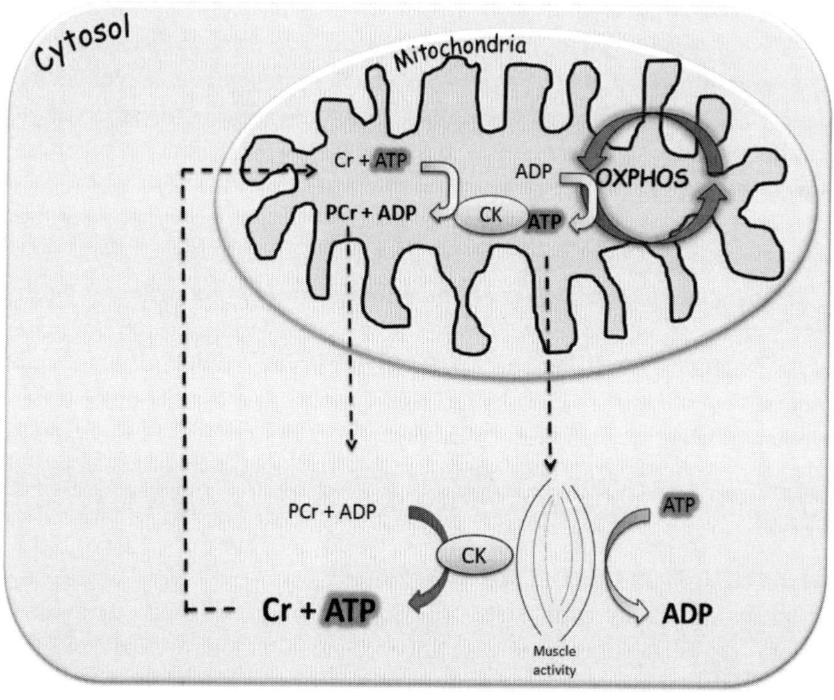

Figure 6. Schematic model of the creatine kinase energy shuttle. The high-energy phosphate bond is transferred from ATP to creatine to form PCr and ADP inside the mitochondria, a reaction catalysed by CK. PCr diffuses to the site of energy utilization, for example the muscles during muscle activity, where the reverse reaction takes place, to maintain adequately high ATP.

Melatonin

Melatonin is produced by the pineal gland, a small endocrine gland located in the center of the brain. The major function of melatonin signal is a part of the system that regulates the sleep vs. wake cycle, done by chemically causing drowsiness and lowering the body temperature [244]. However beside melatonin's main function it has been found to mediate a neuroprotective role in Alzheimer's by scavenging ROS and RNS generated in mitochondria [245-249], as it easily crosses cellular membranes [245, 250]. One of the mechanisms underlying the neuroprotective effects of melatonin is a counter-action against mitochondrial apoptosis-inducing pathways. Melatonin activates the survival signal Bcl-2 dependent pathway, which stabilizes mitochondrial function [251]. Melatonin prevents oxidative stress-induced mitochondrial calcium overload, $\Delta\Psi m$ depolarization, opening of mtPTP, ROS formation, and cytochrome c release in rat astrocytes in a chemical model of Parkinson's disease [251]. Studies showed that even when small amounts of melatonin were administered to mice, it reduced the oxidative damage caused by aging and delayed the inflammatory process, which in turn increased the longevity of the mice [252]. As compared to creatine, melatonin appears to cause very few side-effects in the short term, up to three months, when healthy people take it at low doses [253].

CoQ10

Coenzyme Q10 (CoQ10) is essential for the energy production of the cells as it functions as an electron transporter in the mitochondrial respiratory chain. CoQ10 functions as an electron carrier from enzyme complex I and enzyme complex II to complex III in this process. This is crucial in the process, since no other molecule can perform this function. CoQ10 furthermore links the mitochondrial fatty acid β-oxidation to the respiratory chain by accepting electrons from electron transfer flavoprotein-ubiquinone oxidoreductase (ETF-QO), which resides in the inner mitochondrial membrane, and passing them onto the electron transport complex III [29].

There are three redox states of CoQ10: fully oxidized (ubiquinone), semiquinone (ubisemiquinone), and fully reduced (ubiquinol). The capacity of this molecule to exist in a completely oxidized form and a completely reduced form enables it to perform its functions in the electron transport chain and as an antioxidant respectively. CoQ10 is composed of a benzoquinone ring derived from the aromatic amino acids phenylalanine and tyrosine and ten isoprenoid units synthesized from acetyl-CoA. It is synthesized inside mitochondria by a multienzyme complex [254-256]. We recently revealed moderate CoQ10 deficiency and increased mitochondrial ROS in patient fibroblasts carrying variant ETF-QO proteins with impaired CoQ10 binding affinity, and showed that CoQ10 treatment could decrease the amount of ROS in the cells [23]. Studies showing moderate CoQ10 deficiency in fibroblasts from patients with ETF or VLCAD deficiency [124], suggest that CoQ10 treatment could be beneficial also for patients with other FAO disorders. The causes of CoQ10 deficiency in patients with primary defects in FAO genes or in other genes, not directly involved in CoQ10 synthesis like APTX (aprataxin) and mtDNA, are not known. Common to these patients are mitochondrial energy deficiency and it has been suggested that this could impair mitochondrial import of CoQ10 proteins thereby causing CoQ10 deficiency. CoQ10 also protects against iron-induced apoptosis in dopaminergic neurons [257]. Pretreatment of neuronal cells with CoQ10 maintains mitochondrial membrane potential during oxidative stress and reduces the amount of mitochondrial ROS generation [258]. It was shown that supplementation of CoQ10 could decrease the level of malondialdehyde, an indicator of oxidative stress, and increase the activity of SOD, in a transgenic mice model of Alzheimer's [259].

The efficiency of absorption of orally administered CoQ10 is poor because of its insolubility in water, limited solubility in lipids, and relatively large molecular weight [260]. Idebenone is a short-chain analog of CoQ10, which penetrates membranes and enters mitochondria much more efficiently than CoQ10. It reduces membrane lipids peroxidation and carries electrons from complexes I/II to complex III as well as rescue CoQ10 deficient cells [261]. Idebenone is reduced by ROS and releases electrons to the respiratory chain to be restored in its quinone form, promoting OXPHOS. In addition, it decreases lipoperoxidation in heart homogenates from patients with valvular stenosis [262]. A study with FA patients has reported that idebenone treatment at early stages of the disease seems to reduce the progression of cerebellar manifestations [263]. Furthermore, the effect of idebenone on oxidative markers has also been evaluated. An open-label trial in FA patients has shown a decrease of 8-hydroxy-2′-deoxyguanosine levels after eight weeks of treatment with idebenone [264]. However, study on FA adolescents treated for six months with idebenone, from low to high concentrations, has not revealed any difference in the urinary levels of 8-hydroxy-2′-deoxyguanosine [265]. There are many other contradicting results with idebenone treatment and therefore results should be carefully evaluated and further investigated, because of the technical difficulties in evaluating a marker of oxidative stress.

However it might be likely that the contradicting effect on early vs later progression of disease is due to the accumulation of oxidative damage.

3.2. Mitochondrial-Targeting Antioxidants

While a wide range of lipophilic cations could in principle be utilized for drug targeting purposes, to date, only one such compound has been extensively characterized in this context; triphennylphosphonium (TPP+) cation. Several mitochondrial targeting antioxidants have been developed by conjugating the lipophilic TPP+ to an antioxidant moiety, such as CoQ10 (MitoQ) and α-tocopherol (MitoE) [266]. This approach makes use of the proton gradient across the mitochondrial inner membrane. As a result of the proton gradient, a negative potential to 150 to 180 mV is generated across the inner membrane. Lipophilic cations may therefore accumulate 100- to 1000-fold inside the mitochondria [267].

To date most intervention studies have focused on MitoQ. Within mitochondria, MitoQ is believed to be located primarily within the inner mitochondrial membrane, where the TPP group faces the matrix side of the inner mitochondrial membrane and the ubiquinol moiety is positioned in the hydrophobic interior of the inner membrane [268-270].

MitoE protects mitochondria from isolated rat liver from iron/ascorbate- and *tert*-butylhydroperoxide-induced oxidative damage, measured by decreased lipid peroxidation.

The effect of MitoE on mitochondrial ROS in TNF-induced apoptosis has been investigated in Junkat and U937 cells, where MitoE reduces H_2O_2-induced caspase 3 activity. The cleavage and activation of caspase-8 after incubation with TNF were not affected by MitoE, but the activation of caspase-3 was increased. In addition, increased cleavage of Bid, a pro-apoptotic member of the Bcl-2 protein family, and an increased release of cytochrome c from mitochondria were observed in cells incubated with TNF in the presence of MitoE. Further studies showed that MitoE accelerated TNF-induced apoptosis by increasing the nuclear localization of NF-kB. These findings demonstrate that mitochondrial ROS generation is a component of the TNF signal-transduction pathway during apoptosis [271]. MitoE prevents oxidative-stress-induced cell death in cultured fibroblasts from FA subjects [272].

Mitochondrial-Targeting Peptides – SS-Peptides

An alternative approach to the use of the lipophilic cations (TPP+) to direct antioxidants to the mitochondria is the use of mitochondrial targeting peptides. Szeto Schiller (SS) peptides was some of the first mitochondrial targeting peptides to be found [273, 274] Unlike TPP-based small molecules antioxidants, SS-peptide uptake into mitochondria is largely independent of the membrane potential and is not self-limiting because accumulation of the peptides does not decrease mitochondrial membrane potential [274]. The structural motif of these SS peptides centers on alternating aromatic residues and basic amino acids. The antioxidant properties of these tetrapeptides apparently originate from the presence of Dmt (2',6'-dimethyltyrosine) residue, which has been demonstrated by analysis of SS peptide SS-20 (Phe-D-Arg-Phe-Lys-NH_2), which lack the Dmt residue. Studies showed that this SS-peptide did not demonstrate antioxidant activity compared to other SS-peptides containing the Dmt residue. Two other SS-peptides both containing the Dmt residue; SS-02 (Dmt-D-Arg-Phe-Lys-NH2) and SS-31 (D-Arg-Dmt-Lys-Phe-NH2) have both been shown to exhibit great antioxidant properties. SS-02 has been shown to scavenge H_2O_2 and inhibits the oxidation of linoleic acid and low-density lipoproteins (LDL) [274-276].

Transcriptional Targeting

Targeting transcriptional regulation, as a treatment for oxidative stress, has come increasingly into focus recent years, both because of the lack of effective treatment by the traditional treatments, as antioxidants, but also because of the increasing acknowledgement of the important/essential function of transcriptional signaling pathways in the recent years. One of the transcriptional regulators which have gain much interest, as a target for treatment, is Nrf2. Induction of Nrf2 by drugs has become a potential therapeutic target for especially neurodegenerative diseases. Many new Nrf2 inducers have been found from a variety of sources, including natural products and derivates, clinical drugs and endogenous compounds. Among the inducers, the isothiocyanates (ITCs), present in cruciferous vegetables, have gained attention as potential neuroprotective compounds with indirect antioxidant properties involved in the activation of Nrf2 [277, 278]. Another inducer of Nrf2 is Bardoxolone methyl (methyl 2-cyano-3,12-dioxooleana-1,9(11)dien-28-oate, CDDO-Me, or RTA 402), which is a synthetic triterpenoid derived from the natural product oleanolic acid and member of a class of antioxidant inflammation modulators and are one of the most potent activators of Nrf2 known [279-281].

Conclusion

We have in the present chapter discussed to what extent oxidative stress contribute to the pathogenesis of neuromuscular disorders such as IEM and FA. Even though the data presented do not allow a final answer to the question mark, raised by the chapter title, they do provide evidence that oxidative stress play a key role in modulating the mitochondrial dysfunction and cellular processes associated with the diseases, such as metabolic reprogramming, changes in mitochondrial dynamic and altered regulation of antioxidant systems. Interestingly, in both IEM and FA there is growing evidence that common survival signaling pathways activates such cellular mechanisms to allow the cell to escape ROS-induced apoptosis/necrosis resulting in a growth-promoting and cell degenerative phenotype. As many of these signaling pathways are controlled by redox-sensitive phosphatases/kinases and transcription factors, it seems obvious to suggest that they could directly be oxidized and activated by the ROS/RNS produced as a consequence of the primary genetic defects in IEM and FA as discussed in this chapter. Unravelling the precise molecular triggers and sequence of events that lead to mitochondrial dysfunction and oxidative stress in neuromuscular disorders is certainly a challenge for future research. However, if successful, such studies will add important knowledge to the further development and fine-tuning of mitochondrial targeted therapies for neuromuscular disorders. Monogenetic disorders, like IEM and FA, are seen as attractive models for such studies due to their relatively simple and well-defined etiology.

References

[1] Lin, M.T., Beal, M.F. (2006) Mitochondrial Dysfunction And Oxidative Stress In Neurodegenerative Diseases. *Nature*, 443, 787-795.

[2] Circu, M.L., Aw, T.Y. (2010) Reactive Oxygen Species, Cellular Redox Systems, And Apoptosis. *Free Radic. Biol. Med.*, 48, 749-762.

[3] Echtay, K.S. (2007) Mitochondrial Uncoupling Proteins--What Is Their Physiological Role? *Free Radic. Biol. Med.*, 43, 1351-1371.

[4] St-Pierre, J., Buckingham, J.A., Roebuck, S.J., Brand, M.D. (2002) Topology Of Superoxide Production From Different Sites In The Mitochondrial Electron Transport Chain. *J Biol. Chem*, 277, 44784-44790.

[5] Drose, S., Brandt, U. (2012) Molecular Mechanisms Of Superoxide Production By The Mitochondrial Respiratory Chain. *Adv. Exp. Med. Biol.*, 748, 145-169.

[6] Chance, B., Sies, H., Boveris, A. (1979) Hydroperoxide Metabolism In Mammalian Organs. *Physiol Rev.*, 59, 527-605.

[7] Valko, M., Leibfritz, D., Moncol, J., Cronin, M.T., Mazur, M., Telser, J. (2007) Free Radicals And Antioxidants In Normal Physiological Functions And Human Disease. *Int. J Biochem. Cell Biol.*, 39, 44-84.

[8] Jezek, P., Hlavata, L. (2005) Mitochondria In Homeostasis Of Reactive Oxygen Species In Cell, Tissues, And Organism. *Int. J Biochem. Cell Biol.*, 37, 2478-2503.

[9] Olsen, R.K., Cornelius, N., Gregersen, N. (2013) Genetic And Cellular Modifiers Of Oxidative Stress: What Can We Learn From Fatty Acid Oxidation Defects? *Mol. Genet. Metab*, 110 Suppl, S31-S39.

[10] Cup, E.H., Pieterse, A.J., Ten Broek-Pastoor, J.M., Munneke, M., Van Engelen, B.G., Hendricks, H.T., Van Der Wilt, G.J., Oostendorp, R.A. (2007) Exercise Therapy And Other Types Of Physical Therapy For Patients With Neuromuscular Diseases: A Systematic Review. *Arch. Phys. Med. Rehabil.*, 88, 1452-1464.

[11] Sadeghian, H., Wolfe, G.I. (2010) Therapy Update In Nerve, Neuromuscular Junction And Myopathic Disorders. *Curr. Opin. Neurol.*, 23, 496-501.

[12] Gomes, C.M., Santos, R. (2013) Neurodegeneration In Friedreich's Ataxia: From Defective Frataxin To Oxidative Stress. *Oxid. Med. Cell Longev.*, 2013, 487534.

[13] Berg, J.M., Tymoczko, J.L., Stryer, L. (2002) *Biochemistry*. W.H. Freeman, New York.

[14] Mcbride, H.M., Neuspiel, M., Wasiak, S. (2006) Mitochondria: More Than Just A Powerhouse. *Curr. Biol.*, 16, R551-R560.

[15] Fischer, F., Hamann, A., Osiewacz, H.D. (2012) Mitochondrial Quality Control: An Integrated Network Of Pathways. *Trends Biochem. Sci.*, 37, 284-292.

[16] Ray, P.D., Huang, B.W., Tsuji, Y. (2012) Reactive Oxygen Species (ROS) Homeostasis And Redox Regulation In Cellular Signaling. *Cell Signal.*, 24, 981-990.

[17] Martindale, J.L., Holbrook, N.J. (2002) Cellular Response To Oxidative Stress: Signaling For Suicide And Survival. *J. Cell Physiol*, 192, 1-15.

[18] Murphy, M.P. (2009) How Mitochondria Produce Reactive Oxygen Species. *Biochem. J*, 417, 1-13.

[19] Mates, J.M. (2000) Effects Of Antioxidant Enzymes In The Molecular Control Of Reactive Oxygen Species Toxicology. *Toxicology*, 153, 83-104.

[20] Andreyev, A.Y., Kushnareva,Y.E., Starkov, A.A. (2005) Mitochondrial Metabolism Of Reactive Oxygen Species. *Biochemistry (Mosc.)*, 70, 200-214.

[21] Starkov, A.A., Fiskum, G., Chinopoulos, C., Lorenzo, B.J., Browne, S.E., Patel, M.S., Beal, M.F. (2004) Mitochondrial Alpha-Ketoglutarate Dehydrogenase Complex Generates Reactive Oxygen Species. *J. Neurosci.*, 24, 7779-7788.

[22] Tretter, L., Takacs, K., Hegedus, V., Adam-Vizi, V. (2007) Characteristics Of Alpha-Glycerophosphate-Evoked H2O2 Generation In Brain Mitochondria. *J. Neurochem.*, 100, 650-663.

[23] Cornelius, N., Byron, C., Hargreaves, I., Guerra, P.F., Furdek, A.K., Land, J., Radford, W.W., Frerman, F., Corydon, T.J., Gregersen, N., Olsen, R.K. (2013) Secondary Coenzyme Q10 Deficiency And Oxidative Stress In Cultured Fibroblasts From Patients With Riboflavin Responsive Multiple Acyl-Coa Dehydrogenation Deficiency. *Hum. Mol. Genet.*, 22, 3819-3827.

[24] Rodrigues, J.V., Gomes, C.M. (2012) Mechanism Of Superoxide And Hydrogen Peroxide Generation By Human Electron-Transfer Flavoprotein And Pathological Variants. *Free Radic. Biol. Med.*, 53, 12-19.

[25] Zeevalk, G.D., Bernard, L.P., Song, C., Gluck, M., Ehrhart, J. (2005) Mitochondrial Inhibition And Oxidative Stress: Reciprocating Players In Neurodegeneration. *Antioxid. Redox. Signal.*, 7, 1117-1139.

[26] Otterbein, L.E., Soares, M.P., Yamashita, K., Bach, F.H. (2003) Heme Oxygenase-1: Unleashing The Protective Properties Of Heme. *Trends Immunol.*, 24, 449-455.

[27] Bentinger, M., Brismar, K., Dallner, G. (2007) The Antioxidant Role Of Coenzyme Q. *Mitochondrion.*, 7 Suppl, S41-S50.

[28] Quinzii, C.M., Hirano, M. (2011) Primary And Secondary Coq(10) Deficiencies In Humans. *Biofactors*, 37, 361-365.

[29] Quinzii, C.M., Lopez, L.C., Naini, A., Dimauro, S., Hirano, M. (2008) Human Coq10 Deficiencies. *Biofactors*, 32, 113-118.

[30] Manthey, K.C., Chew, Y.C., Zempleni, J. (2005) Riboflavin Deficiency Impairs Oxidative Folding And Secretion Of Apolipoprotein B-100 In Hepg2 Cells, Triggering Stress Response Systems. *J Nutr.*, 135, 978-982.

[31] Itoh, K., Wakabayashi, N., Katoh, Y., Ishii, T., Igarashi, K., Engel, J.D., Yamamoto, M. (1999) Keap1 Represses Nuclear Activation Of Antioxidant Responsive Elements By Nrf2 Through Binding To The Amino-Terminal Neh2 Domain. *Genes Dev.*, 13, 76-86.
[32] Kobayashi, A., Kang, M.I., Okawa, H., Ohtsuji, M., Zenke, Y., Chiba, T., Igarashi, K., Yamamoto, M. (2004) Oxidative Stress Sensor Keap1 Functions As An Adaptor For Cul3-Based E3 Ligase To Regulate Proteasomal Degradation Of Nrf2. *Mol. Cell Biol.*, 24, 7130-7139.
[33] Yamamoto, T., Suzuki, T., Kobayashi, A., Wakabayashi, J., Maher, J., Motohashi, H., Yamamoto, M. (2008) Physiological Significance Of Reactive Cysteine Residues Of Keap1 In Determining Nrf2 Activity. *Mol. Cell Biol.*, 28, 2758-2770.
[34] Sekhar, K.R., Rachakonda, G., Freeman, M.L. (2010) Cysteine-Based Regulation Of The CUL3 Adaptor Protein Keap1. *Toxicol. Appl. Pharmacol.*, 244, 21-26.
[35] Ma, Q. (2013) Role Of Nrf2 In Oxidative Stress And Toxicity. *Annu. Rev. Pharmacol. Toxicol.*, 53, 401-426.
[36] Itoh, K., Chiba, T., Takahashi, S., Ishii, T., Igarashi, K., Katoh, Y., Oyake, T., Hayashi, N., Satoh, K., Hatayama, I., et al. (1997) An Nrf2/Small Maf Heterodimer Mediates The Induction Of Phase II Detoxifying Enzyme Genes Through Antioxidant Response Elements. *Biochem. Biophys. Res. Commun.*, 236, 313-322.
[37] Seppet, E., Gruno, M., Peetsalu, A., Gizatullina, Z., Nguyen, H.P., Vielhaber, S., Wussling, M.H., Trumbeckaite, S., Arandarcikaite, O., Jerzembeck, D., et al. (2009) Mitochondria And Energetic Depression In Cell Pathophysiology. *Int. J. Mol. Sci.*, 10, 2252-2303.
[38] Kant, R., Bali, A., Singh, N., Jaggi, A.S. (2013) Prolyl 4 Hydroxylase: A Critical Target In The Pathophysiology Of Diseases. *Korean J. Physiol Pharmacol.*, 17, 111-120.
[39] Fogg, V.C., Lanning, N.J., Mackeigan, J.P. (2011) Mitochondria In Cancer: At The Crossroads Of Life And Death. *Chin J Cancer*, 30, 526-539.
[40] Semenza, G.L. (2010) HIF-1: Upstream And Downstream Of Cancer Metabolism. *Curr. Opin. Genet Dev.*, 20, 51-56.
[41] Semenza, G.L. (2010) Defining The Role Of Hypoxia-Inducible Factor 1 In Cancer Biology And Therapeutics. *Oncogene*, 29, 625-634.
[42] WARBURG, O. (1956) On The Origin Of Cancer Cells. *Science*, 123, 309-314.

[43] Smolkova, K., Plecita-Hlavata, L., Bellance, N., Benard, G., Rossignol, R., Jezek, P. (2011) Waves Of Gene Regulation Suppress And Then Restore Oxidative Phosphorylation In Cancer Cells. *Int. J Biochem. Cell Biol.*, 43, 950-968.

[44] Guppy, M. (2002) The Hypoxic Core: A Possible Answer To The Cancer Paradox. *Biochem. Biophys. Res. Commun.*, 299, 676-680.

[45] Altenberg, B., Greulich,K.O. (2004) Genes Of Glycolysis Are Ubiquitously Overexpressed In 24 Cancer Classes. *Genomics*, 84, 1014-1020.

[46] Bonnet, S., Archer, S.L., Allalunis-Turner, J., Haromy, A., Beaulieu, C., Thompson, R., Lee, C.T., Lopaschuk, G.D., Puttagunta, L., Bonnet, S., et al. (2007) A Mitochondria-K+ Channel Axis Is Suppressed In Cancer And Its Normalization Promotes Apoptosis And Inhibits Cancer Growth. *Cancer Cell*, 11, 37-51.

[47] Xie, H., Valera, V.A., Merino, M.J., Amato, A.M., Signoretti, S., Linehan, W.M., Sukhatme, V.P., Seth, P. (2009) LDH-A Inhibition, A Therapeutic Strategy For Treatment Of Hereditary Leiomyomatosis And Renal Cell Cancer. *Mol. Cancer Ther.*, 8, 626-635.

[48] Hatzivassiliou, G., Zhao, F., Bauer, D.E., Andreadis, C., Shaw, A.N., Dhanak, D., Hingorani, S.R., Tuveson, D.A., Thompson, C.B. (2005) ATP Citrate Lyase Inhibition Can Suppress Tumor Cell Growth. *Cancer Cell*, 8, 311-321.

[49] Koppenol, W.H., Bounds, P.L., Dang, C.V. (2011) Otto Warburg's Contributions To Current Concepts Of Cancer Metabolism. *Nat. Rev. Cancer*, 11, 325-337.

[50] Lopez-Lazaro, M. (2008) The Warburg Effect: Why And How Do Cancer Cells Activate Glycolysis In The Presence Of Oxygen? *Anticancer Agents Med. Chem*, 8, 305-312.

[51] Moreno-Sanchez, R., Rodriguez-Enriquez, S., Marin-Hernandez, A., Saavedra, E. (2007) Energy Metabolism In Tumor Cells. *FEBS J*, 274, 1393-1418.

[52] Gatenby, R.A., Gillies, R.J. (2004) Why Do Cancers Have High Aerobic Glycolysis? *Nat. Rev. Cancer*, 4, 891-899.

[53] Bonuccelli, G., Tsirigos, A., Whitaker-Menezes, D., Pavlides, S., Pestell, R.G., Chiavarina, B., Frank, P.G., Flomenberg, N., Howell, A., Martinez-Outschoorn, U.E., et al. (2010) Ketones And Lactate "Fuel" Tumor Growth And Metastasis: Evidence That Epithelial Cancer Cells Use Oxidative Mitochondrial Metabolism. *Cell Cycle*, 9, 3506-3514.

[54] Hirschhaeuser, F., Sattler, U.G., Mueller-Klieser, W. (2011) Lactate: A Metabolic Key Player In Cancer. *Cancer Res.*, 71, 6921-6925.

[55] Vaughn, A.E., Deshmukh, M. (2008) Glucose Metabolism Inhibits Apoptosis In Neurons And Cancer Cells By Redox Inactivation Of Cytochrome C. *Nat. Cell Biol.*, 10, 1477-1483.

[56] Chandel, N.S., Maltepe, E., Goldwasser, E., Mathieu, C.E., Simon, M.C., Schumacker, P.T. (1998) Mitochondrial Reactive Oxygen Species Trigger Hypoxia-Induced Transcription. *Proc. Natl. Acad. Sci. U. S. A*, 95, 11715-11720.

[57] Mansfield, K.D., Guzy, R.D., Pan, Y., Young, R.M., Cash, T.P., Schumacker, P.T., Simon, M.C. (2005) Mitochondrial Dysfunction Resulting From Loss Of Cytochrome C Impairs Cellular Oxygen Sensing And Hypoxic HIF-Alpha Activation. *Cell Metab*, 1, 393-399.

[58] Guzy, R.D., Hoyos, B., Robin, E., Chen, H., Liu, L., Mansfield, K.D., Simon, M.C., Hammerling, U., Schumacker, P.T. (2005) Mitochondrial Complex III Is Required For Hypoxia-Induced ROS Production And Cellular Oxygen Sensing. *Cell Metab*, 1, 401-408.

[59] Brunelle, J.K., Bell, E.L., Quesada, N.M., Vercauteren, K., Tiranti,V., Zeviani, M., Scarpulla, R.C., Chandel, N.S. (2005) Oxygen Sensing Requires Mitochondrial ROS But Not Oxidative Phosphorylation. *Cell Metab*, 1, 409-414.

[60] Kaelin, W.G., Jr. (2005) ROS: Really Involved In Oxygen Sensing. *Cell Metab*, 1, 357-358.

[61] Ma, Q., Cavallin, L.E., Yan, B., Zhu, S., Duran, E.M., Wang, H., Hale, L.P., Dong, C., Cesarman, E., Mesri, E.A., Goldschmidt-Clermont,P.J. (2009) Antitumorigenesis Of Antioxidants In A Transgenic Rac1 Model Of Kaposi's Sarcoma. *Proc. Natl. Acad. Sci. U. S. A*, 106, 8683-8688.

[62] Guzy, R.D., Sharma, B., Bell, E., Chandel, N.S., Schumacker, P.T. (2008) Loss Of The Sdhb, But Not The Sdha, Subunit Of Complex II Triggers Reactive Oxygen Species-Dependent Hypoxia-Inducible Factor Activation And Tumorigenesis. *Mol. Cell Biol.*, 28, 718-731.

[63] Yuan, H.X., Xiong, Y., Guan, K.L. (2013) Nutrient Sensing, Metabolism, And Cell Growth Control. *Mol. Cell*, 49, 379-387.

[64] Hagen, T. (2012) Oxygen Versus Reactive Oxygen In The Regulation Of HIF-1alpha: The Balance Tips. *Biochem. Res. Int.*, 2012, 436981.

[65] Page, E.L., Chan, D.A., Giaccia, A.J., Levine, M., Richard, D.E. (2008) Hypoxia-Inducible Factor-1alpha Stabilization In Nonhypoxic Conditions: Role Of Oxidation And Intracellular Ascorbate Depletion. *Mol. Biol. Cell*, 19, 86-94.

[66] Finkel, T. (2012) Signal Transduction By Mitochondrial Oxidants. *J. Biol. Chem.*, 287, 4434-4440.

[67] Huang, C., Han, Y., Wang, Y., Sun, X., Yan, S., Yeh, E.T., Chen, Y., Cang, H., Li, H., Shi, G., et al. (2009) SENP3 Is Responsible For HIF-1 Transactivation Under Mild Oxidative Stress Via P300 De-Sumoylation. *EMBO J.*, 28, 2748-2762.

[68] Wang, Y., Yang, J., Yang, K., Cang, H., Huang, X.Z., Li, H., Yi, J. (2012) The Biphasic Redox Sensing Of SENP3 Accounts For The HIF-1 Transcriptional Activity Shift By Oxidative Stress. *Acta Pharmacol. Sin.*, 33, 953-963.

[69] Fijalkowska, I., Xu, W., Comhair, S.A., Janocha, A.J., Mavrakis, L.A., Krishnamachary, B., Zhen, L., Mao, T., Richter, A., Erzurum, S.C., Tuder, R.M. (2010) Hypoxia Inducible-Factor1alpha Regulates The Metabolic Shift Of Pulmonary Hypertensive Endothelial Cells. *Am. J Pathol.*, 176, 1130-1138.

[70] Sasabe, E., Yang, Z., Ohno, S., Yamamoto, T. (2010) Reactive Oxygen Species Produced By The Knockdown Of Manganese-Superoxide Dismutase Up-Regulate Hypoxia-Inducible Factor-1alpha Expression In Oral Squamous Cell Carcinoma Cells. *Free Radic. Biol. Med.*, 48, 1321-1329.

[71] Kaewpila, S., Venkataraman, S., Buettner, G.R., Oberley, L.W. (2008) Manganese Superoxide Dismutase Modulates Hypoxia-Inducible Factor-1 Alpha Induction Via Superoxide. *Cancer Res.*, 68, 2781-2788.

[72] Shaw, P.J. (2005) Molecular And Cellular Pathways Of Neurodegeneration In Motor Neurone Disease. *J. Neurol. Neurosurg. Psychiatry*, 76, 1046-1057.

[73] Shaw, P.J. (1999) Motor Neurone Disease. *BMJ*, 318, 1118-1121.

[74] Gandhi, S., Abramov, A.Y. (2012) Mechanism Of Oxidative Stress In Neurodegeneration. *Oxid. Med. Cell Longev.*, 2012, 428010.

[75] Kann, O., Kovacs, R. (2007) Mitochondria And Neuronal Activity. *Am. J. Physiol Cell Physiol*, 292, C641-C657.

[76] Shaw, P.J., Eggett, C.J. (2000) Molecular Factors Underlying Selective Vulnerability Of Motor Neurons To Neurodegeneration In Amyotrophic Lateral Sclerosis. *J. Neurol.*, 247 Suppl 1, I17-I27.

[77] Berridge, M.J. (1998) Neuronal Calcium Signaling. *Neuron*, 21, 13-26.

[78] Bilsland, L.G., Sahai, E., Kelly, G., Golding, M., Greensmith, L., Schiavo, G. (2010) Deficits In Axonal Transport Precede ALS Symptoms In Vivo. *Proc. Natl. Acad. Sci. U. S. A*, 107, 20523-20528.

[79] Williamson, T.L., Cleveland, D.W. (1999) Slowing Of Axonal Transport Is A Very Early Event In The Toxicity Of ALS-Linked SOD1 Mutants To Motor Neurons. *Nat. Neurosci.*, 2, 50-56.

[80] Saha, A.R., Hill, J., Utton, M.A., Asuni, A.A., Ackerley, S., Grierson, A.J., Miller, C.C., Davies, A.M., Buchman, V.L., Anderton, B.H., Hanger, D.P. (2004) Parkinson's Disease Alpha-Synuclein Mutations Exhibit Defective Axonal Transport In Cultured Neurons. *J. Cell Sci.*, 117, 1017-1024.

[81] Trimmer, P.A., Schwartz, K.M., Borland, M.K., De, T.L., Streeter, J., Oron, U. (2009) Reduced Axonal Transport In Parkinson's Disease Cybrid Neurites Is Restored By Light Therapy. *Mol. Neurodegener.*, 4, 26.

[82] Utton, M.A., Noble, W.J., Hill, J.E., Anderton, B.H., Hanger, D.P. (2005) Molecular Motors Implicated In The Axonal Transport Of Tau And Alpha-Synuclein. *J. Cell Sci.*, 118, 4645-4654.

[83] Her, L.S., Goldstein, L.S. (2008) Enhanced Sensitivity Of Striatal Neurons To Axonal Transport Defects Induced By Mutant Huntingtin. *J. Neurosci.*, 28, 13662-13672.

[84] Fang, C., Bourdette, D., Banker, G. (2012) Oxidative Stress Inhibits Axonal Transport: Implications For Neurodegenerative Diseases. *Mol. Neurodegener.*, 7, 29.

[85] Shidara, Y., Hollenbeck, P.J. (2010) Defects In Mitochondrial Axonal Transport And Membrane Potential Without Increased Reactive Oxygen Species Production In A Drosophila Model Of Friedreich Ataxia. *J. Neurosci.*, 30, 11369-11378.

[86] Tobon, A. (2013) Metabolic Myopathies. *Continuum (Minneap. Minn.)*, 19, 1571-1597.

[87] Koopman, W.J., Distelmaier, F., Smeitink, J.A., Willems, P.H. (2013) OXPHOS Mutations And Neurodegeneration. *EMBO J*, 32, 9-29.

[88] Koopman, W.J., Willems, P.H., Smeitink, J.A. (2012) Monogenic Mitochondrial Disorders. *N. Engl. J Med.*, 366, 1132-1141.

[89] Wei, Y.H., Lee, H.C. (2003) Mitochondrial DNA Mutations And Oxidative Stress In Mitochondrial Diseases. *Adv. Clin. Chem.*, 37, 83-128.

[90] Olsen, R.K., Cornelius, N., Gregersen, N. (2013) Genetic And Cellular Modifiers Of Oxidative Stress: What Can We Learn From Fatty Acid Oxidation Defects? *Mol Genet Metab*, 110 Suppl, S31-S39.

[91] Gregersen, N., Andresen, B.S., Pedersen, C.B., Olsen, R.K., Corydon, T.J., Bross, P. (2008) Mitochondrial Fatty Acid Oxidation Defects--Remaining Challenges. *J Inherit. Metab Dis*, 31, 643-657.
[92] Gregersen, N., Olsen, R.K. (2010) Disease Mechanisms And Protein Structures In Fatty Acid Oxidation Defects. *J Inherit. Metab Dis*, 33, 547-553.
[93] Wajner, M., Goodman, S.I. (2011) Disruption Of Mitochondrial Homeostasis In Organic Acidurias: Insights From Human And Animal Studies. *J Bioenerg. Biomembr.*, 43, 31-38.
[94] Kolker, S., Burgard, P., Sauer, S.W., Okun, J.G. (2013) Current Concepts In Organic Acidurias: Understanding Intra- And Extracerebral Disease Manifestation. *J Inherit. Metab Dis*, 36, 635-644.
[95] Ribas, G.S., Vargas, C.R., Wajner, M. (2014) L-Carnitine Supplementation As A Potential Antioxidant Therapy For Inherited Neurometabolic Disorders. *Gene*, 533, 469-476.
[96] Tein, I. (1999) Neonatal Metabolic Myopathies. *Semin. Perinatol.*, 23, 125-151.
[97] Laforet, P., Vianey-Saban, C. (2010) Disorders Of Muscle Lipid Metabolism: Diagnostic And Therapeutic Challenges. *Neuromuscul. Disord.*, 20, 693-700.
[98] Wu, S.B., Wei, Y.H. (2012) AMPK-Mediated Increase Of Glycolysis As An Adaptive Response To Oxidative Stress In Human Cells: Implication Of The Cell Survival In Mitochondrial Diseases. *Biochim. Biophys. Acta*, 1822, 233-247.
[99] Wu, S.B., Ma, Y.S., Wu, Y.T., Chen, Y.C., Wei, Y.H. (2010) Mitochondrial DNA Mutation-Elicited Oxidative Stress, Oxidative Damage, And Altered Gene Expression In Cultured Cells Of Patients With MERRF Syndrome. *Mol Neurobiol.*, 41, 256-266.
[100] Andresen, B.S., Olpin, S., Poorthuis, B.J., Scholte, H.R., Vianey-Saban, C., Wanders, R., Ijlst, L., Morris, A., Pourfarzam,M., Bartlett,K., et al. (1999) Clear Correlation Of Genotype With Disease Phenotype In Very-Long-Chain Acyl-Coa Dehydrogenase Deficiency. *Am. J Hum Genet*, 64, 479-494.
[101] Olsen, R.K., Andresen, B.S., Christensen, E., Bross, P., Skovby, F., Gregersen, N. (2003) Clear Relationship Between ETF/ETFDH Genotype And Phenotype In Patients With Multiple Acyl-Coa Dehydrogenation Deficiency. *Hum Mutat.*, 22, 12-23.
[102] Gregersen, N., Andresen, B.S., Corydon, M.J., Corydon, T.J., Olsen, R.K., Bolund, L., Bross, P. (2001) Mutation Analysis In Mitochondrial

Fatty Acid Oxidation Defects: Exemplified By Acyl-Coa Dehydrogenase Deficiencies, With Special Focus On Genotype-Phenotype Relationship. *Hum Mutat.*, 18, 169-189.

[103] Gregersen, N., Bross, P., Andresen, B.S. (2004) Genetic Defects In Fatty Acid Beta-Oxidation And Acyl-Coa Dehydrogenases. Molecular Pathogenesis And Genotype-Phenotype Relationships. *Eur. J Biochem.*, 271, 470-482.

[104] Bonnefont, J.P., Djouadi, F., Prip-Buus, C., Gobin, S., Munnich, A., Bastin, J. (2004) Carnitine Palmitoyltransferases 1 And 2: Biochemical, Molecular And Medical Aspects. *Mol Aspects Med.*, 25, 495-520.

[105] Spiekerkoetter, U. (2010) Mitochondrial Fatty Acid Oxidation Disorders: Clinical Presentation Of Long-Chain Fatty Acid Oxidation Defects Before And After Newborn Screening. *J Inherit. Metab Dis*, 33, 527-532.

[106] Pedersen, C.B., Kolvraa, S., Kolvraa, A., Stenbroen, V., Kjeldsen, M., Ensenauer, R., Tein, I., Matern, D., Rinaldo, P., Vianey-Saban, C., et al. (2008) The ACADS Gene Variation Spectrum In 114 Patients With Short-Chain Acyl-Coa Dehydrogenase (SCAD) Deficiency Is Dominated By Missense Variations Leading To Protein Misfolding At The Cellular Level. *Hum Genet*, 124, 43-56.

[107] Pedersen, C.B., Zolkipli, Z., Vang, S., Palmfeldt, J., Kjeldsen, M., Stenbroen, V., Schmidt, S.P., Wanders, R.J., Ruiter, J.P., Wibrand, F., et al. (2010) Antioxidant Dysfunction: Potential Risk For Neurotoxicity In Ethylmalonic Aciduria. *J Inherit. Metab Dis*, 33, 211-222.

[108] Schmidt, S.P., Corydon, T.J., Pedersen, C.B., Vang, S., Palmfeldt, J., Stenbroen, V., Wanders, R.J., Ruiter, J.P., Gregersen, N. (2011) Toxic Response Caused By A Misfolding Variant Of The Mitochondrial Protein Short-Chain Acyl-Coa Dehydrogenase. *J Inherit. Metab Dis*, 34, 465-475.

[109] Rocha, H., Ferreira, R., Carvalho, J., Vitorino, R., Santa, C., Lopes, L., Gregersen, N., Vilarinho, L., Amado, F. (2011) Characterization Of Mitochondrial Proteome In A Severe Case Of ETF-QO Deficiency. *J Proteomics.*, 75, 221-228.

[110] Edhager, A.V., Stenbroen, V., Nielsen, N.S., Bross, P., Olsen, R.K.J., Gregersen, N., Palmfeldt,J. (2014).

[111] Schmidt, S.P., Corydon, T.J., Pedersen, C.B., Bross, P., Gregersen, N. (2010) Misfolding Of Short-Chain Acyl-Coa Dehydrogenase Leads To Mitochondrial Fission And Oxidative Stress. *Mol Genet Metab*, 100, 155-162.

[112] Rodrigues, J.V., Gomes, C.M. (2012) Mechanism Of Superoxide And Hydrogen Peroxide Generation By Human Electron-Transfer Flavoprotein And Pathological Variants. *Free Radic. Biol. Med.*, 53, 12-19.

[113] Cornelius, N., Frerman, F.E., Corydon, T.J., Palmfeldt, J., Bross, P., Gregersen, N., Olsen, R.K. (2012) Molecular Mechanisms Of Riboflavin Responsiveness In Patients With ETF-QO Variations And Multiple Acyl-Coa Dehydrogenation Deficiency. *Hum Mol Genet*, 21, 3435-3448.

[114] Cornelius, N., Byron, C., Hargreaves, I., Guerra, P.F., Furdek, A.K., Land, J., Radford, W.W., Frerman, F., Corydon, T.J., Gregersen, N., Olsen, R.K. (2013) Secondary Coenzyme Q10 Deficiency And Oxidative Stress In Cultured Fibroblasts From Patients With Riboflavin Responsive Multiple Acyl-Coa Dehydrogenation Deficiency. *Hum Mol Genet.*

[115] Schmidt, S.P., Corydon, T.J., Pedersen, C.B., Bross, P., Gregersen, N. (2010) Misfolding Of Short-Chain Acyl-Coa Dehydrogenase Leads To Mitochondrial Fission And Oxidative Stress. *Mol Genet Metab*, 100, 155-162.

[116] Ashrafi, G., Schwarz, T.L. (2013) The Pathways Of Mitophagy For Quality Control And Clearance Of Mitochondria. *Cell Death. Differ.*, 20, 31-42.

[117] Gempel, K., Topaloglu, H., Talim, B., Schneiderat, P., Schoser, B.G., Hans, V.H., Palmafy, B., Kale, G., Tokatli, A., Quinzii, C., et al. (2007) The Myopathic Form Of Coenzyme Q10 Deficiency Is Caused By Mutations In The Electron-Transferring-Flavoprotein Dehydrogenase (ETFDH) Gene. *Brain*, 130, 2037-2044.

[118] Olsen, R.K., Olpin, S.E., Andresen, B.S., Miedzybrodzka, Z.H., Pourfarzam, M., Merinero, B., Frerman, F.E., Beresford, M.W., Dean, J.C., Cornelius, N., et al. (2007) ETFDH Mutations As A Major Cause Of Riboflavin-Responsive Multiple Acyl-Coa Dehydrogenation Deficiency. *Brain*, 130, 2045-2054.

[119] Wolfe, L.A., He, M., Vockley, J., Payne, N., Rhead, W., Hoppel, C., Spector, E., Gernert, K., Gibson, K.M. (2010) Novel ETF Dehydrogenase Mutations In A Patient With Mild Glutaric Aciduria Type II And Complex II-III Deficiency In Liver And Muscle. *J Inherit. Metab Dis.*

[120] Wen, B., Dai, T., Li, W., Zhao, Y., Liu, S., Zhang, C., Li, H., Wu, J., Li, D., Yan, C. (2010) Riboflavin-Responsive Lipid-Storage Myopathy

Caused By ETFDH Gene Mutations. *J Neurol. Neurosurg. Psychiatry*, 81, 231-236.

[121] Wen, B., Li, D., Shan, J., Liu, S., Li, W., Zhao, Y., Lin, P., Zheng, J., Li, D., Gong, Y., Yan, C. (2013) Increased Muscle Coenzyme Q10 In Riboflavin Responsive MADD With ETFDH Gene Mutations Due To Secondary Mitochondrial Proliferation. *Mol Genet Metab*, 109, 154-160.

[122] Liang, W.C., Ohkuma, A., Hayashi, Y.K., Lopez, L.C., Hirano, M., Nonaka, I., Noguchi, S., Chen, L.H., Jong, Y.J., Nishino, I. (2009) ETFDH Mutations, Coq10 Levels, And Respiratory Chain Activities In Patients With Riboflavin-Responsive Multiple Acyl-Coa Dehydrogenase Deficiency. *Neuromuscul. Disord.*, 19, 212-216.

[123] Tyni, T., Majander, A., Kalimo, H., Rapola, J., Pihko, H. (1996) Pathology Of Skeletal Muscle And Impaired Respiratory Chain Function In Long-Chain 3-Hydroxyacyl-Coa Dehydrogenase Deficiency With The G1528C Mutation. *Neuromuscul. Disord.*, 6, 327-337.

[124] Bujan, N., Arias, A., Montero, R., Garcia-Villoria, J., Lissens, W., Seneca, S., Espinos, C., Navas, P., De, M.L., Artuch, R., et al. (2014) Characterization Of Coq10 Biosynthesis In Fibroblasts Of Patients With Primary And Secondary Coq10 Deficiency. *J Inherit. Metab Dis*, 37, 53-62.

[125] Tonin, A.M., Ferreira, G.C., Grings, M., Viegas, C.M., Busanello, E.N., Amaral, A.U., Zanatta, A., Schuck, P.F., Wajner, M. (2010) Disturbance Of Mitochondrial Energy Homeostasis Caused By The Metabolites Accumulating In LCHAD And MTP Deficiencies In Rat Brain. *Life Sci.*, 86, 825-831.

[126] Tonin, A.M., Amaral, A.U., Busanello, E.N., Grings, M., Castilho, R.F., Wajner, M. (2013) Long-Chain 3-Hydroxy Fatty Acids Accumulating In Long-Chain 3-Hydroxyacyl-Coa Dehydrogenase And Mitochondrial Trifunctional Protein Deficiencies Uncouple Oxidative Phosphorylation In Heart Mitochondria. *J Bioenerg. Biomembr.*, 45, 47-57.

[127] Scaini, G., Simon, K.R., Tonin, A.M., Busanello, E.N., Moura, A.P., Ferreira, G.C., Wajner, M., Streck, E.L., Schuck, P.F. (2012) Toxicity Of Octanoate And Decanoate In Rat Peripheral Tissues: Evidence Of Bioenergetic Dysfunction And Oxidative Damage Induction In Liver And Skeletal Muscle. *Mol Cell Biochem.*, 361, 329-335.

[128] Song, Y., Selak, M.A., Watson, C.T., Coutts, C., Scherer, P.C., Panzer, J.A., Gibbs, S., Scott, M.O., Willer, G., Gregg, R.G., et al. (2009) Mechanisms Underlying Metabolic And Neural Defects In Zebrafish

And Human Multiple Acyl-Coa Dehydrogenase Deficiency (MADD). *Plos. One.*, 4, E8329.

[129] Kim, S.H., Scott, S.A., Bennett, M.J., Carson, R.P., Fessel, J., Brown, H.A., Ess, K.C. (2013) Multi-Organ Abnormalities And Mtorc1 Activation In Zebrafish Model Of Multiple Acyl-Coa Dehydrogenase Deficiency. *Plos. Genet*, 9, E1003563.

[130] Yuan, H.X., Xiong, Y., Guan, K.L. (2013) Nutrient Sensing, Metabolism, And Cell Growth Control. *Mol Cell*, 49, 379-387.

[131] Sena, L.A., Chandel, N.S. (2012) Physiological Roles Of Mitochondrial Reactive Oxygen Species. *Mol Cell*, 48, 158-167.

[132] Fischer, F., Hamann, A., Osiewacz, H.D. (2012) Mitochondrial Quality Control: An Integrated Network Of Pathways. *Trends Biochem. Sci.*, 37, 284-292.

[133] Zolkipli, Z., Pedersen, C.B., Lamhonwah, A.M., Gregersen, N., Tein, I. (2011) Vulnerability To Oxidative Stress In Vitro In Pathophysiology Of Mitochondrial Short-Chain Acyl-Coa Dehydrogenase Deficiency: Response To Antioxidants. *Plos. One.*, 6, E17534.

[134] Desquiret-Dumas, V., Gueguen, N., Leman, G., Baron, S., Nivet-Antoine, V., Chupin, S., Chevrollier, A., Vessieres, E., Ayer, A., Ferre, M., et al. (2013) Resveratrol Induces A Mitochondrial Complex I-Dependent Increase In NADH Oxidation Responsible For Sirtuin Activation In Liver Cells. *J Biol. Chem.*, 288, 36662-36675.

[135] Djouadi, F., Aubey, F., Schlemmer, D., Ruiter, J.P., Wanders, R.J., Strauss, A.W., Bastin, J. (2005) Bezafibrate Increases Very-Long-Chain Acyl-Coa Dehydrogenase Protein And Mrna Expression In Deficient Fibroblasts And Is A Potential Therapy For Fatty Acid Oxidation Disorders. *Hum Mol Genet*, 14, 2695-2703.

[136] Bonnefont, J.P., Bastin, J., Behin, A., Djouadi, F. (2009) Bezafibrate For An Inborn Mitochondrial Beta-Oxidation Defect. *N. Engl. J Med.*, 360, 838-840.

[137] Yamaguchi, S., Li, H., Purevsuren, J., Yamada, K., Furui, M., Takahashi, T., Mushimoto, Y., Kobayashi, H., Hasegawa, Y., Taketani, T., et al. (2012) Bezafibrate Can Be A New Treatment Option For Mitochondrial Fatty Acid Oxidation Disorders: Evaluation By In Vitro Probe Acylcarnitine Assay. *Mol Genet Metab*, 107, 87-91.

[138] Bastin, J., Lopes-Costa, A., Djouadi, F. (2011) Exposure To Resveratrol Triggers Pharmacological Correction Of Fatty Acid Utilization In Human Fatty Acid Oxidation-Deficient Fibroblasts. *Hum Mol Genet*, 20, 2048-2057.

[139] Bonnefont, J.P., Bastin, J., Laforet, P., Aubey, F., Mogenet, A., Romano, S., Ricquier, D., Gobin-Limballe, S., Vassault, A., Behin, A., et al. (2010) Long-Term Follow-Up Of Bezafibrate Treatment In Patients With The Myopathic Form Of Carnitine Palmitoyltransferase 2 Deficiency. *Clin. Pharmacol. Ther.*, 88, 101-108.

[140] Orngreen, M.C., Madsen, K.L., Preisler, N., Andersen, G., Vissing, J., Laforet, P. (2014) Bezafibrate In Skeletal Muscle Fatty Acid Oxidation Disorders: A Randomized Clinical Trial. *Neurology.*

[141] Lopes, C.A., Le, B.C., Mathieu, L., Rotig, A., Boneh, A., De, L.P., Tarnopolsky, M.A., Thorburn, D.R., Bastin, J., Djouadi, F. (2013) Beneficial Effects Of Resveratrol On Respiratory Chain Defects In Patients' Fibroblasts Involve Estrogen Receptor And Estrogen-Related Receptor Alpha Signaling. *Hum Mol Genet.*

[142] Zhang, Z., Tsukikawa, M., Peng, M., Polyak, E., Nakamaru-Ogiso, E., Ostrovsky, J., Mccormack, S., Place, E., Clarke, C., Reiner, G., et al. (2013) Primary Respiratory Chain Disease Causes Tissue-Specific Dysregulation Of The Global Transcriptome And Nutrient-Sensing Signaling Network. *Plos. One.*, 8, E69282.

[143] Wakabayashi, M., Kamijo, Y., Nakajima, T., Tanaka, N., Sugiyama, E., Yangyang, T., Kimura, T., Aoyama, T. (2012) Fatty Acid Accumulation And Resulting Pparalpha Activation In Fibroblasts Due To Trifunctional Protein Deficiency. *PPAR. Res.*, 2012, 371691.

[144] Tucci, S., Herebian, D., Sturm, M., Seibt, A., Spiekerkoetter, U. (2012) Tissue-Specific Strategies Of The Very-Long Chain Acyl-Coa Dehydrogenase-Deficient (VLCAD-/-) Mouse To Compensate A Defective Fatty Acid Beta-Oxidation. *Plos. One.*, 7, E45429.

[145] Hoffmann, L., Seibt, A., Herebian, D., Spiekerkoetter, U. (2014) Monounsaturated 14:1n-9 And 16:1n-9 Fatty Acids But Not 18:1n-9 Induce Apoptosis And Necrosis In Murine HL-1 Cardiomyocytes. *Lipids*, 49, 25-37.

[146] Sharma, L.K., Fang, H., Liu, J., Vartak, R., Deng, J., Bai, Y. (2011) Mitochondrial Respiratory Complex I Dysfunction Promotes Tumorigenesis Through ROS Alteration And AKT Activation. *Hum Mol Genet*, 20, 4605-4616.

[147] Guo, J., Lemire, B.D. (2003) The Ubiquinone-Binding Site Of The Saccharomyces Cerevisiae Succinate-Ubiquinone Oxidoreductase Is A Source Of Superoxide. *J Biol. Chem.*, 278, 47629-47635.

[148] Huang, J., Lemire, B.D. (2009) Mutations In The C. Elegans Succinate Dehydrogenase Iron-Sulfur Subunit Promote Superoxide Generation And Premature Aging. *J Mol Biol.*, 387, 559-569.

[149] Maranzana, E., Barbero, G., Falasca, A.I., Lenaz, G., Genova, M.L. (2013) Mitochondrial Respiratory Supercomplex Association Limits Production Of Reactive Oxygen Species From Complex I. *Antioxid. Redox. Signal.*.

[150] Lopez-Erauskin, J., Galino, J., Ruiz, M., Cuezva, J.M., Fabregat, I., Cacabelos, D., Boada, J., Martinez, J., Ferrer, I., Pamplona ,R., et al. (2013) Impaired Mitochondrial Oxidative Phosphorylation In The Peroxisomal Disease X-Linked Adrenoleukodystrophy. *Hum Mol Genet*, 22, 3296-3305.

[151] Guzy, R.D., Sharma, B., Bell, E., Chandel, N.S., Schumacker, P.T. (2008) Loss Of The Sdhb, But Not The Sdha, Subunit Of Complex II Triggers Reactive Oxygen Species-Dependent Hypoxia-Inducible Factor Activation And Tumorigenesis. *Mol Cell Biol.*, 28, 718-731.

[152] Schmitz-Hubsch, T., Klockgether, T. (2008) An Update On Inherited Ataxias. *Curr. Neurol. Neurosci. Rep.*, 8, 310-319.

[153] Embirucu, E.K., Martyn, M.L., Schlesinger, D., Kok, F. (2009) Autosomal Recessive Ataxias: 20 Types, And Counting. *Arq Neuropsiquiatr.*, 67, 1143-1156.

[154] Araujo, J., Breuer, P., Dieringer, S., Krauss, S., Dorn, S., Zimmermann, K., Pfeifer, A., Klockgether, T., Wuellner, U., Evert, B.O. (2011) FOXO4-Dependent Upregulation Of Superoxide Dismutase-2 In Response To Oxidative Stress Is Impaired In Spinocerebellar Ataxia Type 3. *Hum. Mol. Genet.*, 20, 2928-2941.

[155] Chen, P., Peng, C., Luff, J., Spring, K., Watters, D., Bottle, S., Furuya, S., Lavin, M.F. (2003) Oxidative Stress Is Responsible For Deficient Survival And Dendritogenesis In Purkinje Neurons From Ataxia-Telangiectasia Mutated Mutant Mice. *J. Neurosci.*, 23, 11453-11460.

[156] Pallardo, F.V., Lloret, A., Lebel, M., d'Ischia, M., Cogger, V.C., Le Couteur, D.G., Gadaleta, M.N., Castello, G., Pagano, G. (2010) Mitochondrial Dysfunction In Some Oxidative Stress-Related Genetic Diseases: Ataxia-Telangiectasia, Down Syndrome, Fanconi Anaemia And Werner Syndrome. *Biogerontology.*, 11, 401-419.

[157] Wang, Y.C., Lee, C.M., Lee, L.C., Tung, L.C., Hsieh-Li, H.M., Lee-Chen, G.J., Su, M.T. (2011) Mitochondrial Dysfunction And Oxidative Stress Contribute To The Pathogenesis Of Spinocerebellar Ataxia Type 12 (SCA12). *J. Biol. Chem.*, 286, 21742-21754.

[158] Watters, D.J. (2003) Oxidative Stress In Ataxia Telangiectasia. *Redox. Rep.*, 8, 23-29.
[159] Marmolino, D. (2011) Friedreich's Ataxia: Past, Present And Future. *Brain Res. Rev.*, 67, 311-330.
[160] Pandolfo, M. (2009) Introduction. Idebenone In The Treatment Of Friedreich Ataxia. *J. Neurol.*, 256 Suppl 1, 1-2.
[161] Campuzano, V., Montermini, L., Molto, M.D., Pianese, L., Cossee, M., Cavalcanti, F., Monros, E., Rodius, F., Duclos, F., Monticelli, A., et al. (1996) Friedreich's Ataxia: Autosomal Recessive Disease Caused By An Intronic GAA Triplet Repeat Expansion. *Science*, 271, 1423-1427.
[162] Parkinson, M.H., Boesch, S., Nachbauer, W., Mariotti, C., Giunti P. (2013) Clinical Features Of Friedreich's Ataxia: Classical And Atypical Phenotypes. *J. Neurochem.*, 126 Suppl 1, 103-117.
[163] Schmucker, S., Puccio, H. (2010) Understanding The Molecular Mechanisms Of Friedreich's Ataxia To Develop Therapeutic Approaches. *Hum. Mol. Genet.*, 19, R103-R110.
[164] Martelli, A., Napierala, M., Puccio, H. (2012) Understanding The Genetic And Molecular Pathogenesis Of Friedreich's Ataxia Through Animal And Cellular Models. *Dis. Model. Mech.*, 5, 165-176.
[165] Babcock, M., De, S.D., Oaks, R., Davis-Kaplan, S., Jiralerspong, S., Montermini, L., Pandolfo, M., Kaplan, J. (1997) Regulation Of Mitochondrial Iron Accumulation By Yfh1p, A Putative Homolog Of Frataxin. *Science*, 276, 1709-1712.
[166] Foury, F., Cazzalini, O. (1997) Deletion Of The Yeast Homologue Of The Human Gene Associated With Friedreich's Ataxia Elicits Iron Accumulation In Mitochondria. *FEBS Lett.*, 411, 373-377.
[167] Foury, F. (1999) Low Iron Concentration And Aconitase Deficiency In A Yeast Frataxin Homologue Deficient Strain. *FEBS Lett.*, 456, 281-284.
[168] Gonzalez-Cabo, P., Bolinches-Amoros, A., Cabello, J., Ros, S., Moreno, S., Baylis, H.A., Palau, F., Vazquez-Manrique, R.P. (2011) Disruption Of The ATP-Binding Cassette B7 (ABTM-1/ABCB7) Induces Oxidative Stress And Premature Cell Death In Caenorhabditis Elegans. *J. Biol. Chem.*, 286, 21304-21314.
[169] Ramirez, R.L., Qian, J., Santambrogio, P., Levi, S., Koeppen, A.H. (2012) Relation Of Cytosolic Iron Excess To Cardiomyopathy Of Friedreich's Ataxia. *Am. J. Cardiol.*, 110, 1820-1827.
[170] Whitnall, M., Suryo, R.Y., Huang, M.L., Saletta, F., Lok, H.C., Gutierrez, L., Lazaro, F.J., Fleming, A.J., St Pierre, T.G., Mikhael, M.R.,

et al. (2012) Identification Of Nonferritin Mitochondrial Iron Deposits In A Mouse Model Of Friedreich Ataxia. *Proc. Natl. Acad. Sci. U. S. A*, 109, 20590-20595.

[171] Muhlenhoff, U., Richhardt, N., Gerber, J., Lill, R. (2002) Characterization Of Iron-Sulfur Protein Assembly In Isolated Mitochondria. A Requirement For ATP, NADH, And Reduced Iron. *J. Biol. Chem.*, 277, 29810-29816.

[172] Duby, G., Foury, F., Ramazzotti, A., Herrmann, J., Lutz, T. (2002) A Non-Essential Function For Yeast Frataxin In Iron-Sulfur Cluster Assembly. *Hum. Mol. Genet.*, 11, 2635-2643.

[173] Gerber, J., Muhlenhoff, U., Lill, R. (2003) An Interaction Between Frataxin And Isu1/Nfs1 That Is Crucial For Fe/S Cluster Synthesis On Isu1. *EMBO Rep.*, 4, 906-911.

[174] Ramazzotti,A., Vanmansart,V., Foury,F. (2004) Mitochondrial Functional Interactions Between Frataxin And Isu1p, The Iron-Sulfur Cluster Scaffold Protein, In Saccharomyces Cerevisiae. *FEBS Lett.*, 557, 215-220.

[175] Shan, Y., Napoli, E., Cortopassi, G. (2007) Mitochondrial Frataxin Interacts With ISD11 Of The NFS1/ISCU Complex And Multiple Mitochondrial Chaperones. *Hum. Mol. Genet.*, 16, 929-941.

[176] Yoon, T., Cowan, J.A. (2003) Iron-Sulfur Cluster Biosynthesis. Characterization Of Frataxin As An Iron Donor For Assembly Of [2Fe-2S] Clusters In ISU-Type Proteins. *J. Am. Chem. Soc.*, 125, 6078-6084.

[177] Shan, Y., Cortopassi, G. (2012) HSC20 Interacts With Frataxin And Is Involved In Iron-Sulfur Cluster Biogenesis And Iron Homeostasis. *Hum. Mol. Genet.*, 21, 1457-1469.

[178] Richardson, D.R., Lane, D.J., Becker, E.M., Huang, M.L., Whitnall, M., Suryo, R.Y., Sheftel, A.D., Ponka, P. (2010) Mitochondrial Iron Trafficking And The Integration Of Iron Metabolism Between The Mitochondrion And Cytosol. *Proc. Natl. Acad. Sci. U. S. A*, 107, 10775-10782.

[179] Lill, R., Kispal, G. (2000) Maturation Of Cellular Fe-S Proteins: An Essential Function Of Mitochondria. *Trends Biochem. Sci.*, 25, 352-356.

[180] Richardson, D.R., Ponka, P. (1997) The Molecular Mechanisms Of The Metabolism And Transport Of Iron In Normal And Neoplastic Cells. *Biochim. Biophys. Acta*, 1331, 1-40.

[181] Ganz, T. (2007) Molecular Control Of Iron Transport. *J. Am. Soc. Nephrol.*, 18, 394-400.

[182] Yoon, T., Cowan, J.A. (2004) Frataxin-Mediated Iron Delivery To Ferrochelatase In The Final Step Of Heme Biosynthesis. *J. Biol. Chem.*, 279, 25943-25946.

[183] Schoenfeld, R.A., Napoli, E., Wong, A., Zhan, S., Reutenauer, L., Morin, D., Buckpitt, A.R., Taroni, F., Lonnerdal, B., Ristow, M., et al. (2005) Frataxin Deficiency Alters Heme Pathway Transcripts And Decreases Mitochondrial Heme Metabolites In Mammalian Cells. *Hum. Mol. Genet.*, 14, 3787-3799.

[184] Lu, C., Cortopassi, G. (2007) Frataxin Knockdown Causes Loss Of Cytoplasmic Iron-Sulfur Cluster Functions, Redox Alterations And Induction Of Heme Transcripts. *Arch. Biochem. Biophys.*, 457, 111-122.

[185] Lill, R. (2009) Function And Biogenesis Of Iron-Sulphur Proteins. *Nature*, 460, 831-838.

[186] Gerber, J., Lill, R. (2002) Biogenesis Of Iron-Sulfur Proteins In Eukaryotes: Components, Mechanism And Pathology. *Mitochondrion.*, 2, 71-86.

[187] Horowitz, M.P., Greenamyre, J.T. (2010) Mitochondrial Iron Metabolism And Its Role In Neurodegeneration. *J. Alzheimers. Dis.*, 20 Suppl 2, S551-S568.

[188] Bradley, J.L., Blake, J.C., Chamberlain, S., Thomas, P.K., Cooper, J.M., Schapira, A.H. (2000) Clinical, Biochemical And Molecular Genetic Correlations In Friedreich's Ataxia. *Hum. Mol. Genet.*, 9, 275-282.

[189] Rotig, A., De, L.P., Chretien, D., Foury, F., Koenig, M., Sidi, D., Munnich, A., Rustin, P. (1997) Aconitase And Mitochondrial Iron-Sulphur Protein Deficiency In Friedreich Ataxia. *Nat. Genet.*, 17, 215-217.

[190] Gonzalez-Cabo, P., Vazquez-Manrique, P., Garcia-Gimeno, M.A., Sanz, P., Palau, F. (2005) Frataxin Interacts Functionally With Mitochondrial Electron Transport Chain Proteins. *Hum. Mol. Genet.*, 14, 2091-2098.

[191] Vazquez-Manrique, R.P., Gonzalez-Cabo, P., Ros, S., Aziz, H., Baylis, H.A., Palau, F. (2006) Reduction Of Caenorhabditis Elegans Frataxin Increases Sensitivity To Oxidative Stress, Reduces Lifespan, And Causes Lethality In A Mitochondrial Complex II Mutant. *FASEB J.*, 20, 172-174.

[192] Wagner, G.R., Pride, P.M., Babbey, C.M., Payne, R.M. (2012) Friedreich's Ataxia Reveals A Mechanism For Coordinate Regulation Of Oxidative Metabolism Via Feedback Inhibition Of The SIRT3 Deacetylase. *Hum. Mol. Genet.*, 21, 2688-2697.

[193] Weir, H.J., Lane, J.D., Balthasar, N. (2013) SIRT3: A Central Regulator Of Mitochondrial Adaptation In Health And Disease. *Genes Cancer*, 4, 118-124.

[194] Krebs, H.A., Veech, R.L. (1969) Equilibrium Relations Between Pyridine Nucleotides And Adenine Nucleotides And Their Roles In The Regulation Of Metabolic Processes. *Adv. Enzyme Regul.*, 7, 397-413.

[195] Ventura-Clapier, R., Garnier, A., Veksler, V. (2004) Energy Metabolism In Heart Failure. *J. Physiol*, 555, 1-13.

[196] Hafner, A.V., Dai,J., Gomes, A.P., Xiao, C.Y., Palmeira, C.M., Rosenzweig, A., Sinclair, D.A. (2010) Regulation Of The Mptp By SIRT3-Mediated Deacetylation Of Cypd At Lysine 166 Suppresses Age-Related Cardiac Hypertrophy. *Aging (Albany. NY)*, 2, 914-923.

[197] Bause, A.S., Haigis, M.C. (2013) SIRT3 Regulation Of Mitochondrial Oxidative Stress. *Exp. Gerontol.*, 48, 634-639.

[198] Chen, Y., Zhang, J., Lin, Y., Lei, Q., Guan, K.L., Zhao, S., Xiong, Y. (2011) Tumour Suppressor SIRT3 Deacetylates And Activates Manganese Superoxide Dismutase To Scavenge ROS. *EMBO Rep.*, 12, 534-541.

[199] Qiu, X., Brown, K., Hirschey, M.D., Verdin, E., Chen, D. (2010) Calorie Restriction Reduces Oxidative Stress By SIRT3-Mediated SOD2 Activation. *Cell Metab*, 12, 662-667.

[200] Tao, R., Coleman, M.C., Pennington, J.D., Ozden, O., Park, S.H., Jiang, H., Kim, H.S., Flynn, C.R., Hill, S., Hayes, M.W., et al. (2010) Sirt3-Mediated Deacetylation Of Evolutionarily Conserved Lysine 122 Regulates Mnsod Activity In Response To Stress. *Mol. Cell*, 40, 893-904.

[201] Bradley, J.L., Blake, J.C., Chamberlain, S., Thomas, P.K., Cooper, J.M., Schapira, A.H. (2000) Clinical, Biochemical And Molecular Genetic Correlations In Friedreich's Ataxia. *Hum. Mol. Genet.*, 9, 275-282.

[202] Al-Mahdawi, S., Pinto, R.M., Varshney, D., Lawrence, L., Lowrie, M.B., Hughes, S., Webster, Z., Blake, J., Cooper, J.M., King, R., Pook, M.A. (2006) GAA Repeat Expansion Mutation Mouse Models Of Friedreich Ataxia Exhibit Oxidative Stress Leading To Progressive Neuronal And Cardiac Pathology. *Genomics*, 88, 580-590.

[203] Yan, L.J., Levine, R.L., Sohal, R.S. (1997) Oxidative Damage During Aging Targets Mitochondrial Aconitase. *Proc. Natl. Acad. Sci. U. S. A*, 94, 11168-11172.

[204] Llorens, J.V., Navarro, J.A., Martinez-Sebastian, M.J., Baylies, M.K., Schneuwly, S., Botella, J.A., Molto, M.D. (2007) Causative Role Of

Oxidative Stress In A Drosophila Model Of Friedreich Ataxia. *FASEB J.*, 21, 333-344.
[205] Swarup, V., Srivastava, A.K., Padma, M.V., Rajeswari, M.R. (2013) Quantitative Profiling And Identification Of Differentially Expressed Plasma Proteins In Friedreich's Ataxia. *J. Neurosci. Res.*, 91, 1483-1491.
[206] Schiavi, A., Torgovnick, A., Kell, A., Megalou, E., Castelein, N., Guccini, I., Marzocchella, L., Gelino, S., Hansen, M., Malisan, F., et al. (2013) Autophagy Induction Extends Lifespan And Reduces Lipid Content In Response To Frataxin Silencing In C. Elegans. *Exp. Gerontol.*, 48, 191-201.
[207] Navarro, J.A., Ohmann, E., Sanchez, D., Botella, J.A., Liebisch, G., Molto, M.D., Ganfornina,M.D., Schmitz,G., Schneuwly,S. (2010) Altered Lipid Metabolism In A Drosophila Model Of Friedreich's Ataxia. *Hum. Mol. Genet.*, 19, 2828-2840.
[208] Ross, B.M., Eder, K., Moszczynska, A., Mamalias, N., Lamarche, J., Ang, L., Pandolfo, M., Rouleau, G., Kirchgessner, M., Kish, S.J. (2000) Abnormal Activity Of Membrane Phospholipid Synthetic Enzymes In The Brain Of Patients With Friedreich's Ataxia And Spinocerebellar Atrophy Type-1. *Mov Disord.*, 15, 294-300.
[209] Eder, K., Kish, S.J., Kirchgessner, M., Ross ,B.M. (1998) Brain Phospholipids And Fatty Acids In Friedreich's Ataxia And Spinocerebellar Atrophy Type-1. *Mov Disord.*, 13, 813-819.
[210] Feki, M., Belal, S., Feki, H., Souissi, M., Frih-Ayed, M., Kaabachi, N., Hentati, F., Ben, H.M., Mebazaa, A. (2002) Serum Vitamin E And Lipid-Adjusted Vitamin E Assessment In Friedreich Ataxia Phenotype Patients And Unaffected Family Members. *Clin. Chem.*, 48, 577-579.
[211] Iorio, L., De, M.G., Filla, A., Di, M.L., Postiglione, A., Patti, L., Campanella, G. (1993) Serum Lipoprotein Fatty Acid Profile In Hereditary Ataxias. *Can. J. Neurol. Sci.*, 20, 206-209.
[212] Puccio, H., Simon, D., Cossee, M., Criqui-Filipe, P., Tiziano,F., Melki, J., Hindelang, C., Matyas, R., Rustin, P., Koenig, M. (2001) Mouse Models For Friedreich Ataxia Exhibit Cardiomyopathy, Sensory Nerve Defect And Fe-S Enzyme Deficiency Followed By Intramitochondrial Iron Deposits. *Nat. Genet.*, 27, 181-186.
[213] Adibhatla, R.M., Hatcher, J.F. (2008) Altered Lipid Metabolism In Brain Injury And Disorders. *Subcell. Biochem.*, 49, 241-268.
[214] Shoichet, S.A., Baumer, A.T., Stamenkovic, D., Sauer, H., Pfeiffer, A.F., Kahn, C.R., Muller-Wieland, D., Richter, C., Ristow, M. (2002) Frataxin Promotes Antioxidant Defense In A Thiol-Dependent Manner

Resulting In Diminished Malignant Transformation In Vitro. *Hum. Mol. Genet.*, 11, 815-821.

[215] Piemonte, F., Pastore, A., Tozzi, G., Tagliacozzi, D., Santorelli, F.M., Carrozzo, R., Casali, C., Damiano, M., Federici, G., Bertini, E. (2001) Glutathione In Blood Of Patients With Friedreich's Ataxia. *Eur. J. Clin. Invest*, 31, 1007-1011.

[216] Paupe, V., Dassa, E.P., Goncalves, S., Auchere, F., Lonn, M., Holmgren, A., Rustin, P. (2009) Impaired Nuclear Nrf2 Translocation Undermines The Oxidative Stress Response In Friedreich Ataxia. *Plos. One.*, 4, E4253.

[217] Jiralerspong, S., Ge, B., Hudson, T.J., Pandolfo, M. (2001) Manganese Superoxide Dismutase Induction By Iron Is Impaired In Friedreich Ataxia Cells. *FEBS Lett.*, 509, 101-105.

[218] Warner, B.B., Stuart, L., Gebb, S., Wispe, J.R. (1996) Redox Regulation Of Manganese Superoxide Dismutase. *Am. J. Physiol*, 271, L150-L158.

[219] Kiningham, K.K., Xu, Y., Daosukho, C., Popova, B., St Clair, D.K. (2001) Nuclear Factor Kappab-Dependent Mechanisms Coordinate The Synergistic Effect Of PMA And Cytokines On The Induction Of Superoxide Dismutase 2. *Biochem. J.*, 353, 147-156.

[220] Shi, X., Dong, Z., Huang, C., Ma, W., Liu, K., Ye, J., Chen, F., Leonard, S.S., Ding, M., Castranova, V., Vallyathan, V. (1999) The Role Of Hydroxyl Radical As A Messenger In The Activation Of Nuclear Transcription Factor NF-Kappab. *Mol. Cell Biochem.*, 194, 63-70.

[221] Busi, M.V., Maliandi, M.V., Valdez, H., Clemente, M., Zabaleta, E.J., Araya, A., Gomez-Casati, D.F. (2006) Deficiency Of Arabidopsis Thaliana Frataxin Alters Activity Of Mitochondrial Fe-S Proteins And Induces Oxidative Stress. *Plant J.*, 48, 873-882.

[222] Emond, M., Lepage, G., Vanasse, M., Pandolfo, M. (2000) Increased Levels Of Plasma Malondialdehyde In Friedreich Ataxia. *Neurology*, 55, 1752-1753.

[223] Bradley, J.L., Homayoun, S., Hart, P.E., Schapira, A.H., Cooper, J.M. (2004) Role Of Oxidative Damage In Friedreich's Ataxia. *Neurochem. Res.*, 29, 561-567.

[224] Santos, M.M., Ohshima, K., Pandolfo, M. (2001) Frataxin Deficiency Enhances Apoptosis In Cells Differentiating Into Neuroectoderm. *Hum. Mol. Genet.*, 10, 1935-1944.

[225] Irazusta, V., Cabiscol, E., Reverter-Branch, Ros, J., Tamarit, J. (2006) Manganese Is The Link Between Frataxin And Iron-Sulfur Deficiency In

The Yeast Model Of Friedreich Ataxia. *J. Biol. Chem.*, 281, 12227-12232.

[226] Napoli, E., Taroni, F., Cortopassi, G.A. (2006) Frataxin, Iron-Sulfur Clusters, Heme, ROS, And Aging. *Antioxid. Redox. Signal.*, 8, 506-516.

[227] Seguin, A., Bayot, A., Dancis, A., Rogowska-Wrzesinska,A., Auchere, F., Camadro, J.M., Bulteau, A.L., Lesuisse, E. (2009) Overexpression Of The Yeast Frataxin Homolog (Yfh1): Contrasting Effects On Iron-Sulfur Cluster Assembly, Heme Synthesis And Resistance To Oxidative Stress. *Mitochondrion.*, 9, 130-138.

[228] Chantrel-Groussard, K., Geromel, V., Puccio, H., Koenig, M., Munnich, A., Rotig, A., Rustin, P. (2001) Disabled Early Recruitment Of Antioxidant Defenses In Friedreich's Ataxia. *Hum. Mol. Genet.*, 10, 2061-2067.

[229] Jiralerspong, S., Ge, B., Hudson, T.J., Pandolfo, M. (2001) Manganese Superoxide Dismutase Induction By Iron Is Impaired In Friedreich Ataxia Cells. *FEBS Lett.*, 509, 101-105.

[230] Lin, J., Handschin, C., Spiegelman, B.M. (2005) Metabolic Control Through The PGC-1 Family Of Transcription Coactivators. *Cell Metab*, 1, 361-370.

[231] Garcia-Gimenez, J.L., Gimeno, A., Gonzalez-Cabo, P., Dasi, F., Bolinches-Amoros, A., Molla, B., Palau, F., Pallardo, F.V. (2011) Differential Expression Of PGC-1alpha And Metabolic Sensors Suggest Age-Dependent Induction Of Mitochondrial Biogenesis In Friedreich Ataxia Fibroblasts. *Plos. One.*, 6, E20666.

[232] Moreira, P.I., Santos, M.S., Oliveira, C.R. (2007) Alzheimer's Disease: A Lesson From Mitochondrial Dysfunction. *Antioxid. Redox. Signal.*, 9, 1621-1630.

[233] Finkel, T. (2005) Radical Medicine: Treating Ageing To Cure Disease. *Nat. Rev. Mol. Cell Biol.*, 6, 971-976.

[234] Gruber, J., Fong, S., Chen, C.B., Yoong, S., Pastorin, G., Schaffer, S., Cheah, I., Halliwell ,B. (2013) Mitochondria-Targeted Antioxidants And Metabolic Modulators As Pharmacological Interventions To Slow Ageing. *Biotechnol. Adv.*, 31, 563-592.

[235] Moreira, P.I., Zhu, X., Wang, X., Lee, H.G., Nunomura, A., Petersen, R.B., Perry, G., Smith, M.A. (2010) Mitochondria: A Therapeutic Target In Neurodegeneration. *Biochim. Biophys. Acta*, 1802, 212-220.

[236] Wallimann, T., Tokarska-Schlattner, M., Schlattner, U. (2011) The Creatine Kinase System And Pleiotropic Effects Of Creatine. *Amino. Acids*, 40, 1271-1296.

[237] Wallimann, T., Wyss, M., Brdiczka, D., Nicolay, K., Eppenberger, H.M. (1992) Intracellular Compartmentation, Structure And Function Of Creatine Kinase Isoenzymes In Tissues With High And Fluctuating Energy Demands: The 'Phosphocreatine Circuit' For Cellular Energy Homeostasis. *Biochem. J.*, 281 (Pt 1), 21-40.

[238] Bessman, S.P., Geiger, P.J. (1981) Transport Of Energy In Muscle: The Phosphorylcreatine Shuttle. *Science*, 211, 448-452.

[239] O'Gorman, E., Beutner, G., Dolder, M., Koretsky, A.P., Brdiczka, D., Wallimann, T. (1997) The Role Of Creatine Kinase In Inhibition Of Mitochondrial Permeability Transition. *FEBS Lett.*, 414, 253-257.

[240] Andres, R.H., Ducray, A.D., Perez-Bouza, A., Schlattner, U., Huber, A.W., Krebs, S.H., Seiler, R.W., Wallimann, T., Widmer, H.R. (2005) Creatine Supplementation Improves Dopaminergic Cell Survival And Protects Against MPP+ Toxicity In An Organotypic Tissue Culture System. *Cell Transplant.*, 14, 537-550.

[241] Andres, R.H., Ducray, A.D., Huber, A.W., Perez-Bouza, A., Krebs, S.H., Schlattner, U., Seiler, R.W., Wallimann, T., Widmer, H.R. (2005) Effects Of Creatine Treatment On Survival And Differentiation Of GABA-Ergic Neurons In Cultured Striatal Tissue. *J. Neurochem.*, 95, 33-45.

[242] Andres, R.H., Huber, A.W., Schlattner, U., Perez-Bouza, A., Krebs, S.H., Seiler, R.W., Wallimann, T., Widmer, H.R. (2005) Effects Of Creatine Treatment On The Survival Of Dopaminergic Neurons In Cultured Fetal Ventral Mesencephalic Tissue. *Neuroscience*, 133, 701-713.

[243] Hersch, S.M., Gevorkian, S., Marder, K., Moskowitz, C., Feigin, A., Cox, M., Como, P., Zimmerman, C., Lin, M., Zhang, L., et al. (2006) Creatine In Huntington Disease Is Safe, Tolerable, Bioavailable In Brain And Reduces Serum 8OH2'dG. *Neurology*, 66, 250-252.

[244] Reiter, R.J. (1991) Melatonin: The Chemical Expression Of Darkness. *Mol. Cell Endocrinol.*, 79, C153-C158.

[245] Tan, D.X., Hardeland, R., Manchester, L.C., Galano, A., Reiter, R.J. (2013) Cyclic-3-Hydroxymelatonin (C3HOM), A Potent Antioxidant, Scavenges Free Radicals And Suppresses Oxidative Reactions. *Curr. Med. Chem.*.

[246] Poeggeler, B., Saarela, S., Reiter, R.J., Tan, D.X., Chen, L.D., Manchester, L.C., Barlow-Walden, L.R. (1994) Melatonin--A Highly Potent Endogenous Radical Scavenger And Electron Donor: New

Aspects Of The Oxidation Chemistry Of This Indole Accessed In Vitro. *Ann. N. Y. Acad. Sci.*, 738, 419-420.

[247] Rosales-Corral, S.A., Acuna-Castroviejo, D., Coto-Montes, A., Boga, J.A., Manchester, L.C., Fuentes-Broto, L., Korkmaz, A., Ma, S., Tan, D.X., Reiter, R.J. (2012) Alzheimer's Disease: Pathological Mechanisms And The Beneficial Role Of Melatonin. *J. Pineal Res.*, 52, 167-202.

[248] Cheng, Y., Feng, Z., Zhang, Q.Z., Zhang, J.T. (2006) Beneficial Effects Of Melatonin In Experimental Models Of Alzheimer Disease. *Acta Pharmacol. Sin.*, 27, 129-139.

[249] Feng, Z., Chang, Y., Cheng, Y., Zhang, B.L., Qu, Z.W., Qin, C., Zhang, J.T. (2004) Melatonin Alleviates Behavioral Deficits Associated With Apoptosis And Cholinergic System Dysfunction In The APP 695 Transgenic Mouse Model Of Alzheimer's Disease. *J. Pineal Res.*, 37, 129-136.

[250] Pohanka, M., Bandouchova, H., Pikula, J. (2012) Melatonin Influences Antioxidant Homeostasis And Basal Metabolism In The BALB/C Mouse Model. *Neuro. Endocrinol. Lett.*, 33 Suppl 3, 183-189.

[251] Wang, X. (2009) The Antiapoptotic Activity Of Melatonin In Neurodegenerative Diseases. *CNS. Neurosci. Ther.*, 15, 345-357.

[252] Acuna-Castroviejo, D., Martin, M., Macias, M., Escames, G., Leon, J., Khaldy, H., Reiter, R.J. (2001) Melatonin, Mitochondria, And Cellular Bioenergetics. *J. Pineal Res.*, 30, 65-74.

[253] Buscemi, N., Vandermeer, B., Hooton, N., Pandya, R., Tjosvold, L., Hartling, L., Vohra, S., Klassen, T.P., Baker, G. (2006) Efficacy And Safety Of Exogenous Melatonin For Secondary Sleep Disorders And Sleep Disorders Accompanying Sleep Restriction: Meta-Analysis. *BMJ*, 332, 385-393.

[254] Orsucci, D., Mancuso, M., Ienco, E.C., Logerfo, A., Siciliano, G. (2011) Targeting Mitochondrial Dysfunction And Neurodegeneration By Means Of Coenzyme Q10 And Its Analogues. *Curr. Med. Chem.*, 18, 4053-4064.

[255] Hargreaves, I.P. (2003) Ubiquinone: Cholesterol's Reclusive Cousin. *Ann. Clin. Biochem.*, 40, 207-218.

[256] Lenaz, G., Fato, R., Formiggini, G., Genova, M.L. (2007) The Role Of Coenzyme Q In Mitochondrial Electron Transport. *Mitochondrion.*, 7 Suppl, S8-33.

[257] Kooncumchoo, P., Sharma, S., Porter, J., Govitrapong, P., Ebadi, M. (2006) Coenzyme Q(10) Provides Neuroprotection In Iron-Induced Apoptosis In Dopaminergic Neurons. *J. Mol. Neurosci.*, 28, 125-141.

[258] Somayajulu, M., Mccarthy, S., Hung, M., Sikorska, M., Borowy-Borowski, H., Pandey, S. (2005) Role Of Mitochondria In Neuronal Cell Death Induced By Oxidative Stress; Neuroprotection By Coenzyme Q10. *Neurobiol. Dis.*, 18, 618-627.

[259] Yang, X., Yang, Y., Li, G., Wang, J., Yang, E.S. (2008) Coenzyme Q10 Attenuates Beta-Amyloid Pathology In The Aged Transgenic Mice With Alzheimer Presenilin 1 Mutation. *J. Mol. Neurosci.*, 34, 165-171.

[260] Bhagavan, H.N., Chopra, R.K. (2006) Coenzyme Q10: Absorption, Tissue Uptake, Metabolism And Pharmacokinetics. *Free Radic. Res.*, 40, 445-453.

[261] Meier, T., Buyse, G. (2009) Idebenone: An Emerging Therapy For Friedreich Ataxia. *J. Neurol.*, 256 Suppl 1, 25-30.

[262] Rustin, P., Von Kleist-Retzow, J.C., Chantrel-Groussard, K., Sidi, D., Munnich, A., Rotig, A. (1999) Effect Of Idebenone On Cardiomyopathy In Friedreich's Ataxia: A Preliminary Study. *Lancet*, 354, 477-479.

[263] Artuch, R., Aracil, A., Mas, A., Colome, C., Rissech, M., Monros ,E., Pineda, M. (2002) Friedreich's Ataxia: Idebenone Treatment In Early Stage Patients. *Neuropediatrics*, 33, 190-193.

[264] Schulz, J.B., Dehmer, T., Schols, L., Mende, H., Hardt, C., Vorgerd, M., Burk, K., Matson, W., Dichgans, J., Beal, M.F., Bogdanov ,M.B. (2000) Oxidative Stress In Patients With Friedreich Ataxia. *Neurology*, 55, 1719-1721.

[265] Di Prospero, N.A., Baker, A., Jeffries, N., Fischbeck, K.H. (2007) Neurological Effects Of High-Dose Idebenone In Patients With Friedreich's Ataxia: A Randomised, Placebo-Controlled Trial. *Lancet Neurol.*, 6, 878-886.

[266] Murphy, M.P., Smith, R.A. (2000) Drug Delivery To Mitochondria: The Key To Mitochondrial Medicine. *Adv. Drug Deliv. Rev.*, 41, 235-250.

[267] Smith, R.A., Porteous, C.M., Coulter, C.V., Murphy, M.P. (1999) Selective Targeting Of An Antioxidant To Mitochondria. *Eur. J. Biochem.*, 263, 709-716.

[268] Asin-Cayuela, J., Manas, A.R., James, A.M., Smith, R.A., Murphy, M.P. (2004) Fine-Tuning The Hydrophobicity Of A Mitochondria-Targeted Antioxidant. *FEBS Lett.*, 571, 9-16.

[269] James, A.M., Cocheme, H.M., Murphy, M.P. (2005) Mitochondria-Targeted Redox Probes As Tools In The Study Of Oxidative Damage And Ageing. *Mech. Ageing Dev.*, 126, 982-986.

[270] Kelso, G.F., Porteous, C.M., Coulter, C.V., Hughes, G., Porteous, W.K., Ledgerwood, E.C., Smith, R.A., Murphy, M.P. (2001) Selective

Targeting Of A Redox-Active Ubiquinone To Mitochondria Within Cells: Antioxidant And Antiapoptotic Properties. *J. Biol. Chem.*, 276, 4588-4596.

[271] Hughes, G., Murphy, M.P., Ledgerwood, E.C. (2005) Mitochondrial Reactive Oxygen Species Regulate The Temporal Activation Of Nuclear Factor Kappab To Modulate Tumour Necrosis Factor-Induced Apoptosis: Evidence From Mitochondria-Targeted Antioxidants. *Biochem. J.*, 389, 83-89.

[272] Hart, P.E., Lodi, R., Rajagopalan, B., Bradley, J.L., Crilley, J.G., Turner, C., Blamire, A.M., Manners, D., Styles, P., Schapira, A.H., Cooper, J.M. (2005) Antioxidant Treatment Of Patients With Friedreich Ataxia: Four-Year Follow-Up. *Arch. Neurol.*, 62, 621-626.

[273] Szeto, H.H. (2006) Cell-Permeable, Mitochondrial-Targeted, Peptide Antioxidants. *AAPS. J.*, 8, E277-E283.

[274] Zhao, K., Zhao, G.M., Wu, D., Soong, Y., Birk, A.V., Schiller, P.W., Szeto, H.H. (2004) Cell-Permeable Peptide Antioxidants Targeted To Inner Mitochondrial Membrane Inhibit Mitochondrial Swelling, Oxidative Cell Death, And Reperfusion Injury. *J. Biol. Chem.*, 279, 34682-34690.

[275] Szeto, H.H. (2008) Development Of Mitochondria-Targeted Aromatic-Cationic Peptides For Neurodegenerative Diseases. *Ann. N. Y. Acad. Sci.*, 1147, 112-121.

[276] Szeto, H.H. (2008) Mitochondria-Targeted Cytoprotective Peptides For Ischemia-Reperfusion Injury. *Antioxid. Redox. Signal.*, 10, 601-619.

[277] Calkins, M.J., Johnson, D.A., Townsend, J.A., Vargas, M.R., Dowell, J.A., Williamson, T.P., Kraft, A.D., Lee, J.M., Li, J., Johnson, J.A. (2009) The Nrf2/ARE Pathway As A Potential Therapeutic Target In Neurodegenerative Disease. *Antioxid. Redox. Signal.*, 11, 497-508.

[278] Joshi, G., Johnson, J.A. (2012) The Nrf2-ARE Pathway: A Valuable Therapeutic Target For The Treatment Of Neurodegenerative Diseases. *Recent Pat CNS. Drug Discov.*, 7, 218-229.

[279] Honda, T., Rounds, B.V., Bore, L., Finlay, H.J., Favaloro, F.G., Jr., Suh, N., Wang, Y., Sporn, M.B., Gribble, G.W. (2000) Synthetic Oleanane And Ursane Triterpenoids With Modified Rings A And C: A Series Of Highly Active Inhibitors Of Nitric Oxide Production In Mouse Macrophages. *J. Med. Chem.*, 43, 4233-4246.

[280] Dinkova-Kostova, A.T., Liby, K.T., Stephenson, K.K., Holtzclaw, W.D., Gao, X., Suh, N., Williams, C., Risingsong, R., Honda, T., Gribble, G.W., et al. (2005) Extremely Potent Triterpenoid Inducers Of The

Phase 2 Response: Correlations Of Protection Against Oxidant And Inflammatory Stress. *Proc. Natl. Acad. Sci. U. S. A*, 102, 4584-4589.

[281] Sporn, M.B., Liby, K.T., Yore, M.M., Fu, L., Lopchuk, J.M., Gribble, G.W. (2011) New Synthetic Triterpenoids: Potent Agents For Prevention And Treatment Of Tissue Injury Caused By Inflammatory And Oxidative Stress. *J. Nat. Prod.*, 74, 537-545.

In: Oxidative Stress
Editor: Cassidy Croft
ISBN: 978-1-63117-578-7

Chapter 2

Oxidative Stress in Biofilms: Causes, Role in Diseases and Biological Effects

María Gabriela Paraje *

IMBIV (CONICET) y Departamento de Farmacia, Facultad de Ciencias Químicas, Universidad Nacional de Córdoba, Córdoba, Argentina

Abstract

Active oxygen species are produced as inescapable by-products of a normal aerobic metabolism, and their production is further enhanced by exposure to certain environmental conditions, or as a result of some diseases. Oxidative stress is defined as an imbalance between the production of free radicals (FR) and antioxidant defenses in favor of the former, which can result from an excess of prooxidant, antioxidant deficiency or both factors. There are many kinds of FR, but these can be grouped together under the name of reactive oxygen species (ROS) or reactive nitrogen species (RNS), determined by the ability of each species according to the four basic characteristics: reactivity, specificity, selectivity and diffusivity.

---

* IMBIV (CONICET) y Departamento de Farmacia, Facultad de Ciencias Químicas, Universidad Nacional de Córdoba, Haya de la Torre y Medina Allende, 5000 Córdoba, Argentina. Tel: +54-0351-5353865 int. 53354 Fax: +54-0351-5353865 int. 53364, E-mail: paraje@fcq.unc.edu.ar; gabrielaparaje@gmail.com.

The defense mechanisms of living organisms have developed antioxidant physiological defenses that prevent the formation of FR, recognize oxidative damage and repair. Antioxidant defenses can be classified according to their nature as enzymatic or non-enzymatic antioxidants, and depending on their origin, as endogenous or exogenous antioxidants. The reactive species not neutralized by antioxidant defenses can damage the cellular membranes by oxidation lipids, critical enzymes of the intermediary metabolism or other proteins, and also break DNA chains.

Oxidative stress is involved in various disease processes such as cardiovascular and neurological disorders, diabetes, ischemia and cancer; it being one of the most important causative agents of mutagenesis, tumorigenesis and even aging. Furthermore, it has been also associated with the chronic inflammation caused by the biofilms of the FR that are generated during bactericidal attack of macrophages and neutrophils.

Biofilms are microbial communities containing sessile cells embedded in a self-produced extracellular polymeric matrix (containing polysaccharides, DNA and other components). In comparison with their planktonic (free-living) counterparts, sessile cells are often much more resistant to various stress conditions, with this increased resistance having a considerable impact on the treatment of biofilm-related infections.

In the first part of this review, the reactivates of active species of oxygen and the antioxidant system of the oxidative stress responses will be highlighted briefly, and their physiological role in biofilms discussed. Subsequently, the similarities and differences between oxidative stress responses in bacteria and eukaryotic microorganism biofilms will be reviewed, and finally the phenotypic adaptation of microbial biofilms is discussed in response to stress resulting from exposure to environmental pollutants, disinfectants and antibiotics is discussed Despite some progress, better understanding of the genotypic and phenotypic adaptation of sessile (biofilm-associated) microorganisms to various forms of stress is still required in order to develop more effective anti-biofilm strategies.

Keywords: Stress; reactive oxygen species (ROS); reactive nitrogen species (RNS); biofilms; sessile cells; antibiotics

All excesses are bad; everything has its place and time, in the right measure.

1. Oxidative Stress: Brief History

Oxygen is absolutely necessary for life on our planet. However, under physiological conditions, the use of oxygen by the cells of living organisms can generate harmful reactive oxygen species (ROS).

In the late 1950's, free radical (FR) and antioxidants were almost unheard of in the clinical and biological sciences despite chemists having known about them for years in the context of radiation, polymer and combustion technology. In a pioneering paper in 1954, Rebecca Gerschman, an Argentinian researcher, published her famous article 'oxygen poisoning' in Science relating to the toxic effects of elevated oxygen levels on aerobes to those of ionizing radiation, and proposed that oxygen toxicity is due to FR formation [1].

Dr. Gerschman et al. first suggested that ROS were toxic agents and generated pathologies, and established three basic postulates:

- the molecular mechanism can produce FR common injury when animals are under high pressure from oxygen and ionizing radical.
- an imbalance between oxidants and antioxidants favoring FR produces toxic effects.
- FR production is a phenomenon with implications for aging and carcinogenesis.

Although these postulates are still the basis of many investigations, they did not capture the imagination of most life scientists until the discovery of superoxide dismutase enzymes (SOD) by McCord and Fridovich in 1968 [2]. These authors had previously observed the ability of several proteins to inhibit the reduction of cytochrome C by xanthine oxidase, and in a sudden flash of inspiration it was realized that these inhibitory effects were due to a novel protein contaminating the other proteins tested. On purifying this contaminant, they identified the first enzyme (copper and zinc-containing SOD) known to act on a FR substrate [3] and at the same time observed that illuminated chloroplasts reduced cytochrome C, which was inhibited by catalase (CAT). However, they could not understand how removing hydrogen peroxide (H_2O_2) was able to prevent a reduction reaction [4, 5].

2. Reactive Oxygen Species: The Main Actor

It has been estimated that approximately 2% of the oxygen consumed by a normal organism leads to the formation of ROS, of which several are FR or are involved in their formation. A FR is defined as oxygen molecules or fragments of molecules containing one or more unpaired electrons in a higher energy level. This condition, chemically very unstable, becomes extremely active since the odd electron or one "desperately seeking a pair" exits the atomic imbalance. To achieve its objective, it subtracts an electron from any neighboring molecule, i.e., through oxidation altering its structure, and converts it into another free radical anxious to capture an electron, thus creating a chain reaction. The FR character of molecular oxygen is established by two unpaired electrons and the ensuing chemistry –involving one-electron transfers supports the concept of oxidative stress [5].

This mismatch provides electronic paramagnetic properties, giving them a high and indiscriminate reactivity, with the loss of electrons in different molecules destabilizing biological processes. FR randomly forms different ROS inside a cell normally not exceeding 3-5% of oxygen transformations in the breathing chain. Active oxygen species are produced as an inescapable by-product of normal aerobic metabolism, thereby fulfilling an essential role in ATP synthesis and other physiological reactions. However their excess is highly damaging to the cell, with their production being further enhanced by exposure to certain environmental conditions, through diet, or as a result of some diseases [6].

Sies H, in 1985, defined oxidative stress as an imbalance between the production of FR and antioxidant defenses in favor of the former, which can result from an excess of pro-oxidant FR, antioxidant deficiency or both factors [7].

In biological systems, in addition to FR other chemical species are generated that are not reactive themselves, but produce highly reactive FR in the presence of transition metals (iron and copper) or other radicals. There are many kinds of FR, but these can be grouped together under the name of ROS or nitrogen species (RNS), determined by the ability of each species according to the four basic characteristics: reactivity, specificity, selectivity and diffusivity [6-8].

The major ROS generated during respiration are those in which the unpaired electron belongs to an oxygen atom: peroxyl radical or peroxide radical (ROO•), hydroxyl radical (HO•) or superoxide anion ($O_2^{\bullet-}$). $O_2^{\bullet-}$ and HO• are highly reactive FR, being able to oxidize many biological structures indiscriminately and damage them, which in turn gives rise to OH• [8-11].

H_2O_2 is not a free radical, but is a precursor of FR. UV radiation causes the hemolytic cleavage of the oxygen–oxygen bond to form HO•. Redox metal ions (Fe^{2+} or Fe^{3+} or Cu^+) react with H_2O_2 to generate HO• (Fenton reaction). H_2O_2 is relatively stable (half-life, minutes -months) when protected against light and trace metal contamination. H_2O_2 is, however, rapidly destroyed by antioxidant enzymes (CAT, glutathione peroxidase). Singlet oxygen is not a free radical and is a photo-excited oxygen species. Hypochlorous acid (HOCl) is formed from myeloperoxidase/ H_2O_2-dependent oxidation of chloride anion. HOCl has intermediate reactivity-more reactive than H_2O_2 but considerably less reactive than HO• [12].

Although $O_2^{\bullet-}$ production is essential for bacterial cell killing, $O_2^{\bullet-}$ alone is not responsible, H_2O_2 in the presence of released iron could form HO•, a potent oxidant, *via* the Fenton mechanism (Equation 1) or the Haber–Weiss mechanism (Equation 2). HO• is a potent antimicrobial oxidant [12, 13]. The three most diffusive components are $O_2^{\bullet-}$, H_2O_2 and OH•, and these are capable of reacting with molecules that are remote from the source, even those with capacity to cross the cell membranes [7, 12, 14] (Fig. 1, see also Table 1).

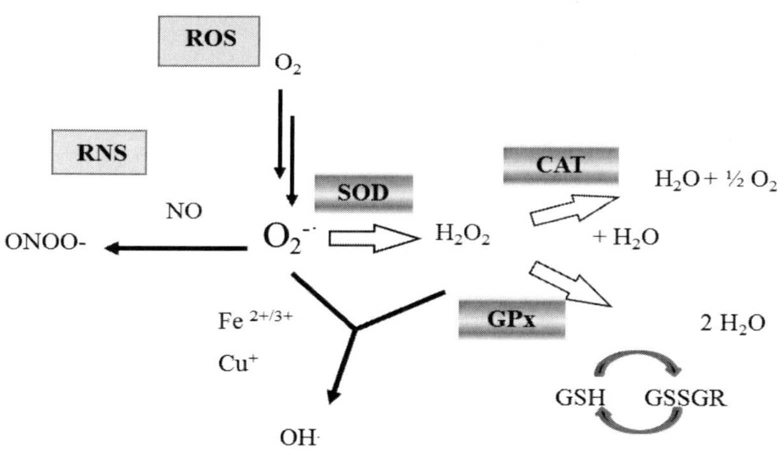

Figure 1. The main pathways of ROS and RNS production and the antioxidant system of defense. SOD is an enzyme that catalyzes the dismutation of superoxide into H_2O_2. H_2O_2 is removed by glutathione peroxidase (GPx) and CAT.

$$Fe^{2+} + H_2O_2 \rightarrow Fe^{3+} + HO\bullet + OH^- \quad (1)$$

Table 1. Characteristics and biological half-lives of Reactive Oxygen Species (ROS)

Reactive Oxygen Species (ROS)				
	Symbol	**Prooxidant**	**Description**	**Half-Lives (s)**
Free radical	$O_2\bullet^-$	superoxide anion radical	- poor oxidant, the largest reducer, the simple addition of a proton leads to the formation of the ROO• that becomes a very active, selective and specific oxidant. - not particularly reactive to lipids, carbohydrates or nucleic acids, and shows limited reactivity with certain proteins. - reacts with proteins contains metals in its prosthetic group.	10^{-6}
Free radical	HO•	hydroxyl radical	- extremely reactive. - diffuses only to low distance - formed by the *Fenton reaction* and decomposition of *peroxynitrite.* - extremely reactive, reacts with any molecule that is close, without any specificity, will attack most cellular components.	10^{-9}
Free radical	RO•	alkoxy radicals	-less reactive than HO•, but more than ROO•.	10^{-6}
Free radical	ROO•	peroxyl radicals	-oxygen-centred organic radicals. -lipid forms participate in *lipid peroxidation* reactions. -produced in the presence of oxygen by radical addition to double bonds or hydrogen abstraction. -weak oxidant, high diffusability.	10^{-2}
Free radical	$Q\bullet^-$	semiquinone radical	- a free radical resulting from the removal of one hydrogen atom with its electron during the process of dehydrogenation of a hydroquinone toquinone, or alternatively through the addition of a single hydrogen atom to a quinone.	highly unstable
No free radical	H_2O_2	hydrogen peroxide	-oxidant. -can be formed by dismutation of $O_2\bullet^-$ or by direct reduction of O_2. - is lipid soluble and thus able to diffuse across membranes.	minute-months
No free radical	$^1O_2$	singlet oxygen	-powerful oxidizing agent.	10^{-5}
No free radical	ROOH	*organic hydroperoxide*	-formed by radical reactions with cellular components such as *lipids* and *nucleobases*	function of temperature
No free radical	HOCl	*hypochlorous acid*	-formed from H_2O_2 by *myeloperoxidase.* -lipid soluble and highly reactive. -will readily oxidize protein constituents, including *thiol groups*, *amino* and *methionine.*	*minutes*

$$O_2\bullet^- + H_2O_2 \rightarrow Fe^3 \rightarrow OH + OH- + O_2 \quad (2)$$

ROS can also be produced by a host of exogenous sources such as xenobiotic, chlorinated compounds, environmental agents, metals (redox and non-redox), ions, and radiation.

3. Nitric Oxide: The Supporting Actor?

Another form of stress is termed nitrosative stress, with nitrate (NO_3^-) and nitrites (NO_2^-) are being used as terminal electron acceptors under anaerobic conditions. On increasing $O_2^{\bullet-}$, this reacts with the nitric oxide (NO•) leading to the formation of peroxynitrite (ONOO-), which is highly reactive and damaging [15]. Therefore, NO• decreases the oxidative stress available to exert its physiological function and also generates even more harmful species. NO• as free radical has an intermediate reactivity with a half-life from 1 to 10 seconds [16], but the reversible redox conversion of nitrite and NO• in a physiological setting is now widely accepted. NO_2^- has long been identified as a stable intermediate of NO• oxidation but several lines of evidence support the reduction of nitrite to NO• *in vivo* [15, 16]. NO• is synthesized from *L-arginine* by the *action* of *nitric oxide synthase* (NOS) *in* a two-step oxidation process (Equation 3) This is actually the fastest know nonenzymatic reaction in biology proceeding at diffusion-controlled rates of 1.9 x 10^{10} $M^{-1}s^{-1}$ and is given by:

$$\text{Arginine} + O_2 + 1\tfrac{1}{2}\,\text{NADPH} \rightarrow \text{hydroxyl-arginine} + O_2 + \tfrac{1}{2}\,\text{NADPH} \rightarrow \text{citrulline} + \text{NO}\bullet \quad (3)$$

NO• is not necessarily short lived and is intrinsically no more reactive than oxygen. The reactivity of NO• *per se* has been greatly overestimated *in vitro* because no drain is provided to remove NO•. NO• persists in solution for several minutes in micromolar concentrations before it reacts with oxygen to form much stronger oxidants like nitrogen dioxide ($NO_2\bullet$) [17].

The reaction of NO• and $O_2^{\bullet-}$ being biologically significant for at least two reasons [17]:

- First, NO• and $O_2^{\bullet-}$ can antagonize each other's biological action. It has been well known for a long time that NO•-mediated effects are often enhanced by adding SOD to physiological preparations, which may be understood as a competition for $O_2^{\bullet -}$ between SOD and NO•. Therefore, NO• can protect itself by removing $O_2^{\bullet -}$

- Second, the consequences of ONOO– generation deserve special consideration, with one molecular form of protonated ONOO– (ONOOH) being a very powerful oxidizing cytotoxic species.

In addition, NO• directly promotes the CAT activity that converts H_2O_2 to O_2 and H_2O.

Today, NO• is additionally formed in biological processes. Typically, in eukaryotes, NO• is a versatile molecule that has many functions in both eukaryotic and prokaryotic cells, with the occurrence and function of NOS having been well investigated in eukaryotic cells. NO• is detected in nanomolar concentrations, with the reactive nature of NO•, its hydrophobicity and fast diffusion making NO• an ideal messenger molecule that can easily cross cell boundaries and quickly disappear again [17, 18]. NO• is as an important signaling molecule for vasodilatation, as a neurotransmitter for brain cells and as an antimicrobial agent produced by macrophages.

4. Nitric Oxide, Superoxide, and Peroxynitrite: The Good, the Bad, and the Ugly [17]

Peroxynitrous acid (ONOOH) decomposes within a cage that contains two powerful radical species: HO• and NO_2•. Under physiological conditions ONOO– has a half-life of less than one second, and it is converted to its protonated form ONOOH, ONOOH, which in turn decays to generate multiple toxic products with reactivity similar to those of NO_2• and HO• [17, 19]. In fact, ONOO– reacts rather specifically with tyrosine residues in proteins, leading to the formation of nitro-tyrosine, which may be considered to be a fingerprint of ONOO– reactivity in a cellular setting, and can it also oxidize lipids, proteins, DNA, and carbohydrates [19, 20].

ONOO– reacts relatively slowly with most biological molecules, and modifies tyrosine in proteins to create nitrotyrosines, leaving a footprint detectable *in vivo*. Nitration of structural proteins, including neurofilaments and actin, can disrupt filament assembly with major pathological consequences [17, 20].

The past ten years have revealed that crucial features of neuronal communication, blood vessel modulation and immune response are mediated by the remarkably simple chemical NO•, which is released by different cell types, mainly macrophages, is involved in a great variety of processes, for example, in infectious diseases, liberation of NO• by cells of the innate immune system contributes to early control of infections [21]. In addition, induction of this molecule has been reported to have beneficial effects in the treatment of acute myocardial infarction, to be necessary for the maintenance of homeostasis in the kidney and to have cytotoxic effects on tumor cells [22]. On the other hand, production of the same molecule at high concentrations or under certain specific conditions can have detrimental effects on health [21, 23]. Thus, overproduction of NO• has been implicated in autoimmune disorders such as rheumatoid arthritis and multiple sclerosis, chronic inflammation and neurodegeneration [21-24]. NO• has also been shown to be involved in the apoptotic process, production of this metabolite inducing apoptosis of some cell types, including macrophages, neurons and human neutrophils [25,26]. Macrophages are very important in the control of infections. These cells are capable of phagocytosing and killing microorganisms and secrete an array of cytotoxic products such as H_2O_2 and NO. In addition to its functions as a messenger molecule, it has been shown that NO• is released by macrophages upon stimulation with bacterial toxins to mediate the innate immune response [24-29].

During the last decade it has become apparent that NOS is also encoded and expressed in certain prokaryotes, but only recently have studies suggested *in vivo* functions for the enzyme [30]. In contrast to eukaryotes, the formation of NO• in prokaryotes has been mainly attributed to catabolic processes, with NO• having been described as an intermediate of denitrification and nitrification. During denitrification, NO• is formed in the reduction of NO_2^- by nitrite reductase (NIR) as a free intermediate that reaches a certain steady state concentration in liquid culture. In further steps, NO• is reduced to N_2O by the integral membrane protein nitric oxide reductase (NOR). The phylogenetic analysis of the enzyme has shown that NOR is a member of the family of respiratory heam-copper oxidases, and the abundance of NO• in the atmosphere of the early earth has led to the hypothesis that mitochondrial cytochrome aa_3 oxidase evolved from an ancient NOR. Similar to denitrifiying bacteria, ammonia oxidizing bacteria (AOB) also produce NO• during catabolic reactions. However, the production and function of NO• in AOB is not clearly attributed to a specific enzymatic mechanism and represents a long-standing and unsolved question in the biology of nitrifying bacteria [29].

In the 1990s, NOS was also shown to be present in bacteria [31]. NO• is produced by microorganisms as a physiological response to medium oxidants, with the effect of NO• being also beneficial. However, with NO• has been also observed to be able to immediately protect bacteria from ROS, thus playing a critical role in the adaptation to oxidative stress associated with rapid metabolic changes [32].

Table 2. Characteristics and biological half-lives of Reactive Nitrogen Species (RNS)

Reactive nitrogen species (RNS)				
	Symbol	**Prooxidant**	**Description**	**Half-Lives (s)**
Free radical	NO•	nitric oxide radical	- an important cellular signaling molecule involved in many physiological and pathological processes. - a versatile molecule that has many functions in eukaryotic and prokaryotic cells.	1-10
No free radical	ONOO-	<u>*peroxynitrite*</u>	- formed in a rapid reaction between $O_2•^-$ and NO•. - lipid soluble and similar in reactivity to hypochlorous acid. - protonation forms ONOOH, which can undergo homolytic cleavage to form HO• and NO_2•	0.05-1

Although the roles of ROS and RNS have been extensively studied in planktonic bacterial physiology, there is still only limited information available, with more research being necessary to determine the precise role of cellular stress in biofilms, and it could be also useful to study the different factors that participate in the physiological characteristics of microorganisms [33]. However, whereas substantial research efforts have been made to elucidate the various functions of NO• in multicellular eukaryotes, little is known about its role in communities of prokaryotic organisms (biofilms). An aim of future work will be to adapt *in situ* detection techniques for use in microbial ecology and elucidate the functions of NO• in microbial communities of different complexities. NO• formation in bacteria poses new questions concerning the function of NO• in microbial communities and their interaction with each other and with eukaryotic hosts.

5. Oxidative Stress: A Loss if Balance

The defense mechanisms of living organisms have developed antioxidant physiological defenses that prevent the formation of FR, recognize oxidative damage and repair. These defenses are called antioxidants and are considered at normal levels as substances that possess a greater affinity than any other molecule for interaction with RL [12, 34].

The antioxidant defenses can be classified according to their nature as enzymatic or non-enzymatic antioxidants, and depending on their origin, as endogenous or exogenous antioxidants. After collision with RL, the antioxidant gives up an oxidized electron and is transformed into a non-toxic weak RL [35]. However, not all antioxidants act in this manner, with the ones called enzymes catalyzing chemical reactions through substrates that react with RL [34].

An antioxidant substance is one which, at relatively low concentrations, is able to compete with other oxidizable substrates and, therefore, retard or inhibit oxidation of these substrates [36]. This definition includes enzymatic and non- enzymatic antioxidants. An ideal antioxidant should be readily absorbed and quench FR, and chelate redox metals at physiologically relevant levels with interact with other antioxidants for regeneration of the antioxidant [12, 35].

These are classified as endogenous (found in organisms and are synthesized by their cells) and exogenous (entering through the nutrient). The main enzymes, involved in the detoxification of ROS are SOD, CAT, GPx and glutathione reductase (GSSGR) [12, 34-37].

Non-enzymatic antioxidants include Vitamin E and C, thiol antioxidants (glutathione, thioredoxin and lipoic acid), melatonin, carotenoids, natural flavonoids, and other compounds. Some antioxidants can interact with other antioxidants regenerating their original properties; this mechanism is often referred to as the "antioxidant network" [35, 36] (Table 3).

Table 3. Antioxidants in Biological Systems

Antioxidants		
	Non-enzymatic	
Enzymatic	**Endogenous**	**Exogenous**
Superoxide Dismutase (SOD)	Glutatione (GSH)	Tocopherols (Vitamin E)
Catalase (Cat)	Coenzyme Q	Ascorbate (Vitamin C)
Glutathione peroxidase (GPx)	Tioctic acid	Carotenoids
Glutathione reductase (GSSGR)	Melatonin	Flavonoids

The ROS/RNS not neutralized by antioxidant defenses can damage the cellular membranes by oxidation lipids, critical enzymes of the intermediary metabolism or other proteins, and also break DNA chains. Oxidative damage caused by these species in biological macromolecules can have critical consequences, it being one of the most important causative agents of mutagenesis, tumorigenesis and even aging.

6. All Excesses Are Bad: The Cell Damage

The production of ROS, including FR, is a natural, inevitable and ongoing process referred to as a biological continuum. All cells, regardless of their types, are constantly producing molecules with unpaired electrons, with the damage that FR cause in different tissues depending on the balance between ROS and antioxidant defenses [35, 36] (Fig. 2).

Under physiological conditions, a critical balance between the production of prooxidants and the antioxidant system exists. However, when this balance is broken, through an increase in the ROS/RNS production and/or a reduction in the antioxidant defenses, an overproduction of prooxidant is induced resulting in a process denominated oxidative stress [4, 7, 11, 22, 38]. In this situation, the overproduction of ROS can lead to the damage of cellular components including lipids, proteins, and DNA [34-39]. If this damage is not repaired, mutagenesis and cellular death can occur, which probably participate in the pathogenesis of various illnesses such as Alzheimer, multiple sclerosis, diabetes, as well as in infectious diseases including Chagas disease, bacterial meningitis and hepatitis [22, 24, 29, 34, 39].

FR reacts with lipids, proteins, carbohydrates and nucleic acids within cells and with extracellular matrix components [33]. Furthermore, it been also associated with the chronic inflammation caused by microorganisms (biofilms) of the FR that are generated during bactericidal attack of macrophages and neutrophils [25-28, 40]. Toxins too induces too an oxidative imbalance in blood cells, with an overproduction of FR and a decrease in the antioxidant defenses [41-44].

The following different biomarkers are examples that have been used to follow the development of the oxidative stress [45, 46] (Fig. 3).

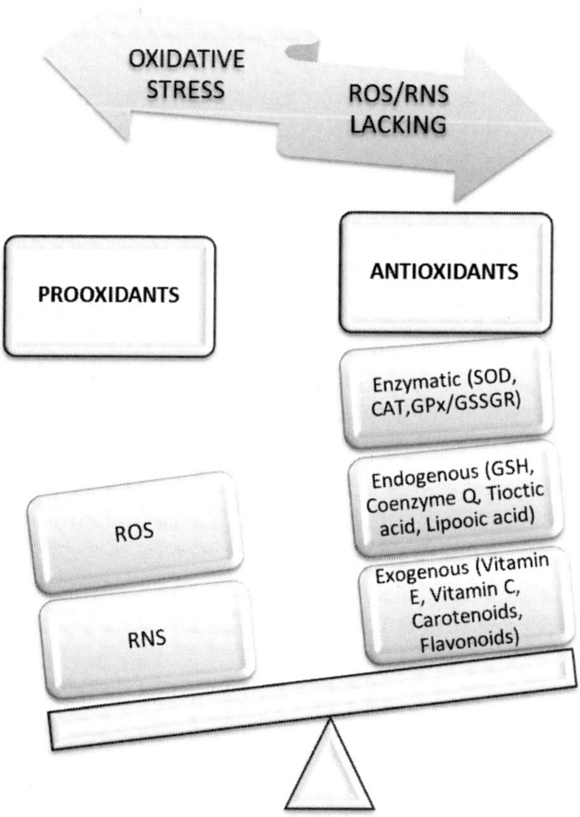

Figure 2. The loss of balance: as a consequence of imbalance between prooxidant and antioxidant in favor of the prooxidants, leading to potential damage.

Lipidic Damage

The damage observed due to an oxidative attack of lipids in biological membranes is called lipid peroxidation, and primarily occurs on the polyunsaturated fatty acid chain with the resulting membranes having a loss of flexibility, secretory functions and gradient breaking transmembrane ions. This is a chain reaction, taking place in the three phases of initiation, propagation and termination, which react with molecular oxygen yielding a hydroperoxyl radical. This radical can in turn remove a hydrogen atom from a methylene carbon of another polyunsaturated fatty acid to form a new radical and lipid hydroperoxide.

The lipid radical then combines with another molecule of oxygen and the chain reaction continues. The end products of this lipid peroxidation process are aldehydes, hydrocarbonates, various gases and chemical waste, including malondialdehyde (MDA) and 4 -hydroxy-2 -nonenal (HNE), with MDA also being a well-known biomarker of the lipidic damage induced by oxidizing stress [46, 47]. Lipid peroxidation may have profound effects on cell functions, by affecting the membranes and producing changes in the flow, leading to increased permeability, reduced membrane potential and finally rupture.

MDA can react with lipids and proteins in lipid peroxidation to form conjugated Shiff bases, which are insoluble products. Moreover, while MDA molecules react with DNA, causing a number of genetic mutations, HNE is capable of reacting with protein and causing major alterations that directly affect various signaling pathways as well as the proteins directly involved in cell death mechanisms, or through protein modification of carboxylation and sulfhydryl functions causing, for example, loss of enzyme inactivation [48, 49].

Protein Damage

The action of FR on proteins may be reversible or irreversible, depending on the purpose and form of oxidative damage exerted mainly on the unsaturated bonds, aromatic rings and the thiol groups (-SH). Thus, certain proteins rich in amino acids (tryptophan, tyrosine, phenylalanine, histidine, methionine and cysteine) may be structurally and functionally modified. Tryptophan, tyrosine, histidine and cysteine are particularly sensitive to ROS, and sulfhydryl groups may be converted into disulfide (S = S) to produce an inactivation enzyme (if the protein is an enzyme) [45, 49-51].

Interaction with Carbohydrates

The FR interacts with carbohydrates in different ways. Glucose is a scavenger of superoxide radical whereas mannose and mannitol are HO• scavengers. However, polysaccharides are depolymerized by FR, as hyaluronic acid and proteinglicanos. Carbonyl residues and advanced oxidation protein products (AOPP) are the two parameters normally used to evaluate the level of oxidative damage to proteins [33, 50- 52].

DNA Damage

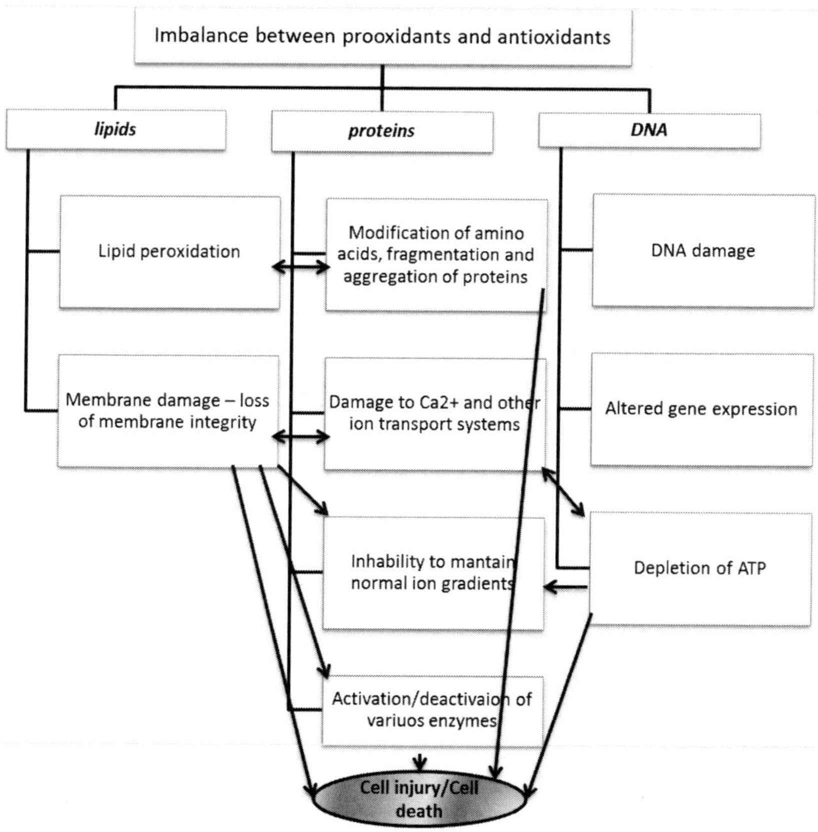

Figure 3. Markers of oxidative damage, proteins, lipids and DNA are the main targets of ROS and RNS.

FR can react with all components of the DNA. In the presence of oxygen, peroxyl radicals are formed by the addition of oxygen to the bases of DNA. The subsequent reactions of the radicals formed in the DNA lead to a large number of effects, including strand breaks and a basic site and base modifications. Cross-bridges are also formed from DNA protein. When a free radical attacks a deoxyribose of DNA, a strand break is produced; with the number of products resulting from the oxidation of the nitrogenous bases of DNA by FR exceeding twenty. These include 8 - hydroxy - deoxyguanine (8-OH- dG), which is the most frequently seen alteration., and is used as a biomarker of oxidative stress by being able to reflect small changes in oxidative damage to DNA. Furthermore, its importance resides in its high mutagenic effect, as 8-OH- dG in DNA replication pairs with adenine instead of cytosine. A moderate DNA damage can arrest the cell cycle or repair mechanisms to maintain DNA integrity. However, if this damage is excessive, it can set in motion processes that induce apoptosis and cell death [45, 49-52].

7. Understanding Biofilms: What are These?

In 1684, Antonie van Leeuwenhoek, was the first to display the "animalcules" (bacteria) found in plaque scraped from his teeth plaque, and described that: "The numbers of these animalcules in the scurf of a man's teeth are so many that I believe they exceed the number of men in a kingdom". Zobell (1943) noted an "effect" in seawater and described many of the fundamental characteristics of attached microbial communities. In the years which followed, researchers have concentrated primarily on planktonic (free-floating) bacteria, the kinds of microbes studied by the likes of Louis Pasteur and Robert Koch. It was not until the 1970s that scientists began to appreciate that bacteria in the biofilm mode of existence constitute such a major component of the bacterial biomass in most environments. JW Costerton at the Center for Biofilm Engineering in Montana used the name "biofilms" as a more generic term for microorganisms adhering to wet surfaces in freshwater ecosystems [53]. Donald (2002) [54] made a widely accepted description of biofilms. A biofilm is generally defined as microbial communities containing sessile cells embedded in a self-produced extracellular polymeric matrix (containing polysaccharides, DNA and other components) and adherent to an inert or living surface [33, 55,56].

Bacteria exist in two principal forms, as free-floating planktonic replicating cells and in biofilms. However, it is now generally acknowledged that the majority of microbial cells on earth are living in spatially distinct communities, referred to as biofilms, a form in which they behave very differently. In fact, it is now known that 99 % of all bacteria exist in biofilms, with only 1 % living in the planktonic state. Biofilms constituting a microbial multicellular lifestyle and are defined as organized communities of bacteria, collaborating among themselves and being attached to an inert or living surface contained in a self-produced polymeric matrix made principally of exopolysaccharide [53, 56]. This matrix contains polysaccharides, proteins and DNA and is bisected by ramifying the water channels that carry the bulk fluid into the community by convective flow [57]. Biofilms can be composed of a population developed from a single species, or from a community derived of multiple microbial species. Hypotheses about the ecological advantages of forming biofilms include protection from the environment, nutrient availability, metabolic cooperation, and the acquisition of new genetic traits [54-57].

Microbial multicellular communities or biofilms come in a great variety of sizes and shapes, with some of the most common types containing mushroom-like, pillar-like, hilly, or flat multicellular structures, which allow cells to form long-term relationships, interact with each other and establish metabolic cooperation [56-57].

The association of bacteria with a surface and the development of a biofilms can be viewed as a survival mechanism, with bacteria benefiting by acquiring nutrients and protection from biocides. In cases of adverse conditions such as desiccation, osmotic shock, or exposure to toxic compounds, UV radiation, or predators, the microbial community as a whole can provide protection. Moreover, biofilms are also sites where genetic material is easily exchanged because of the proximity of the cells, thus maintaining a large gene pool. [54, 56, 58]. Biofilms are permeated at all levels by a network of channels through which water, bacterial garbage, nutrients, enzymes, metabolites and oxygen move to and fro, with gradients of chemicals to providing the power to shunt the substances around the biofilms. Oxygen may be depleted within only 30-40 μm of the water/biofilm interface. Although the precise depth of the oxygen gradient in the biofilm varies depending on the oxygen content in the bulk water, water temperature, and water flow, this gives a rough idea of how far oxygen can diffuse [59].

Although research on biofilms has surged in the last 20-30 years, the majority of biofilm research to date has focused on external biofilms, or those that form on various surfaces in our natural environment. A better tool to analyze external biofilms has realized they cause a wide range of problems in industrial environments. For example, biofilms can develop on the interiors of pipes, which can lead to clogging and corrosion. Biofilms on floors and counters can make sanitation difficult in food preparation areas [54-56].

Since biofilms have the ability to clog pipes, watersheds, storage areas, and contaminate food products, large companies with facilities that are negatively impacted by their presence have naturally taken an interest in supporting biofilm research, particularly research that specifies how biofilms can be eliminated [53, 56-59].

This means that many recent advances in biofilm detection have resulted from collaborations between microbial ecologists, environmental engineers, and mathematicians.

8. Are Microorganisms Living in the Community Stressed?

In comparison with their planktonic (free-living) counterparts, the sessile cells that form biofilms are often more resistant to various stresses, including antibacterial agents [11, 49-52, 60, 61]. Hence, biofilms can cause serious problems during antibiotics (ATBs) therapies and it has been reported that sub-inhibitory levels of ATBs may induce or inhibit bacterial biofilm formation [60-62]. This increased resistance has a considerable impact on the treatment of biofilm-related infections. There is growing evidence that the mechanism of cell death initiated by some ATBs includes the production of ROS [11, 64-66].

Like in eukaryotes, NO• is also recognized as a signal by bacteria. NO• is obtained from a product of the anaerobic reduction, with this process resulting in a switch from O_2 to NO_3^-, NO_2^- or nitrous oxide (N_2O) as the electron acceptor.

In *Escherichia coli*, NO• can act as a signaling molecule with effect regulator proteins like SoxR (superoxide regulator) and FNR (fumarate-nitrate reduction) influencing the response to stress [67]. In addition, the role of the periplasmic antioxidant enzymes of the Shiga toxin-producing *Escherichia coli* O157:H7 (STEC) in the formation of biofilms was studied by proteomic analyses, and significantly higher expression levels of zinc SOD and thiol peroxidase were found in STEC cells grown under biofilm conditions than under planktonic conditions [68]. In *Bacillus subtilis*, NO• can induce the transcription of genes via the two-component regulatory system and leads to the expression of Hmp, a flavohemoglobin that has been shown to function in the detoxification of NO• [69]. Falsetta et al. showed that NO• plays a dual role in *Neisseria gonorrhoeae* biofilm formation. In the predominately anaerobic environment of the human cervix, NO• plays a role as an electron acceptor in a respiratory pathway necessary for the survival of the gonococcus. The NOR is critical for production of a biofilm and is involved in the reduction of NO• to N_2O. Mutants in *norB* can accumulate NO•, thus resulting in biofilm dispersal, which can be reversed by an NO• scavenger, with NO• being involved in biofilm dispersal [70]. In *Streptomyces turgidiscabie* (a plant pathogenic bacterium) NOS is involved in a biosynthesis pathway rather than in producing free NO•.

Barraud et al. (2006) detected $ONOO^-$ inside microcolonies in *Pseudomonas aeruginosa* biofilms, with $ONOO^-$ being formed from NO• oxidation only in the presence of ROS [71]. Although it is not clear how $ONOO^-$ is produced inside the microcolonies, O_2 gradients can occur, with simultaneous O_2 and NO_3^- respiration having recently been demonstrated for *P. aeruginosa* populations. Schlag et al. have reported interplay between respiratory nitrate reduction and biofilm formation in *Staphylococcus aureus* SA113 and *Staphylococcus epidermidis* RP62A and have shown that the presence of nitrite, a product of nitrate respiration, causes a stress response, which concomitantly involves impairment of PIA-mediated biofilm formation. They have also provided data suggesting that the acidified nitrite derivative NO•, widely used as a defense or signaling molecule in biological systems, is directly or indirectly involved in the inhibition of *S. aureus* biofilm formation [67].

They are also provided evidence that nitrite-derived NO• played a role in the inhibition of biofilm formation and that biofilm-embedded staphylococci could be efficiently killed by nitrite in an acidic environment. Despite NO• exposure being able to reduce staphylococcal viability, *S. aureus* has been described as being relatively resistant to growth inhibition by NO•, principally by the observation of efficient NO• scavenging mechanisms, where flavohemoprotein Hmp was shown to play a crucial role in counteracting NO• toxicity [73].

The oxidative and nitrosative stress could be produced inside biofilms, thereby affecting their growth under different conditions and resulting in ROS and RNS production, with a decrease of the extracellular matrix [33, 42, 74]. Although *S. aureus* it is now established that produces biofilms little is known about the environmental factors that trigger this formation. Arce Miranda y col (2011) observed that biofilm formation was influenced by different conditions, with there being a close relation with extracellular stress (ROS and NO•) and suggest a strong relation between the nutrients as sugars, pH and biofilm formation [33]. When was compared the effect of microaerobiosis, it was evident that the strains exhibited maximum extracellular stress, with the reduced culture possibly increasing the shelf life of these species and their derivatives in these conditions. In *S. aureus* biofilm the extracellular stress (eROS and NO•) was more significant than that of intracellular ROS (iROS). Although no other report was found in the literature about this effect, the oxidative stress stimuli should now be incorporated into the list of factors involved in the formation of biofilm [33, 42, 74].

NO•, as a simple molecule and free intermediate in the primary metabolism, may have been an ancient signal for cell-cell communication before the evolution of highly sophisticated, specialized molecules. It is very likely that NO• has not only a versatile role in multicellular eukaryotic systems, but also in organized prokaryotic systems.

9. How Do Biofilms Provide Protection from Antibiotics?

Biofilms in nature are generally beneficial and are frequently established on hydrous solid and semi-solid surfaces, such as soil and rock material, or on the surfaces of animals and plants [53, 54]. Microbial communities natively populate human mucous membranes and epithelial surfaces, for example, the gastrointestinal tract, oral cavity, and skin. However, despite our bodies being colonized with a mixed microbial community of characteristic compositions, they are important and beneficial to us as they can degrade nutrients and thereby make these accessible [33, 55, 77, 78]. In addition, they can synthesize certain vitamins which we are unable to synthesize on our own. In particular, these communities play key roles in the development of our immune systems and in the anatomy of the mucosal surfaces, as well as providing protective functions against exogenous pathogens [56, 75, 78].

The relationship between the host and its microbial communities is delicately balanced, but under certain conditions it can break down and result in infectious diseases. According to a recent public announcement from the National Institutes of Health (USA), more than 60% of all microbial infections are caused by biofilms [56, 75]. Related to this, although the planktonic form of bacteria has been very useful in understanding acute infections, chronic ones are more related to the presence of biofilms, with current research indicating an important role for bacterial biofilms in recurrent or chronic infections, including those which are not responsive to a culture-appropriate ATB therapy [56, 74, 75 79].

Surface-associated microorganisms are responsible for several chronic infections such as: periodontitis, heart valve inflammation, in lung infections in patients with cystic fibrosis [55, 56, 71, 74, 75] child middle-ear infections [80], in chronic rhinosinusitis [81], in chronic osteomyelitis and infections caused by a variety of surgical implants, wound infections in burn patients, urinary tract infections, in intravenous catheters and stents, among others [82]. This link between the concept of biofilms and chronic infectious disease is still the subject of a many studies.

The traditional ATBs resistance of planktonic bacteria usually involves inactivation of the ATBs, modification of targets, and exclusion of the ATB, actions that typically require the acquisition of specific genetic factors, such as genes for β-lactamase or efflux pumps [56, 83]. One of the most important aspects of bacterial biofilm formation is the increased resistance of the constituent microbes to ATBs and other stressors, with the structural nature of the biofilms and the characteristics of the sessile cells producing resistance towards the antimicrobial agents, leading to a protected environment against adverse conditions and the host´s defenses [55, 56, 84]. Free living bacteria, on the other hand, are generally susceptible to ATBs treatment and to host defense mechanisms. However, the minimal inhibitory concentration (MIC) and minimal bactericidal concentration (MBC) of ATBs to biofilm-growing bacteria is up to 100–1000 fold higher than for planktonic bacteria, and possibly 150-3000 times more resistant to disinfectant [42, 56, 79,85].

Despite decades of research, very little is known about the molecular mechanisms of ATB resistance in biofilms. Although several theories have been proposed, the precise mechanism of how this sensitivity is altered has still not been clarified. Nevertheless, it is possible to separate these mechanisms into intrinsic (or innate) and extrinsic (or induced) resistance factors to biofilms [56, 77, 85, 86].

The intrinsic factors of resistance are activated as part of the biofilm developmental pathway, which are integral parts of the biofilm structure and physiology resulting from conversion to a biofilm lifestyle. The influences of several different intrinsic biofilm factors affecting ATB resistance have been identified. For example: the biofilm matrix may act as a diffusion barrier;

microenvironments within biofilms can be established; small subpopulations of bacteria within the biofilms may differentiate into persisters; an increased production of oxidative stress causes might changes in the physiology of bacteria; and an antagonist of ATB and degradation mechanisms may be active in some parts of the biofilms [55, 83-86].

Other groups resulting from transcriptional induction by treatment with an ATB agent itself are extrinsic or induced resistance factors. The mutation frequency of biofilm-growing bacteria is significantly increased compared with planktonically growing isogenic bacteria, and there is an increased horizontal gene transmission in biofilms. These physiological conditions may explain why biofilm-growing bacteria easily become multidrug resistant by means of traditional resistance mechanisms against β-lactam ATBs, such as, aminoglycosides and fluoroquinolones, which can be detected by routine susceptibility testing in the clinical microbiology laboratory when planktonic bacterial growth is investigated. Thus, bacterial cells in biofilms may simultaneously produce enzymes that degrade ATBs, have ATB targets of low affinity, and over-expressed efflux pumps that have a broad range of substrates.

ATB treatment can result in an increased production of oxidative stress within a biofilm. Consequently, one would expect that there must be some ATB-regulated genes that can influence ATB resistance or the sensitivity of biofilm bacteria, and it is likely that numerous genetic loci are activated upon treatment with ATBs. These induced factors may work synergistically with intrinsic factors to enhance survival in the face of strong antimicrobial stresses.

Oxidative stress is considered to cause enhanced mutability in biofilms. Recent data suggest that microcolony structures, due to endogenous oxidative stress, are specific sites within biofilms where enhanced genetic adaptation and evolutionary change take place [69-70]. In addition, Boles and Singh showed that endogenous oxidative stress in biofilms promotes ATB resistance, and that the addition of antioxidants reduces the diversity in biofilms [87]. Recently, it was also observed that an increased production of oxidative stress caused change in the extracellular polysaccharides (EPS) in biofilms of *S. aureus* [33].

MICs have long been the standard for ATB susceptibility testing as they can measure the actions of ATBs against planktonic organisms and serve as an important reference in the treatment of many acute infections. The application of MICs in the treatment of infections involving bacterial biofilms is often ineffective, with numerous studies having now demonstrated that biofilm-grown microorganisms have an inherent lack of susceptibility to ATBs, whereas planktonic cultures of this same organism do not [11, 49-52].

In planktonic cells, the induction of ROS following the treatment of bacteria with ATBs has been well documented in the case of quinolones, ampicillin, aminoglycosides, chloramphenicol, trimethoprim and rifampicin, and ciprofloxacin [11, 49-52, 60,61, 76-79, 88]. All these afore mentioned ATBs induce oxidative stress regardless of their specific targets, and the detailed mechanism of ATBs-mediated ROS formation has already been partly revealed, demonstrated that the general mechanism of lethal $OH^{\cdot}$ production in the presence of bactericidal ATB involves the transient depletion of NADH due to changes in the tricarboxylic acid cycle metabolism, destabilization of iron sulfur clusters and iron miss regulation. The role of ROS in ATB mediated cell death is also supported by the fact that mutations in genes belonging to the ROS defense increase drug sensitivity [88,89].

During their evolution, bacteria have been able to develop successful strategies for survival, which include attachment to surfaces and the development of protective biofilms where bacteria behave very differently to the free-floating types. These successful strategies make it difficult to control biofilm growth, with a biofilm providing bacteria with a 10- to 1,000-fold increase in ATB resistance compared to free ones. Some mechanisms of resistance appear to be intrinsic to growth in a biofilm, with inhibited diffusion through the matrix, reduced metabolism by nutrient limitation, formation of dormant persisters, and the increased production of oxidative stress all appearing to impact on the development of a protective environment within the biofilm; in addition to the extrinsic factors such as -induced gene expression by ATBs in biofilm cells. Due to the heterogeneous nature of biofilms, it is likely that multiple mechanisms of antimicrobial resistance are useful in order to explain biofilm survival in a number of cases, with ATB resistance being the result of an intricate mixture of intrinsic and extrinsic factors. However, additional mechanisms must also exist to be able account for increased biofilm ATB resistance. Although several methods to test biofilm-growing bacteria have already been developed, their clinical relevance with regard to the prediction of clinically successful therapies still awaits confirmation.

Conclusion

In conclusion, ROS, RNS and their downstream derivatives could play an important role in biofilm development. This suggests that cellular stress is produced inside biofilms, thereby affecting their growth under different conditions and resulting in ROS and RNS production, with a decrease of the extracellular matrix occurring under unfavorable conditions. These radical oxidizers can then accumulate in an extracellular medium and thus affect the matrix. Although adaptive responses against oxidative stress caused by these ROS/RNI have been extensively studied with planktonic cells, comparatively little is known about biofilm responses, with the basis for this apparent acquired resistance being currently poorly understood. Oxidative imbalance is due to an overproduction of ROS/RNI or through a reduction in the oxidative defenses being insufficient to remove the FR, and therefore the antioxidant system plays a very important role in the control of this process. Since NO is a fast diffusing, reactive molecule with various biological functions, its action might to be expected significant over short distances into biofilms.

A better understanding of the genotypic and phenotypic adaptation of sessile (biofilm-associated) microorganisms to various forms of stress is still required in order to develop more effective anti-biofilm strategies.

Acknowledgments

M Gabriela Paraje is a member of the Research Career (CIC) of CONICET.

The assistance of Inés Albesa, Julio Arce Miranda and Natalia Angel Villegas is gratefully acknowledged. This work was supported by grants from CONICET, SECyT-UNC, MinCyT, and Agencia Nacional de Promoción Científica y Tecnológica. We would like to thank native speaker, Dr. Paul Hobson, for revision of the manuscript.

References

[1] Gerschman R, Gilbert DL, Nye SW, Dwyer P, Fenn WO. Oxygen poisoning and X-irradiation: a mechanism in common. *Science.* 1956;119:623–626.

[2] Mccord JM, Fridovich I. Superoxide dismutase. An enzymic function for erythrocuprein (haemocuprein). *J. Biol. Chem.* 1969;244:6049–6055.

[3] Mccord JM, Fridovich I. The utility of superoxide dismutase in studying free radical reactions. I. Radicals generated by the interaction of sulfite, dimethylsulfoxide and oxygen. *J. Biol. Chem.* 1969;244:6056–6063.

[4] Gutteridge JMC, Halliwell B. Free radicals and antioxidants in the year 2000. A historical look to the future. *Annals of the New York Academy of Sciences A*. 2000;899: 136-147.

[5] Halliwell B, Gutteridge JMC. Reactive species can be poisonous. In: Halliwell B, Gutteridge JMC, eds. *Free Radicals in Biology and Medicine 4th ed.* Oxford University Press; New York. 2007:440–487.

[6] Bergendi L, Benes L, Durackova Z, Ferencik M. Chemistry, physiology and pathology of free radicals. *Life Sciences.* 1999;65:1865-1874.

[7] Sies H. Oxidative stress: introductory remarks. In: H. Sies, eds. *Oxidative Stress.* London: Academic Press Inc,;1985:1-7.

[8] Miller DM, Buettner GR, Aust, SD. Transition metals as catalysts of "autoxidation" reactions. *Free Radical Biology and Medicine.* 1990;8:95-108.

[9] Montoya SC, Comini LR, Sarmiento M, Becerra C, Albesa I, Argüello GA, Cabrera JL. Natural anthraquinones probed as Type I and Type II photosensitizers *J Photochem Photobiol B.* 2005. 14;78(1):77-83.

[10] Fujita M, Tsuruta R, Kasaoka S, Fujimoto K, Tanaka R, Oda Y, Nanba M,Igarashi M, Yuasa M, Yoshikawa T, et al. In vivo real-time measurement of superoxide anion radical with a novel electrochemical sensor. *Free Radical Biology and Medicine.* 2009;47:1039-1048.

[11] Albesa I, Becerra MC, Battán PC, Páez PL. Oxidative stress involved in the antibacterial action of different antibiotics. *Biochem Biophys Res Commun.* 2004;317:605-9.

[12] Kalyanaraman B. Teaching the basics of redox biology to medical and graduate students: oxidants, antioxidants and disease mechanisms. *Redox Biology*. 2013;1(1):244–257.

[13] Grant SS, Kauffman BB, Chand NS, Hasely N, Hung DT. Eradication of bacterial persisters with antibiotic-generated hydroxyl radicals. *Proceedings of the National Academy of Science of USA*. 2012;109:12147–12152.

[14] Inoue, M., Sato, E.F., Nishikawa, M., Park, A.M., Kira, Y., Imada, I., and Utsumi, K. Mitochondrial generation of reactive oxygen species and its role in aerobic life. *Current Medicinal Chemistry.* 2003;10:2495-2505.

[15] Pereira C. The redox interplay between nitrite and nitric oxide: from the gut to the brain. Redox Biology. 2013;1(1):276–284.

[16] Zacharia IG, Deen,WM. Diffusivity and solubility of nitric oxide in water and saline. *Annals of Biomedical Engineering*. 2005;33:214-222.

[17] Beckman JS, Koppenol WH. Nitric oxide, superoxide and peroxynitrite: the good, the bad and the ugly. *Am. J. Physiol*. 1996;271:C1424–C1437.

[18] Bedioui F, Villeneuve,N. Electrochemical nitric oxide sensors for biological samples - Principle, selected examples and applications. *Electroanalysis*. 2003;15:5-18.

[19] Trujillo M., Naviliat M., Alvarez MN, Peluffo G, RadiR. Peroxynitrite biochemistry: formation, reactions and detection. *Analysi.* 2000;28,518-527.

[20] Lundberg J.O., Weitzberg E., Gladwin M.T. The nitrate-nitrite-nitric oxide pathway in physiology and therapeutics. *Nature Reviews Drug Discovery*.2008;7(2):156–167.

[21] Ito S, Ishii KJ, Ihata A, Klinman DM. Contribution of nitric oxide to CpG-mediated protection against *Listeria monocytogenes*. *Infect Immun.* 2005;73:3803–3805.

[22] Kalyanaraman B. Teaching the basics of redox biology to medical and graduate students: Oxidants, antioxidants and disease mechanisms. *Redox Biol.* 2013;8(1):244-257.

[23] Rahman, K. Studies on free radicals, antioxidants, and co-factors. *Clinical Interventions in Aging*. 2007:2(2);219–236.

[24] Rodriguez-Galan MC, Sotomayor CE, Cano R, Porporatto C, Renna MS, Paraje MG, Cejas H, Correa SG. Immune-neuroendocrine interactions during a fungal infection in immune component or immunes suppressed host. *Neuroimmunomodulation.* 2010;17 (3): 188-191.

[25] Paraje MG, Barnes AI, Albesa I. An *Enterobacter cloacae* toxin able to generate oxidative stress and to provoke dose-dependent lysis of leukocytes. *Int J Med Microbiol.* 2005;295:109–116.

[26] Baronetti JL, Angel Villegas N, Paraje, MG, Albesa, I. Nitric oxidemediated apoptosis in rat macrophages subjected to Shiga toxin 2 from Escherichia coli. *Microbiol. Immunol.* 2011;55:231–238.

[27] Baronetti J, Angel Villegas N, Aiassa V, Paraje MG, Albesa I. Hemolysin from *Escherichia coli* induces oxidative stress in blood. *Toxicon.* 2013;70:15–20.

[28] Albesa I, Barnes A, Paraje, MG. Induction of oxidative stress in leukocytes by a *Enterobacter cloacae* toxin able to form oligomers and

binding to proteins. *Biochemical and Biophysical Research Communications*. 2000;274 (3): 649-654.

[29] Paraje MG, Correa SG, Theumer Martin, Renna MS, and CE Sotomayor. Candida albicans-secreted lipase induces injury and steatosis in immune and parenchymal cells. *Canadian Journal of Microbiology*. 2008;54(8):647-59.

[30] Richardson DJ. Bacterial respiration: a flexible process for a changing environment. Microbiology. 2000;146:551-571.

[31] Chen YJ, Rosazza JPN. A Bacterial, Nitric-Oxide synthase from a *Nocardia* species. *Biochemical and Biophysical Research Communications*. 1994;203:1251-1258.

[32] Poole RK. Nitric oxide and nitrosative stress tolerance in bacteria. *Biochemical Society Transactions* 2005;33:176-180.

[33] Arce Miranda JE, Sotomayor CE, Albesa I, Paraje MG. Oxidative and nitrosative stress in *Staphylococcus aureus* biofilm. *FEMS Microbiol Lett*. 2011;1:23–9.

[34] Mayor-Oxilia, R. Oxidative Stress and Antioxidant Defense System. *Rev. Inst. Med. Trop*. 2010;5(2):23-29.

[35] *Sies H*. Strategies of antioxidant defense. *Eur J Biochem 1993;215:213-219*.

[36] Jones DP. Redefining oxidative stress. *Antioxidants & Redox Signaling*. 2006;8:1865–1879.

[37] Páez PL, Becerra MC, Albesa I. Effect of the association of reduced glutathione FEMS Microbiol Lett. 2010;303(1):101-5

[38] Aiassa V, Barnes AI, Smania AM, Albesa I. Sublethal ciprofloxacin treatment leads to resistance via antioxidant systems in *Proteus mirabilis*. *FEMS Microbiol Lett*. 2012;327:25-32.

[39] Guiñazú N, Carrera-Silva EA, Becerra MC, Pellegrini A, Albesa I, Gea S. Induction of NADPH oxidase activity and reactive oxygen Int J Parasitol. 2010;40(13):1531-8.

[40] Paraje, MG; Eraso, AJ and Albesa,I. Pore formation, polymerization, hemolytic and leukotoxic effects of a new *Enterobacter cloacae* toxin neutralized by antiserum. *Microbiol Res*. 2005;160:203-11.

[41] Paraje MG, Correa SG, Albesa I, Sotomayor CE. Lipase of *Candida albicans* induces activation of NADPH oxidase and L-arginine pathways on resting and activated macrophages. *Biochem Biophys Res Commun*. 2009;11:390(2):263-8.

[42] Angel Villegas N, Baronetti J, Albesa I, Polifroni R, Parma A, Etcheverría A, Becerra M, Padola N, Paraje M. Relevance of biofilms

in the pathogen:esis of shiga-toxin-producing *Escherichia coli* Infection. *Scientific World Journal*. 2013;12;607258.

[43] Barnes AI, Paraje MG, Orsilles M, Albesa I. Molecular properties and metabolic effect on blood cells produced by a new toxin of Enterobacter cloacae. *Cell Biology and Toxicology*. 2001;17(6):409-418.

[44] Paraje MG, Iribarren P, Albesa,, I. Interaction of bacterial toxin with leukocytes measured by flow cytometry. *Current Microbiology*. 2002;45(3):171-174.

[45] Correa-Salde V, Albesa I. Reactive oxidant species and oxidation of protein and haemoglobin as biomarkers of susceptibility to stress caused by chloramphenicol. *Biomed Pharmacother*. 2009;63(2):100-4.

[46] Dalle-Donne I, Rossi R, Colombo R, Giustarini D, Milzani A. Biomarkers of oxidative damage in human disease. *Clin Chem* 2006;52:601–623.

[47] Yoshida Y, Umeno A, Shichiri M. Lipid peroxidation biomarkers for evaluating oxidative stress and assessing antioxidant capacity *in vivo. J. Clin. Biochem. Nutr. 2013; (52)1: 9–16.*

[48] Poli G, Schaur RJ, Siems WG, Leonarduzzi G. 4-Hydroxynonenal: a membrane lipid oxidation product of medicinal interest. *Med Re Rev*. 2008;28:569–631.

[49] Becerra MC, Páez PL, Laróvere LE, Albesa I. Lipids and DNA oxidation in *Staphylococcus aureus* as a consequence of oxidative stress generated by ciprofloxacin. *Mol Cell Biochem*. 2006;285(1-2):29-34.

[50] Páez PL, Becerra MC, Albesa I. Comparison of macromolecular oxidation by reactive oxygen species in three bacterial genera exposed to different antibiotics. *Cell Biochem Biophys*. 2011;61(3):467-72.

[51] Aiassa V, Baronetti JL, Paez PL, Barnes AI, Albrecht C, Pellarin G, Eraso AJ, Albesa I. Increased advanced oxidation of protein products and enhanced total antioxidant capacity in plasma by action of toxins of *Escherichia coli* STEC. *Toxicol In Vitro*. 2011;25(1):426-31

[52] Aiassa V, Barnes AI, Albesa I. In vitro oxidant effects of D-glucosamine reduce adhesión and biofilm formation of Staphylococcus epidermidis. *Rev Argent Microbiol*. 2012;44(1):16-20.

[53] Costerton JW, Geesey GG, Cheng GK. How bacteria stick. *Sci. Am*. 1978; 238:86–95.

[54] Donald RM. Biofilms: Microbial life on surfaces. *Emerg Infect Dis*. 2002; 8(9): 881-890.

[55] Costerton W, Veeh R, Shirtliff M, Passmore M, Post C, Ehrlich G. The application of biofilm science to the study and control of chronic bacterial infections. *J Clin Invest.* 2003;112:1466-77.
[56] Paraje MG. Antimicrobial resistance in biofilms. In: Antonio Méndez-Vilas Ed, *Science against microbial pathogens: communicating current research and technological advances* (volume 2). Microbiology Book Series, number # 3 Formatex Research Center. 2011. pag: 736-744.
[57] Pamp SJ, Gjermansen M, Tolker-Nielsen T. The biofilm matrix—A sticky framework. In: Kjelleberg S, Givskov M, eds. *The Biofilm Mode of Life.* Norfolk: Horizon Bioscience. 2007:37–69.
[58] Pamp SJ, Sternberg C, Tolker-Nielsen T. Insight into the microbial multicellular lifestyle via flow-cell technology and confocal microscopy. *Cytometry* Part A. 2009: 75A: 90–103. doi: 10.1002/cyto.a.20685
[59] Wilson M. *Microbial Inhabitants of Humans: Their Ecology and Role in Health and Disease.* Cambridge: Cambridge University Press; 2005.
[60] Aiassa V, Barnes AI, Albesa I. Resistance to ciprofloxacin by enhancement of antioxidant defenses in biofilm and planktonic *Proteus mirabilis.* Biochem Biophys Res Commun. 2010; 26:393(1):84-8
[61] Battán PC, Barnes AI, Albesa I. Resistance to oxidative stress caused by ceftazidime and piperacillin in a biofilm of *Pseudomonas.* Luminescence. 2004;19(5):265-70.
[62] Boehm A, Steiner S, Zaehringer F, Casanova A, Hamburger F, Ritz D, Keck W, Ackermann M, Schirmer T, Jenal U. Second messenger signalling governs *Escherichia coli* biofilm induction upon ribosomal stress. *Mol. Microbiol.* 2009;2: 1500-1516.
[63] Boehm A, Steiner S, Zaehringer F, Casanova A, Hamburger F, Ritz D, Keck W, Ackermann M, Schirmer T, Jenal U. Second messenger signalling governs *Escherichia coli* biofilm induction upon ribosomal stress. *Mol. Microbiol.* 2009;2: 1500-1516.
[64] Kohanski MA, Dwyer DJ, Hayete B, Lawrence CA, Collins JJ. A common mechanism of cellular death induced by bactericidal antibiotics. *Cell.* 2007;130:797-810.
[65] Dwyer DJ, Kohanski MA, Collins JJ. Role of reactive oxygen species in antibiotic action and resistance. *Curr Opin Microbiol.* 2009;12:482-9.
[66] Páez PL, Becerra MC, Albesa I. Antioxidative mechanisms protect resistant strains of *Staphylococcus aureus* against ciprofloxacin oxidative damage. *Fundam Clin Pharmacol.* 2010;24:771-6.
[67] Kiley PJ, BeinertH. The role of Fe-S proteins in sensing and regulation in bacteria. *Current Opinion in Microbiology* 2003;6:181-185.

[68] Kim YH, Lee Y, Kim S, Yeom J, Seok Kim B, Oh S, Park S, Jeon CO, Park W. The role of periplasmic antioxidant enzymes of the Shiga toxin-producing *E. coli* O157:H7 in the formation of biofilms. *Proteomics.* 2006;23:6181-93.

[69] Nakano MM. Induction of ResDE-dependent gene expression in *Bacillus subtilis* in response to nitric oxide and nitrosative stress. *Journal of Bacteriology*. 2002;184: 1783-1787.

[70] Falsetta ML, Steichen CT, McEwan AG, Cho C, Ketterer M, Shao J, Hunt J, Jennings MP, Apicella MA The composition and metabolic phenotype of *Neisseria gonorrhoeae* biofilms. *Front. Microbio.* 2011; 2:75. doi: 10.3389/fmicb.2011.00075.

[71] Barraud N, Hassett DJ, Hwang SH, Rice SA, Kjelleberg S, Webb JS. nvolvement of nitric oxide in biofilm dispersal of *Pseudomonas aeruginosa*. *J Bacteriol*. 2006;188:7344-53.

[72] Schlag S, Nerz C, Birkenstock TA, Altenberend F, Götz F. Inhibition of staphylococcal biofilm formation by nitrite. *J Bacteriol.* 2007;189: 7911-9.

[73] Richardson AR, Dunman P M, Fang FC. The nitrosative stress response of *Staphylococcus aureus* is required for resistance to innate immunity. *Mol Microbiol*. 2006; 61:927–939.

[74] Angel Villegas N, Arce Miranda J, Becerra MC, Baronetti J, Ravetti S, Sotomayor C, Albesa I, Paraje MG. How different culture conditions affect cellular stresses in the biofilms. In: A. Mendez-Vilas, ed. *Microbes in Applied Research: Current Advances and Challenges.* World Scientific Publishing Co. Pte. Ltd. - ISBN: 978-981-4405-03-4. 2012. Pag: 629-635

[75] Paraje MG. Confocal scanning laser microscopy for the study of biofilms in tissues of the upper airway in otolaryngologic diseases. In Antonio Méndez-Vilas and Jesús Díaz Álvarez, ed, *Microscopy: Science, Technology, Applications and Education*. Formatex Research Center. Volume 1 ISBN (13): 978-84-614-6189-9. Badajoz, Spain. 2010. pag: 590-596.

[76] Aiassa V, Barnes AI, Albesa I. Macromolecular oxidation in planktonic population and biofilms of *Proteus mirabilis* exposed to ciprofloxacin. *Cell Biochem Biophys*. 2013; 15.

[77] Pellarín MG, Albrecht C, Rojas MJ, Aguilar JJ, Konigheim BS, Paraje MG, Albesa I, Eraso AJ. Inhibition of Cytotoxicity of Shiga toxin of *Escherichia coli* O157:H7 on Vero cells by *Prosopis alba Griseb* (Fabaceae) and *Ziziphus mistol Griseb* (Rhamnaceae) extracts. *Journal*

of Food Protection. 2013;76 (10): 1733–1739. doi: 10.4315/0362-028X.JFP-13-087.

[78] Dethlefsen L, McFall-Ngai M, Relman DA. An ecological and evolutionary perspective on human-microbe mutualism and disease. *Nature.* 2007; 449(7164):811–818.

[79] Páez PL, Becerra MC, Albesa I. Impact of ciprofloxacin and chloramphenicol on the lipid bilayer of *Staphylococcus aureus*: changes in membrane potential. *Biomed Res Int.* 2013:276524.

[80] Romero Diaz R, Picciafuoco S, Paraje MG, Villegas NA, Arce J, Albesa I, Cremonezzi D, Commisso R, Paglini-Oliva P. Relevance of biofilms in pediatric tonsillar disease. *European Journal of Clinical Microbiology & Infectious Diseases.* 2011,30(12): 1503-1509.

[81] Zernotti ME, Angel Villegas N, Roques Revol M, Baena-Cagnani CE, Arce Miranda JE, Paredes ME, Albesa I, Paraje MG. Evidence of bacterial biofilm i,n nasal polyposis. *J Investig Allergol Clin Immunol.* 2010;20(5): 380-5.

[82] Otto M. Staphylococcal biofilms. *Curr Top Microbiol Immunol.* 2008; 322:207-228.

[83] Patel R. Biofilms and antimicrobial resistance. *Clin Orthop Relat Res.* 2005;41–47.

[84] Vuong C, Kocianova S, Voyich JM, Yao Y, Fischer ER, DeLeo FR, Otto M. A crucial role for exopolysaccharide modification in bacterial biofilm formation, immune evasion, and virulence. *J Biol Chem.* 2004; 279(52):54881-6.

[85] Mah T-FC, O'Toole GA. Mechanisms of biofilm resistance to antimicrobial agents. *Trends Microbiol.* 2001;9:34–39.

[86] Anderson GG, O'Toole GA. Innate and Induced Resistance Mechanisms of Bacterial Biofilms. In: Romeo T eds. *Bacterial Biofilms.* Current Topics in Microbiology and Immunology 322, Springer-Verlag: Berlin Heidelberg, 2008;85-105.

[87] Boles BR, Singh PK. Endogenous oxidative stress produces diversity and adaptability in biofilm communities. *Proc Natl Acad Sci U S A.* 2008;105:12503–12508.

[88] Dwyer DJ, Kohanski MA, Hayete B, Collins JJ. Gyrase inhibitors induce an oxidative damage cellular death pathway in *Escherichia coli. Mol Syst Biol.* 2007;3:91.

In: Oxidative Stress
Editor: Cassidy Croft
ISBN: 978-1-63117-578-7

Chapter 3

Oxidative Stress and Age Related Macular Degeneration

N. Manresa, Ph.D.[2,*], *J. Mulero, Ph.D.*[1], *M. Losada and P. Zafrilla, Ph.D.*[1]
[1]Department of Food Technology and Nutrition, Catholic University of San Antonio. Murcia, Spain
[2]University Hospital Jose Mª Morales Meseguer, Murcia, Span

Abstract

The oxidative stress may cause injury to the retinal pigment epithelium, the Bruch's membrane and the choroid, which are layers in the eye involved in the pathophysiology of age related degeneration macular (AMD). These oxidative processes are thought to contribute to the clinical manifestation of pigment dispersion, accumulation of intracellular lysosomal lipofuscin and extracellular drusen deposits.

The purpose of this chapter is to analyze the possible routes of oxidative stress in the AMD and the biomarkers of oxidative eye damage. The mitochondria may be especially important in this process because the reactive oxygen species (ROS) produced in their electron transport chain can damage cellular components. In several studies, the increase in

* Author to whom correspondence should be addressed: Department of Food Technology and Nutrition, Catholic University of San Antonio, Murcia 30107. Spain. Email: noemi-mr@hotmail.com; Phone: +34968278705. Fax: +34968278622.

mitochondrial DNA (mtDNA) damage and mutations (for example, production of oxidized derivatives of the DNA bases, 8-oxoguanine), and the decrease in the efficacy of DNA repair have been correlated with the occurrence and the stage of AMD. Also, lymphocytes from AMD patients displayed a higher amount of total endogenous basal and oxidative DNA damage, exhibited a higher sensitivity to hydrogen peroxide and UV radiation, and repaired the lesions. Furthermore, there is increasing evidence that constant oxidative stress impairs autophagy and heterophagy, as well as increases protein aggregation and causes inflammaome activation leading to the pathological phenotype of AMD. Other mechanism is the iron accumulation in AMD, that it is a toxic in the visual phototransduction cascade and catalyzes the conversion of hydrogen peroxide to hydroxyl radical, which is the most damaging of the ROS. This has therapeutic potential for diminishing iron-induced oxidative damage to prevent or treat AMD.

Finally, dietary factors play an important role in the control of oxidative stress. In a large clinical trial, dietary supplements of antioxidants including carotenoids, vitamin C, vitamin E and zinc, experienced reduced progression to advanced AMD. The effect of lutein was a significant reduction in malonyldialdehide (MDA) level and increase in the gene expression of antioxidant enzyme activities (SODs and catalase). In the chapter analyzed all antioxidant therapies and future lines of investigation in oxidative stress.

Abbreviations

AMD	Age-related macular degeneration
RPE	Retinal pigment epithelial
CNV	Choroidal new vessels
ROS	Reactive oxygen species
ER	Endoplasmic reticulum
ARPE-19	A human retinal pigment epithelial cell line
8-oxoG	8-Oxo-7,8-dihydroguanine
STAT3	Signal transducer and activator of transcription-3
VEGF	Vascular endothelial growth factor
Nrf2	Nuclear factor erythroid 2 related factor 2
SODs	Superoxide dismutase
GPx-s	Glutathione peroxidase
PON1	Paraoxonase
HDL	High-density lipoprotein
Hcy	Homocysteine

MDA	Malondialdehyde
MsrA	Methionine sulfoxide reductase A
JNKs	Jun kinases
AST	Astaxanthin
ERK	Extracellular signal regulated kinase
GSH	Glutathione
GSSG	Glutathione disulfide
Cys	Cysteine
CySS	Cystine
ox-LDL	Oxidized LDL
CEP	Carboxyethylpyrrole
L	Lutein
Z	Zeaxanthin
LCPUFAs	Long-Chain Polyunsaturated Fatty Acids
DHA	Docosahexaenoic acid
EPA	Eicosapentaenoic acid

Introduction

The age-related macular degeneration (AMD) is the leading cause of blindness in elderly populations. To data, the exact mechanism of macular degeneration has remained elusive. Epidemiological studies over the last two decades have provided the risk factors associated with AMD, including: age, sex, diet, nutrition status, smoking, and genetic markers [1].

Phenotypically, AMD can be divided into two main forms: dry (atrophic) and wet (exudative) type and further subdivided into early and late stage disease.

The early stage of dry AMD is asymptomatic, although pigment mottling, accumulation of intracellular lysosomal lipofuscin, and extracellular drusen deposits can be detected [2]. The late stage of dry AMD, also known as geographic atrophy, is characterized by discrete areas of retinal pigment epithelial (RPE) loss and impairment of the overlying retinal photoreceptor cells. In wet AMD, aberrant blood vessels sprout from the choroidal capillaries (choroidal new vessels, CNV) and penetrate through the Bruch's membrane leading to subretinal membranes, hemorrhage, retinal edema and damage to retinal cells. If left untreated, late stage fibrosis and permanent visual loss may occur.

The prevalence of early AMD is the 18% in the population aged 65 to 74 years and 30% in the population older than 74 years [3]. Findings from 2 population-based studies indicate that the prevalence of geographic atrophy is approximately half the prevalence of CNV studies [4] in persons older than 75 years. Since the population older than 65 years is the fastest growing segment of our society, the burden of disease will increase during the 21st century [5].

The population needs new therapies to prevent and treat exudative and atrophic maculopathy. The use of antioxidant vitamins has been shown to delay disease progression at an intermediate stage, and rapid innovation in the use of antiangiogenic therapies has resulted in new clinical methods to treat the exudative phase of AMD. However, developing new treatment and prevention strategies targeting earlier stages of the disease requires a better understanding of the underlying disease mechanisms.

Oxidative Stress in AMD

The pathogenic mechanism of AMD is poorly understood; recent numerous studies have implicated high levels of oxidative stress in macular photoreceptor cells (rods and cones) and the adjacent RPE cells as causative factors in the development of AMD. The oxidative stress occurs when the level of pro-oxidants exceeds the level of antioxidants in a cell and results in the oxidation of cellular components and consequent loss of cellular function. That depends on genetic predisposition, cumulative light damage, free radical injury, and hemodynamic abnormalities.

The production of reactive oxygen species (ROS) is stimulated by irradiation, aging, inflammation, increased partial pressure of oxygen, air pollutants, cigarette smoke, and reperfusion injury. The oxygen-derived metabolites cause oxidative damage to cytoplasmic and nuclear elements of cells and cause changes in the abnormal extracellular matrix [6].

Routes and Mechanisms of Oxidative Stress

This section of the chapter, we will collect the different routes studied oxidative stress in AMD, and also add recent studies provide important data in this clinical area.

Autophagy and Heterophagy

The RPE constitutes the outermost layer of the retina, and has many important functions in the homeostasis of the eye to maintain normal vision. The RPE is under constant pressure from high metabolic demands in an environment with high levels of oxidative stressors. The photoreceptor outer segments are enriched in polyunsaturated fatty acids, which can undergo lipid peroxidation. Lipid peroxidation is greatest in the macula and increases with factor such as the age or ultraviolet light [7]. It is important to recognize aging changes in the RPE-Bruch membrane-choriocapillaris complex that occur in aged eyes. In vitro evidence [6] indicates that RPE lipofuscin is a photoinducible generator of ROS that can compromise lysosomal integrity, induce lipid peroxidation, reduce phagocytic capacity and cause RPE cell death. Lipofuscin granules are continuously exposed to visible light and high oxygen tension, which cause ROS production and possibly further oxidative damage to the RPE cell proteins and lipid membranes. These oxidative processes are thought to contribute to the clinical manifestation of pigment dispersion, accumulation of intracellular lysosomal lipofuscin and extracellular drusen deposits [8].

The oxidative stress, protein aggregation and immunological events are involved in the pathogenesis of AMD. The autophagy is a cellular housekeeping process that removes damaged organelles and protein aggregates, whereas heterophagy is the phagocytosis of exogenous photoreceptor outer segments. The heterophagy of the photoreceptor outer segments photoreceptor outer segments occurs at the apical side of the RPE cells. When there is damage in the autophagy and/or heterophagy produce the accumulation of auto-oxidative lipofuscin in the lysosomes of RPE cells, as well as drusen formation in the extracellular space between the RPE and the Bruch's membrane, this situation is increased with the aging. Furthermore, the oxidized low-density lipoproteins and lipid peroxidation reduce the degradation of phagocytosed photoreceptor outer segments material, and increase cellular stress in the RPE cell [9].

For example, the reaction product of ethanolamine and 2 retinaldehyde molecules, N-retinylidene-N-retinylethanolamine (A2-E), is the major photosensitizing chromophore in lipofuscin that causes ROS. The A2-E also raises lysosomal pH, thus interfering with lysosomal enzyme activity and reducing lysosomal protein and glycosaminoglycan degradation. When RPE cells are exposed to light, A2-E conjugated to low-density lipoprotein, and causes loss of lysosomal integrity and also inhibits RPE phagolysosomal degradation of photoreceptor phospholipidin vitro [10].

In inmunological events, the oxidized phospholipids in the retinal photoreceptors stimulate to express chemoattractant molecules that recruit monocytes into the subretinal space and differentiate into tissue resident macrophages. The accumulation of oxidatively damaged molecules also leads to retinal apoptosis and inflammation. Apoptotic cells, if not rapidly cleared, undergo secondary necrosis and can also stimulate the innate immune system. Evidence of inflammatory cell involvement in the later stages of AMD includes the presence of multinucleated giant cells and leukocytes in the choroid of AMD. Therefore, there is a strong relation between oxidative stress and inflammatory response in the pathology of the AMD.

The oxidative stress can induce electron leakage from the mitochondrial electron transport chain, followed by formation of hydroxyl radicals, superoxide, hydrogen peroxide and hypochlorite as a consequence of many enzymatic reactions. An imbalance between the generation and the suppression of ROS can lead to undesirable effects, for example, due to protein unfolding and damage, especially in age-related conditions.

It has been speculated that lipofuscin itself could be cytotoxic because of its ability to provide a redox-active surface by incorporating oxidatively labile iron [13]. This could result in the formation of oxygen radicals and cause oxidative modification of proteins, lipids and nucleic acids. For example, many proteins isolated from RPE cell derived lipofuscin have been modified and decorated by the markers of oxidative stress, such as malondialdehyde (MDA), hydroxynonenal and products of glycosylation and product-specific receptor. One of the most toxic products of lipid peroxidation is 4-hydroxy-2-nonenal and it can modify and inactivate proteins. Nineteen proteins that were consistently modified regardless of stage of AMD or retinal region were identified. These proteins are involved in two main functions: energy production and stress response. Modest increases in content of proteins involved in 4-hydroxy-2-nonenal detoxification were observed in patients with AMD [14]. As a result, the high metabolic activity impaired mitochondrial function is assumed to lead to the accelerated degeneration of RPE cells and secondarily to photoreceptor cell death [15].

In the RPE is the αB/A1-crystallin as a novel lysosomal component that could regulate both phagocytosis and autophagy to reduce the oxidative stress [16]. The αB crystallin has been shown to have antiapoptotic properties in RPE cells. In AMD, αB crystallin is expressed in RPE in association with subretinal drusen deposits and it is more prominently expressed in the late stage of the disease. Deficiency of αB crystallin sensitizes RPE cells and other cells to external stress and the αB crystallin overexpression protects RPE from stress induced apoptosis [17].

In conclusion, a failure of the RPE cells to use autophagy can result in accumulation of aggregation-prone proteins, cellular degeneration and finally cell death. There is increasing evidence that constant oxidative stress impairs autophagy and heterophagy, as well as increases protein aggregation and causes inflammasome activation leading to the pathological phenotype of AMD [9].

Apoptosis

The specific mechanisms involved in endoplasmic reticulum (ER) stress-induced apoptosis remain to be fully elucidated. The available evidence suggests that transcriptional induction of CHOP is critical in ER stress induced apoptosis. Overexpression of CHOP can lead to cell cycle arrest and apoptosis, and activation of caspase cascades also occurs in ER stress.

A study to investigate the relation the apoptosis and cigarette smoke. The present study aimed to investigate the role of stress and the unfolded protein response in cigarette smoke related RPE apoptosis. The inhabitation of CHOP activation by pharmacological chaperones or genetic approaches attenuated hydroquinone-induced RPE cell apoptosis. In contrast to enhanced CHOP activation, protein level of active XBP1, a major regulator of the adaptive unfolded protein response, was reduced in hydroquinone-treated cells. Conversely, overexpressing XBP1 protected RPE cells and attenuated oxidative stress-induced RPE apoptosis [18].

Mitochondria are recognized as the central regulator of apoptotic cell death and ER-mitochondrial crosstalk may mediate stress signals between these compartments. Indeed, mitochondrial changes including loss of mitochondrial membrane potential, release of cytochrome c, and activation of caspase 9 and caspase 3 have been observed in ER stress. It has also been reported that CHOP, the ER stress induced transcription factor, not only down regulates Bcl-2 expression but also leads to translocation of Bax from cytosol to mitochondria. The activation and mitochondrial localization of Bax and Apaf 1 (Apoptotic Protease-Activating Factor 1), which is required in post-mitochondrial apoptotic cascades, have been identified to contribute to mitochondrial impairment in ER stress induced apoptosis [19, 20].

Expression of αB crystallin has also been linked to AMD, where its increased expression has been suggested to be a biomarker for the disease. After, we explained that the αB 3/A1-crystallin regulated phagocytosis and autophagy, and in this part, it controls the apoptosis. In the actually study evaluated the role of αB crystallin in ER stress-mediated apoptosis in RPE, and demonstrate that αB crystallin provides critical protection of mitochondrial function in this process [18].

Iron

The iron may be a major source of oxidative stress in AMD. Iron accumulates with age increase and iron is a potent generator of radicals and results in photoreceptor/RPE toxicity when locally elevated in conditions such as ocular siderosis.

Some functions are: ferrous iron can catalyze the conversion of hydrogen peroxide to hydroxyl radical, which is the most damaging of the ROS. Also, photoreceptor cells continuously shed and synthesize their disc membranes, depending on iron-containing enzymes like fatty acid desaturase for biogenesis of lipids…While the mechanism of iron accumulation in AMD is unknown, plausible culprits include inflammation, hypoxia, and oxidative stress, all of which contribute to AMD pathogenesis.

Studies detected increased iron in AMD affected maculas, specifically in the RPE and Bruch's membrane of early AMD, geographic atrophy and exudative AMD patients. In the *study Post-mortem,* AMD eyes have increased levels of iron in retina compared to age-matched healthy donors. The iron chelation protects photoreceptors and RPE in a variety of mouse models. This has therapeutic potential for diminishing iron-induced oxidative damage to prevent or treat AMD [21].

The inflammation can cause cellular iron sequestration through IL- 6 mediated upregulation of hepcidin (anti-microbial activity, and its expression is upregulated by infection, inflammation and iron). Bmpc6 is crucial for regulation of iron homeostasis through hepcidin, and in oxidative stress observed low levels of dBmp6. Study *post-mortem,* RPE from patients with early AMD exhibited decreased Bmp6 levels and contributes to iron build-up in AMD. This may in turn propagate a vicious cycle of oxidative stress and iron accumulation, exacerbating AMD [22].

DNA

The AMD is complex and polygenic, resulting from cooperation of a variety of genes in the initiation and progression of the disease. Therefore, large-scale molecular biological experiments are needed in order to better understand the pathogenesis and progression of AMD and to identify new targets for AMD-directed therapeutics and diagnostics. The study of AMD is complicated by the limitations of animal models. The gradual decline in cellular functions associated with aging is not caused by changes in the expression of a few individual genes, but rather by cumulative alterations in the activity of numerous genes in many tissues. We showed that senescence accelerated OXYS rats are a suitable model for the study of pathogenesis and for investigation of possible therapeutic targets in AMD. Over 600 genes showed significant differences in expression between the two strains. These genes are involved in disease-associated pathways such as immune response, inflammation, apoptosis, Ca2+ homeostasis and oxidative stress [23].

The ROS and nitrogen species produced during stress may damage crucial biomolecules of the RPE cells. These effects have been confirmed in rodent research with the downregulation of DNA repair enzymes involved in repair of oxidative damage occurred in aged RPE and choroid. Therefore, mtDNA damage and repair may contribute to the dysfunction of retina, which in turn, may play a role in AMD. The results of another experiment showing that the mtDNA repair of oxidative damage in RPE cells is slow and inefficient compared to that of nDNA, suggest the general relationship between mutagenesis of mtDNA and nDNA rather than indicate that mtDNA is a preferential target in AMD pathogenesis [24].

The ARPE-19 (a human retinal pigment epithelial cell line) is a commonly accepted model for research in the molecular mechanisms of AMD pathology. When these cells are exposed to the breakdown products of lutein and β-carotene they displayed nDNA damage contributing to an additional systematic oxidative stress [25]. Also, the oxidative stress may be associated with many kinds of DNA damage, including single- and double-strand breaks and oxidative modifications of the DNA bases. For example, 8-Oxo-7,8-dihydroguanine (8-oxoG) is one hallmark of oxidative DNA damage and a major promutagenic component in oxidative stress [26]. The authors observed that the 8-oxoG level in aqueous humor was higher in patients with exudative AMD, and the level was correlated with the area of macular lesion [27]. This led to the conclusion that DNA damage may be one of the mechanisms underlying the action of oxidative stress in AMD.

Today, science is deepening the role of certain genes to know their role well. In addition to wound-response genes, the list of genes with aggravated stage of retinopathy is enriched by oxidation reduction players that consist mostly of oxidative stress-related genes (e.g., Nqo1, Xdh, Cdo1 and Cbr1). Among them, we found decreased expression of antioxidant enzymes catalyzing the reaction with reduced glutathione and oxidoreductases of the thioredoxin family of proteins that regulate the thiol redox state and protect cells and tissues from oxidative stress. The decreased levels of thioredoxins can be linked to the increased oxidative damage of proteins and lipids previously identified in this strain. Increased oxidative stress and the accumulation of oxidatively damaged molecules lead to the dysfunction of various metabolic and signaling pathways, which, in turn, causes retinal cell death or malfunction [23].

The expression of the *RAD51* gene, the product of which plays a crucial role in the repair of DNA double-strand breaks by homologous recombination, was down-regulated in response to an oxidative stimulus in AMD. Also, lymphocytes from AMD patients exhibited a higher sensitivity to hydrogen peroxide and UV radiation, and repaired the lesions induced by these agents less efficiently than the corresponding cells from the control individuals. We postulate that the impaired efficacy of DNA repair may be combined with the enhanced sensitivity of RPE cells to blue and UV light, contributing to the pathogenesis of AMD [28].

The signal transducer and activator of transcription-3 (STAT3) protein are important for the regulation of cell differentiation, proliferation, and angiogenesis. Previous studies have verified that STAT3 is a direct transcriptional activator of the vascular endothelial growth factor (VEGF) gene. Recent findings have suggested that diabetes increases the level of STAT3 activation and thereby contributes to the pathophysiology of vascular injury. In early stages of experimentally induced CNV in diabetic mice and in RPE cells when exposed to hyperglycaemic environments, we provided the first evidence that the level of p-STAT3 was dramatically up-regulated and accompanied by increased oxidative stress and upregulation of VEGF. These results suggest that hyperglycaemia promotes the development of CNV by inducing oxidative stress, which in turn activates STAT3 signalling in RPE cells. Antioxidant supplementation helped attenuate the development of CNV [29].

Also, the tumour inhibitor p53 gene has the ability of triggering proliferation arrest and cellular death by apoptosis subsequent to several factors, among them oxidative stress. The p53 protein is a major regulator of gene expression. Using genetically manipulated mice carrying an extra copy of gene p53 (transgenic mice super p53) versus control mice, we have investigated the generation of ROS and antioxidant activity in the optic nerve of mice in relation to p53 availability. A significant increase in free radical formation, antioxidant activity and nitric oxide synthesis was found in the optic nerves from transgenic super p53 mice compared to respective controls. The presence of an extra copy of the p53 gene correlated with redox status in the mouse optic nerve. This transgenic mouse could be useful as an experimental model to study cell resistance to neurodegenerative processes in relation to oxidative stress and to apoptosis induction, such as AMD [30].

Several lines of evidence have implicated oxidative stress-induced damage to the RPE in the pathogenesis of AMD, suggesting that the aging RPE may exhibit increased susceptibility to cell damage induced by exogenous stressors. The transcription factor, nuclear factor erythroid 2 related factor 2 (Nrf2), serves as the master regulator of a highly coordinated antioxidant response in virtually all cell types. These data indicate that the aging RPE is vulnerable to oxidative damage due to impaired Nrf2 signaling, and that Nrf2 signaling is a promising target for novel pharmacologic or genetic therapeutic strategies [31].

Finally, we want to note that the pathophysiology of oxidative stress in AMD is closely related to the genetic. The activity and the importance of genes in AMD is still a very new science and currently researching this lot. In conclusion, we had studied a small part of the importance of frequency of polymorphisms DNA repair enzyme genes to fight the oxidative stress AMD [32].

Antioxidants: Enzymes and Supplements

Antioxidants fight against any damage caused by oxidative stress and provide a healthy environment for the development of the macula. There are *antioxidant enzymes and antioxidant supplements* to combat AMD, and then explain the functions of these antioxidants. In the final of the chapter, we explain the kind of diet with antioxidants that prevents the AMD. Now, we study the role of the antioxidants and other important studies.

To combat the deleterious effects of ROS, cells have evolved an intrinsic antioxidant defense network that consists of a variety of scavengers, such as superoxide dismutase (SODs), glutathione peroxidase (GPx-s), catalase and glutathione S-transferase. Protection against superoxide radicals is provided by

SODs, which catalyze the dismutation of superoxide to H2O2. Catalase catalyzes the conversion of H2O2 to water (preventing the generation of hydroxyl radicals) and oxygen, and GPx-s catalyze the reduction of H2O2 and reduce lipid hydroperoxides to their corresponding alcohols and free H2O2 to water. The level of the enzymes is decrease in AMD, for example: catalase and glutathione reductase, SODs, metallothionein (an acutephase reactant protein that scavenges hydroxyl radicals), heme oxygenase-1 and heme oxygenase-2), etc. The genetic defects (e.g., in antioxidant enzymes), dietary or uptake deficiencies in antioxidants, or exposure to noxious agents (e.g., cigarette smoking) could enhance oxidative RPE damage during life and predispose to AMD [6].

The computational analysis predicted a number of miRNAs including miR-30b that could putatively target catalase mRNA. Exposure to several stress-inducing agents including H2O2 has been reported to alter miRNA expression profile. The study demonstrated that a sublethal dose of H2O2 up-regulated the expression of miR-30b, a member of the miR-30 family, which inhibited the expression of endogenous catalase both at the transcript and protein levels. However, antisense (antagomirs) of miR-30b was not only found to suppress the miR-30b mimics-mediated inhibitions, but also to dramatically increase the expression of catalase even under an oxidant environment [33].

Other enzyme is the paraoxonase (PON1), a calcium-dependent esterase, is closely associated with the high-density lipoprotein (HDL) subfraction containing apolipoprotein A-I in human serum. A cysteine thiol group contained by the active site of PON1 is essential for PON1-mediated protection of LDL against atherogenic oxidative damage. The homocysteine (Hcy) can be converted into homocysteine thiolactone in all cell types; this leads to potentially harmful protein damage by homocysteineylation that may be involved in the pathology of vascular diseases. PON1 shows homocysteine thiolactonase activity, which might contribute to the detoxification of this metabolite of Hcy. In mice, it has been found that PON1 mRNA is downregulated and there is lower PON1 activity with moderate to severe hyperhomocysteinemia, which is caused by a hyperhomocysteinemic diet or by a genetic deficiency in cystathionine beta-synthase [34]. The patients with exudative-type AMD had significantly higher Hcy concentrations compared to controls. The higher Hcy levels were correlated with higher serum malondialdehyde. and lower PON 1 activity; according to results, it can be stated that Hcy may negatively regulate PON 1 gene expression in active

AMD, which could contribute to lower serum PON1 activity due to enhanced oxidative stress [35].

The antioxidant enzyme methionine sulfoxide reductase A (MsrA) is highly expressed in the RPE. Study tested the effects of acute silencing or overexpression of MsrA on the phagocytosis of photoreceptor outer segment fragments, a demanding, daily function of the RPE that is essential for vision. RPE cells manipulated to express higher or lower levels of MsrA than control cells showed no signs of cell death but increased or decreased, respectively, POS binding as well as engulfment. Furthermore, ATP content directly correlated with MsrA protein levels in RPE cells that used mitochondrial oxidative phosphorylation for ATP synthesis but not in RPE cells that relied on glycolysis alone. The contribution of MsrA to energy metabolism is independent of its function in protection from elevated oxidative stress but contributes to routine but vital photoreceptor support by RPE cells [36].

Enzymes are a strong therapeutic target to treat AMD and many laboratories are currently investigating drugs in this field. An example is the Jun kinases (JNKs) (mitogen-activated protein kinase family). The JNKs regulate key cellular processes such as cell proliferation, migration, survival, and cytokine production. They are activated in response to growth factors, proinflammatory cytokines, microbial components, and a variety of stresses, including oxidative stress. The JNK1 deficiency or total JNK inhibition decreases VEGF expression and reduces CNV in a wet AMD [37].

We have named the most important enzymes in yet further research. Note that many enzymes are used as biomarkers of AMD to assess the degree of AMD disease. This issue will be explained later biomarkers. Now, we study some antioxidants that are good results in clinical departaments.

The astaxanthin (AST) has been reported to possess a wide variety of biologic functions, including anti-inflammatory, antiapoptotic and anticarcinogenic activity, as well as neuroprotective and cardioprotective effects. In addition to these activities, AST has been shown to have a high level of antioxidant activity 10 times higher than that of other carotenoids, such as lutein, canthaxanthin, and β-carotene and 100 times higher than α-tocopherol. The protective effect of AST on ARPE-19 cells against oxidative stress and the possible underlying mechanism. The treatment with AST reduces H2O2-induced cell death and apoptosis in ARPE-19 cells, and that the mechanism by which AST induced cytoprotection could include the Nrf2-antioxidant-response element. These data indicate that AST might provide a valuable therapeutic strategy for early AMD [38].

The canolol is a phenolic compound recently isolated from crude canola oil, which exhibits potent antioxidant activity. In the study, the investigators found that there was an increase in the expression of catalase and glutathione S-transferase-pi upon canolol treatment, which was positively correlated with the protective effects of canolol. In addition, Nrf-2 is a key molecule for the basal and inducible expression of genes regulating the redox state of a cell. By binding to the antioxidant response element, Nrf-2 induces the expression of antioxidant genes. The extracellular signal regulated kinase (ERK) cascade is one of the major mitogen-activated protein kinase pathways and its activation is generally thought to mediate cell survival. ERK was shown to protect against oxidative stress-induced cell injury and death. It has been shown that overexpression of $ERK_{1/2}$ confers resistance against RPE cell death due to serum-depletion–mediated oxidative stress, which suggested that ERK activation may be a general signaling defense against oxidative stress damage [39].

The prevention of telomere shortening by antioxidants may be a useful approach for reducing the cumulative effects of oxidative stress in RPE cells. Melatonin has antioxidant mechanisms because melatonin has receptors localized in the RPE, which act locally as a neurohormone and/or neuromodulator. The melatonin exerts additional benefit through down-regulating hTERT (catalytic subunit if telomerase) expression and stimulated telomerase activity in RPE, which subsequently helps to prevent or treat AMD. We suggest that melatonin therapy as pharmacologic agents and/or melatonin-rich foods, especially in AMD patients with measured low serum melatonin levels or high risk patients would be possibly an alternative approach to prevent and/or treat AMD. The melatonin has potential to prevent telomere shortening in RPE, while not precluding other mechanisms, namely antioxidative properties and/or restoration of inner blood-retina barrier integrity, reduced VEGF, hypoxia and nitric oxide levels [40, 41].

Biomarkers of Oxidative Stress

The use of biomarkers of oxidative stress in AMD is important because it helps us to see the degree of evolution of the disease and whether treatment or prophylaxis is doing an antioxidant effect.

Endogenous antioxidants, including such non-enzymatic scavengers as glutathione (GSH) and such antioxidant enzymes as SODs, GPx-s and catalase, are the first lines of defense against oxidative stress and act by scavenging potentially damaging free radical moieties.

Serum MDA is the end product of the primary reactions that lead to the significant oxidation of such polyunsaturated fatty acids in cellular membranes and, thus, serves as a reliable marker of oxidative stress. The study observed increase in SODs activity in our study may be related to increased MDA levels, as a compensatory regulation in response to oxidative stress in AMD patients [42].

Quantification of oxidative stress by the measurement of cysteine thiol/disulfide couples and lipid peroxidation products in plasma may be an effective tool for identifying patients at risk of developing AMD, progressing to later stages of the disease, or both. The thiolated amino acid cysteine (Cys) and the Cys-derived antioxidant GSH are oxidized to their respective disulfides, cystine (CySS) and glutathione disulfide (GSSG). The redox potentials of Cys/CySS and GSH/GSSG couples reflect the body's overall redox status. In our previous studies, the redox potentials of Cys/CySS and reduced and oxidized Glutathione (GSH/GSSG) showed increased oxidation in association with age and smoking, both risk factors for AMD. Plasma levels of oxidative stress biomarkers were determined in 77 AMD patients and 75 controls recruited from a clinical practice. Cysteine, cystine (CySS), glutathione, isoprostane, and isofuran were measured, and participants were genotyped for polymorphisms in the complement factor H and age-related maculopathy susceptibility 2 genes. Investigation of the gene–environment interaction involved in AMD revealed a relationship between a plasma biomarker of oxidative stress, CySS, and complement factor H genotype. These data suggest a potential association between inflammatory regulators and redox status in AMD pathogenesis [43]. Other study, the following parameters were determined: GSH/GSSH, protein carbonyl groups, total antioxidant activity in plasma and the activity of endogenous antioxidant enzymes, such as, GPx-s, gluthatione reductase and SODs. Values of SODs, gluthatione reductase and GPx-s are higher in control group than in patients with wet AMD. According to the GSH/GSSH results, average values were higher in the control than in patients with wet AMD and data were not significantly different. We have demonstrated that systematic oxidative stress, measured by different biomarkers is closely associated with the wet AMD [44].

Other biomarker of oxidative stress is the hcy. In a study of 58 patients (24 men and 34 women) with a mean age of 76.3 years (the age and sex influence in the hiperhomocysteinemia). The hiperhomocysteinemia was recorded in 44.1%, 22.4 % and 21.4 % of patients with neovascular AMD, atrophic AMD and controls, respectively [45]. It suggests a significant association between elevated plasma Hcy levels and exudative neovascular AMD, but there is a strong association with atrophic AMD. The hcy high levels correlated with increased serum MDA and one lower PON1 activity. According to the results, we can say that Hcy downregulates active gene expression PON 1 in AMD, which helps reduce serum PON1 activity by increasing oxidative stress. Furthermore, related increasing oxidized LDL (ox-LDL) and the ratio ox-LDL/HDL with high levels of Hcy due to low activity of the PON1 [46].

The CRP levels were significantly higher among individuals with intermediate and advanced stages of AMD compared with controls. The risk of AMD was lowest among individuals who had low CRP values and never smoked. In contrast, risk tended to be highest among smokers who also had higher levels of CRP. Even among individuals who never smoked, the risk of AMD was increased 2-fold among those with the highest category of CRP compared with the lowest level of CRP as the referent category [47]. Elevated CRP and hcy levels are associated with AMD and implicate the role of chronic inflammation and atherosclerosis.

In order to reveal an autoantibody profile for AMD and identify biomarkers for progression of this disease, investigators have performed an antigen microarray analysis of serum samples from patients with AMD and healthy controls. Sera from the AMD groups contained high levels of IgG and IgM autoantibodies to some systemic antigens when compared to the normal group. Targeted antigens included cyclic nucleotide phosphodiesterase, phosphatidylserine and proliferating cell nuclear antigen. The IgG/IgM ratio for antibodies to phosphatidylserine was notably elevated in the AMD group compared to the normal group, and this ratio correlated best with the stage of AMD patients with an anti- phosphatidylserine ratio greater than the cut-off value had a 44-fold risk for advanced AMD with choroidal neovascularisation [48]. Others antibodies are related with the carboxyethylpyrrole (CEP) oxidative protein modifications. CEP adducts are uniquely generated from oxidation of docosahexaenoate-containing lipids that are abundant in the retina. In the study measured the CEP autoantibodies by ELISA in 916 AMD and 488 control donors. Mean CEP adduct and autoantibody levels were found to be elevated in AMD plasma by approximately 60 and approximately 30%, respectively. Genotyping was performed for AMD risk polymorphisms associated with age-related maculopathy susceptibility 2, high temperature requirement factor A1, complement factor H, and complement C3, and the risk of AMD was predicted based on genotype alone or in combination with the CEP markers. The AMD risk predicted for those exhibiting elevated CEP markers and risk genotypes was 2-3-fold greater than the risk based on genotype alone. Finally, they concluded that CEP plasma biomarkers, particularly in combination with genomic markers, offer a potential early warning system for assessing susceptibility to this blinding, multifactorial disease.

In conclusion, there are biomarkers of oxidative stress to evaluate and control the evaluation of the AMD. The choice of biomarker is based on our technological and economic possibilities; we highlight especially hcy and antioxidant enzymes such as SODs.

Antioxidant Diet and Supplements

Currently there is no significant cure for AMD. The prevention may be the first and logic approach to reduce vision loss, justifying an intensive search for some kinds of intervention able to prevent the onset of AMD or to delay its progression to more advanced and severe forms.

Since the early 90's, when "large population studies" appeared, several hypotheses have been formulated around the idea that nutritional supplements such as antioxidants, vitamins and/or minerals may be able to reduce the risk of AMD development.

Antioxidants

Vitamin and Mineral Supplements

Antioxidants are recommended for AMD due to oxidative stress on photoreceptors in the retina and the fact that cumulative damage caused by blue light enhances free radical production. It has been proposed that antioxidants may prevent cellular damage in the retina by reacting with free radicals [49]. The substances that possess antioxidant activity are vitamins C and E, beta-carotene and some minerals, such as zinc, copper, selenium and manganese. EDCCS (Eye Disease Case-Control Study) showed that high plasma levels of antioxidants (vitamins A, C, E, selenium and carotenoids) are associated with a lower risk of developing neovascular AMD [50]. In 1994, the Baltimore Longitudinal Study on Aging, reported a protective effect against AMD for high plasma concentrations of Vitamin E [51]. In 1998, the

Beaver Dam Eye Study, showed that a high intake of carotenoids and vitamin E is associated with a lower risk of developing large drusen [52]. In 2001, AREDS report no. 8, a large multicentric, randomised clinical trial, revealed that the risk of progression to advanced AMD was reduced by 28% in patients with intermediate AMD treated with high doses of antioxidant supplements (vitamins C and E, zinc and β-carotene) [53]. In 2004, AREDS report no. 13 showed that mortality was lower in patients taking zinc alone or with antioxidants when compared to those not taking this mineral [54]. The Rotterdam Study showed that an above-average intake of the 4 AREDS trial nutrients protected against AMD development or early AMD, as indicated by large drusen, and was associated with a 35% reduction in the risk of AMD [55]. Chong et al. 2007 showed that antioxidant supplements prevented early AMD [56]. The antioxidant (beta-carotene, vitamin C and E) and zinc supplements were able to delay progression to advanced AMD and prevent loss of visual acuity in individuals displaying signs of the disease [57].

Carotenoids

Macular pigments (MP) consist of two natural xanthophylls from the carotenoid family: lutein (L) and zeaxanthin (Z). Macular pigments are found in photoreceptor axons in the pigment epithelium and in the external segments [58].

Macular concentrations of L and Z decrease with age, which exacerbates the harmful effects of blue light on photoreceptors. Two mechanisms have been proposed: macular pigments may act as an optical filter, due to their ability to absorb blue light, and they are strong antioxidants, neutralising free radicals generated by light. Seddon et al. (1995) [59] concluded that the risk of developing the most severe form of macular degeneration was 43% lower in individuals who consume large amounts of fruits and vegetables rich in L and Z (6mg/day). Delcourt et al. (2006) [60] found that high plasma L and total L and Z concentrations are associated with a reduced risk of age-related maculopathy. Neelan et al. 2008 in the CARMA Study (Carotenoids in Age-related Maculopathy Study) investigated whether administration of 12 mg of L and 2 mg of Z, in combination with antioxidants (120 mg of vitamin C, 15mg of vitamin E, 20mg of zinc and 0.4 mg of copper), had a beneficial effect on visual function and/or was able to delay progression of early to late disease stages. They showed that although no beneficial effects were demonstrated in the primary outcome measure at the stated end point (12 months), secondary outcomes favoured the supplemented group [61].

Protection against AMD from greater L and fish consumption in persons with high genetic risk based on 2 major AMD genes raises the possibility of personalized preventive interventions [62]. The totality of evidence on beneficial and adverse effects from AREDS2 and other studies suggests that lutein/zeaxanthin could be more appropriate than beta carotene in the AREDS-type supplements [63] and reduce the risk for AMD, with an OR of 0.38 and 0.65, respectively [64]. Finally, low L and Z levels in the human macula may represent a pathogenic risk factor for AMD development and the investigators suggest that supplementation may contribute to maintaining eye health.

Dietary Fatty Acids: Docosahexaenoic Acid (DHA) and Eicosapentaenoic Acid (EPA)

The role of fatty acids in AMD was initially investigated because of the hypothesis that AMD and cardiovascular disease may share a similar pathogenesis and fat intake has been associated with atherosclerosis and cardiovascular disease.

Omega-3 fatty acids, also known as Long-Chain Polyunsaturated Fatty Acids (LCPUFAs), are essential to human health. Omega-3 fatty acids include alpha-linolenic acid (a short-chain omega-3 fatty acid) and long-chain omega-3 fatty acids docosahexaenoic acid (DHA) and eicosapentaenoic acid (EPA). Omega -3 are highly concentrated in the brain and appear to be particularly important for cognitive and behavioural function. In fact, infants who do not get enough omega-3 from their mothers during pregnancy are risk for developing vision problems.

Omega-3 fatty acids, especially DHA, have morphological, functional and protective roles in the retina [65]:

1. Morphological role – DHA is the main PUFA found within the outer segments of rods and has anti-apoptotic, anti-inflammatory and antiangiogenic functions.
2. Functional role – DHA provides an adequate environment for conformational changes in rhodopsin.
3. Protective role - DHA protects against aging of the retina and may reduce lipofuscin accumulation in the retinal pigment epithelium and lipid deposits in Bruch's membrane. These accumulations are frequent in AMD pathology.
4. DHA protects photoreceptors from oxidative stress induced apoptosis.

Several epidemiologic studies [66-68] demonstrated that high dietary omega-3 fatty acid intakes were associated with a 38% reduction in the risk of late AMD. Eating fish at least twice a week was associated with a reduced risk of both early AMD. The case-control study conducted by SanGiovanni et al. concluded that higher intake of omega-3 and fish is associated with decreased risk of neovascular AMD [69]. AREDS report n. 20 showed that total dietary intake of total long-chain omega-3 polyunsaturated fatty acids (LCPUFA) was inversely associated with neovascular AMD. Dietary intake of arachidonic acid was directly associated with the prevalence of neovascular AMD70. AREDS report n. 23 suggested that dietary intake, of long-chain omega-3 polyunsaturated fatty acids, is associated with a decreased risk of progression from bilateral drusen [71].

There is an important study "LUTEGA" that included the Supplementation either once (dosage D1) or twice daily (dosage D2) of 10 mg L / 1 mg Z/ O-3-LCPUFAs (thereof 100 mg DHA, 30 mg EPA) / antioxidants, or placebo. They observed that the constant supplementation of L, Z, O-3-LCPUFAs and antioxidants in AMD patients seems to be useful [72].

Two important prospective observational studies reveal that fish consumption and omega-3 fatty acid intake decrease the risk of AMD: The Blue Mountains Eye Study and the Melbourne Collaborative Cohort Study. The objective of this longitudinal study was to investigate the association between baseline dietary fatty acids and 10-year incidence of AMD in an elderly Australian cohort [73, 74].

SanGiovanni et al. (2009) [75], observed that participants reporting the highest baseline omega-3 LCPUFA intakes were approximately 30% less likely to develop advanced AMD by the end of the 12-year follow-up period than those reporting the lowest omega-3 LC-PUFA intakes.

New studies are also assessing the benefices of polyphenols in AMD, such as the resveratrol present in red wine or nuts. The resveratrol exerts protection against acrolein-induced cytotoxicity in human ARPE-19 cells via increases in the mitochondrial bioenergetics [76]. Eating 1 serving per day of any type of nut reduces the risk of progression of macular degeneration by 40%[77]. Epidemiological evidence suggests that moderate wine consumption and antioxidants rich diets may protect against AMD.

Several studies support the benefits of regular dietary fish and omega-3 PUFA intakes on the risk of AMD, especially in individuals with lower omega-6 to omega-3 ratios.

Other studies have also suggested that higher vegetable fat and trans unsaturated fatty acid intakes increase the prevalence of late AMD, while omega-3 fatty acids and olive oil were associated with a reduced prevalence of early and late AMD.

Conclusion

The retina is especially prone to oxidative stress due to high oxygen pressure and exposure to UV and blue light promoting ROS generation. An imbalance between the production and neutralization of ROS by antioxidant defence is associated with oxidative stress, which plays an important role in the pathogenesis of many age-related and degenerative diseases. It is important to control with biomarkers of oxidative stress and prevent the degeneration with antioxidants diet.

References

[1] Jager RD, Mieler WF, Miller JW. Age-related macular degeneration. *The new england Journal of medicine,* 2008; 358: 2607-17.

[2] Kinnunen K, Petrovski G, Moe MC, Berta A, Kaarniranta K. Molecular mechanisms of retinal pigment epithelium damage and development of age related macular degeneration. *Acta Ophthalmol.,* 2012; 90:299-309.

[3] Klein R, Klein BE, Linton KL. Prevalence of age-related maculopathy: the Beaver Dam Eye Study. *Ophthalmology,* 1992; 99:933-943.

[4] Vingerling JR, Dielemans I, Hofman A, et al. The prevalence of age-related maculopathy in the Rotterdam Study. *Ophthalmology,* 1995; 102:205-210.

[5] Evans J, Wormald R. Is the incidence of registrable age-related macular degeneration increasing? *Br. J. Ophthalmol.,* 1996; 80:9-14.

[6] Marco A. Zarbin. Current concepts in the pathogenesis of age-related macular degeneration. *Arch. Ophthalmol.,* 2004; 122: 598-614.

[7] De La Paz M, Anderson RE. Region and age-dependent variation in susceptibility of the human retina to lipid peroxidation. *Invest. Ophthalmol. Vis. Sci.,* 1992; 33:3497-3499.

[8] Wu YL, Li J, Yao K. Structures and biogenetic analysis of lipofuscin bis-retinoids. *J. Zhejiang. Univ. Sci. B,* 2013;14(9):763-73.

[9] Kai Kaarniranta, Debasish Sinha, Janusz Blasiak, Anu Kauppinen, Zoltán Veréb,Antero Salminen, Michael E. Boulton and Goran

Petrovski. Autophagy and heterophagy dysregulation leads to retinal pigment epithelium dysfunction and development of age-related macular degeneration. *Autophagy,* 2013; 9:7, 973–984.

[10] Finnemann SC, Leung LW, Rodriguiez-Boulan E. The lipofuscin component A2E selectively inhibits phagolysosomal degradation of photoreceptor phospholipid by the retinal pigment epithelium. *Proc. Natl. Acad. Sci. USA,* 2002; 99:3842-3847.

[11] Xu H, Chen M, Forrester JV. Para-inflammation in the aging retina. *Prog. Retin. Eye Res.,* 2009; 28(5):348–368.

[12] Ding X, Patel M, Chan CC. Molecular pathology of age-related macular degeneration. *Prog. Retin. Eye Res.,* 2009; 28(1):1–18.

[13] Höhn A, Jung T, Grimm S, Grune T. Lipofuscin-bound iron is a major intracellular source of oxidants: role in senescent cells. *Free Radic. Biol. Med.,* 2010; 48:1100-8.

[14] Ethen CM, Reilly C, Feng X, Olsen TW, Ferrington DA. Age-related macular degeneration and retinal protein modification by 4-hydroxy-2-nonenal. *Invest. Ophthalmol. Vis. Sci.,* 2007; 48(8):3469-79.

[15] Jarrett SG, Boulton ME. Consequences of oxidative stress in age-related macular degeneration. *Mol. Aspects Med.,* 2012; 33(4):399-417.

[16] Zigler JS Jr., Zhang C, Grebe R, Sehrawat G, Hackler L Jr., Adhya S, et al. Mutation in the βA3/A1-crystallin gene impairs phagosome degradation in the retinal pigmented epithelium of the rat. *J. Cell Sci.,* 2011; 124:523-31.

[17] Sreekumar PG, Spee C, Ryan SJ, Cole SP, Kannan R, Hinton DR. Mechanism of RPE Cell Death in Crystallin Deficient Mice: A Novel and Critical Role for MRP1-Mediated GSH Efflux. *PLoS One,* 2012; 3:e33420.

[18] Chen C, Cano M, Wang JJ, Li J, Huang C, Yu Q, Herbert TP, Handa J, Zhang SX. Role of UPR dysregulation in oxidative injury of retinal pigment epithelial cells. Antioxid Redox Signal. 2013.

[19] Obeng EA, Boise LH. Caspase-12 and caspase-4 are not required for caspase-dependent endoplasmic reticulum stress-induced apoptosis. *J. Biol. Chem.,* 2005; 280:29578–29587.

[20] Smith MI, Deshmukh M. Endoplasmic reticulum stress-induced apoptosis requires bax for commitment and Apaf-1 for execution in primary neurons. *Cell Death Differ.,* 2007; 14:1011–1019.

[21] Delu Song and Joshua L. Dunaief. Retinal iron homeostasis in health and disease. Frontiers in aging neuroscience. 2013.

[22] Hadziahmetovic M, Song Y, Wolkow N, Iacovelli J, et al. Bpm6 regulates retinal iron homeostasis and has altered expression in age-related macular degeneration. *Am. J. Pathol.,* 2011;179,335–348.

[23] Oyuna S. Kozhevnikova, Elena E. Korbolina, Nikita I. Ershov and Natalia G. Kolosova. Rat retinal transcriptome: Effects of aging and AMD-like retinopathy. *Cell Cycle,* 2013;12:11, 1745–1761.

[24] Wang, A.L.; Lukas, T.J.; Yuan, M.; Neufeld, A.H. Increased mitochondrial DNA damage and down-regulation of DNA repair enzymes in aged rodent retinal pigment epithelium and choroid. *Mol. Vis.,* 2008; 14, 644–651.

[25] Kalariya, N.M.; Ramana, K.V.; Srivastava, S.K.; van Kuijk, F.J. Genotoxic effects of carotenoid breakdown products in human retinal pigment epithelial cells. *Curr. Eye Res.,* 2009; 3, 737–747.

[26] Delaney, S.; Jarem, D.A.; Volle, C.B.; Yennie, C.J. Chemical and biological consequences of oxidatively damaged guanine in DNA. *Free Radic. Res.,* 2012; 46, 420–441.

[27] Lau LI, Liu CJ, Wei YH. Increase of 8-hydroxy-2'-deoxyguanosine in aqueous humor of patients with exudative age-related macular degeneration. *Invest. Ophthalmol. Vis. Sci.,* 2010; 51(11):5486-90.

[28] Janusz Blasiak, Sylwester Glowacki, Anu Kauppinen, Kai Kaarniranta. Mitochondrial and Nuclear DNA Damage and Repair in Age-Related Macular Degeneration. *Int. J. Mol. Sci.,* 2013; 14, 2996-3010.

[29] Xia Li, Yan Cai, Yu-Sheng Wang, Yuan-Yuan Shi, Wei Hou, et al. Hyperglycaemia Exacerbates Choroidal Neovascularisation in Mice via the Oxidative Stress- Induced Activation of STAT3 Signalling in RPE Cells. *PLoS One,* 2012;7(10):e47600.

[30] Gallego-Pinazo, R. et al. The tumour inhibitor p53 gene has the ability of triggering proliferation arrest and cellular death by apoptosis subsequent to several factors, among them oxidative stress. *Archivos de la Sociedad Española de Oftalmología,* 2008; 83(2): 105-111.

[31] Sachdeva MM, Cano M, Handa JT. Nrf2 signaling is impaired in the aging RPE given an oxidative insult. *Exp. Eye Res.,* 2013; Nov 8. pii: S0014-4835(13)00313-8.

[32] Görgün E, Güven M, Unal M, Batar B, Güven GS, Yenerel M, Tatlipinar S, Seven M, Yüksel A. Polymorphisms of the DNA repair genes XPD and XRCC1 and the risk of age-related macular degeneration. *Invest. Ophthalmol. Vis. Sci.,* 2010; 51(9):4732-7.

[33] Haque R, Chun E, Howell JC, Sengupta T, Chen D, Kim H. MicroRNA-30b-mediated regulation of catalase expression in human ARPE-19 cells. *PLoS One,* 2012;7(8):e42542.

[34] Janel, N., Robert, K., Chabert, C., Ledru, A., Gouédard, C., Barouki, R., Delabar, J.M & Chassé, J.F. Mouse liver paraoxonase-1 gene expression is downregulated in hyperhomocysteinemia. *Thromb. Haemost.,* 2004; 92: 221-222.

[35] Orhan, A., Sedat, A., Hakan, A., Aphmet, K.,Sukru,B., Emine, C., Ibrahim, K., Orhan, B. Decreased serum paraoxonase 1 activity and increased serum homocysteine and malondialdehyde levels in age-related macular degeneration. *Tohoku J. Exp. Med.,* 2009; 217:17-22.

[36] Dun Y, Vargas J, Brot N, Finnemann SC. Independent roles of methionine sulfoxide reductase A in mitochondrial ATP synthesis and as antioxidant in retinal pigment epithelial cells. *Free Radic. Biol. Med.,* 2013; 65C:1340-1351.

[37] Zuhal Yildirim, Nil Irem Ucgun, Filiz Yildirim. The role of oxidative stress and antioxidants in the pathogenesis of age-related macular degeneration. *Clinics,* 2011; 66.

[38] Li Z, Dong X, Liu H, Chen X, Shi H, Fan Y, Hou D, Zhang X. Astaxanthin protects ARPE-19 cells from oxidative stress via upregulation of Nrf2-regulated phase II enzymes through activation of PI3K/Akt. *Molecular Vision,* 2013; 19:1656-1666.

[39] Dong X, Li Z, Wang W, Zhang W, Liu S, Zhang X. Protective effect of canolol from oxidative stress-induced cell damage in ARPE-19 cells via an ERK mediated antioxidative pathway. *Mol. Vis.,* 2011;17:2040-8.

[40] Rastmanesh R. Potential of melatonin to treat or prevent age-related macular degeneration through stimulation of telomerase activity. *Med. Hypotheses,* 2011; 76(1):79-85.

[41] Rosen RB, Hu DN, Chen M, McCormick SA, Walsh J, Roberts JE. Effects of melatonin and its receptor antagonist on retinal pigment epithelial cells against hydrogen peroxide damage. *Mol. Vis.,* 2012;18:1640-8.

[42] Jia L, Dong Y, Yang H, Pan X, Fan R, Zhai L. Serum superoxide dismutase and malondialdehyde levels in a group of Chinese patients with age-related macular degeneration. *Aging Clin. Exp. Res.,* 2011; 23(4):264-7.

[43] Milam A, Brantley JR, Melissa P. et al. Plasma Biomarkers of Oxidative Stress and Genetic Variants in Age-Related Macular Degeneration. *Am. J. Ophthalmol.,* 2012;153:460–467.

[44] Zafrilla P, Losada M, Perez A, Caravaca G, Mulero J. Biomarkers of oxidative stress in patients with wet age related macular degeneration. *J. Nutr. Health Aging,* 2013;17(3):219-22.

[45] Axer-Siegel, R., Bourla, D., Ehrlich, R., Dotan, G., Benjamín, Y., Gañendo, S. Association of Neovascular Age-related Macular Degeneration and Hyperhomocysteinemia, *Am. J. Ophthalmol.,* 2004; 137:84–89.

[46] Javadzadeh, A., Ghorbanihaghjo, A., Bahreini, E., Rashtchizadeh, N., Argani, H., Alizadeh, S. Serum paraoxonase phenotype distribution in exudative age-related macular degeneration and its relationship to homocysteine and oxidized low-density lipoprotein. *Retina,* 2012; 32(4):658-66.

[47] Johanna M. Seddon. et al. Association Between C-Reactive Protein and Age-Related Macular Degeneration. *JAMA,* 2011;291.

[48] Morohoshi K, Patel N, Ohbayashi M, Chong V, Grossniklaus HE, Bird AC, Ono SJ. Serum autoantibody biomarkers for age-related macular degeneration and possible regulators of neovascularization. *Exp. Mol. Pathol.,* 2012;92(1):64-73.

[49] Seddon JM, Hennekens CH. Vitamins, minerals, and macular degeneration. Promising but unproven hypotheses. *Arch. Ophthalmol.,* 1994;112 (2):176-179.

[50] Antioxidant status and neovascular age-related macular degeneration. Eye Disease Case-Control Study Group. *Arch. Ophthalmol.,* 1993; 111 (1): 104-109. Erratum in: Arch Ophthalmol 1993; 111 (11): 1499. Arch Ophthalmol 1993; 111 (9): 1228. *Arch. Ophthalmol.,* 1993; 111 (10): 1366.

[51] West S, Vitale S, Hallfrisch J, Munoz B, Muller D, Bressler S, Bressler NM. Are antioxidants or supplements protective for age-related macular degeneration? *Arch. Ophthalmol.,* 1994; 112 (2): 222-227.

[52] VandenLangenberg GM, Mares-Perlman JA, Klein R, Klein BE, Brady WE, Palta M. Associations between antioxidant and zinc intake and the 5-year incidence of early age-related maculopathy in the Beaver Dam Eye Study. *Am. J. Epidemiol.,* 1998; 148(2): 204-214.

[53] A randomized, placebo-controlled, clinical trial of high-dose supplementation with vitamins C and E, beta carotene, and zinc for age-related macular degeneration and vision loss: AREDS Report No. 8. *Arch. Ophthalmol.,* 2001; 119 (10): 1417-1436. Erratum in: 2008; 126 (9): 1251.

[54] Clemons TE, Kurinij N, Sperduto RD. Associations of mortality with ocular disorders and an intervention of high-dose antioxidants and zinc in the Age-Related Eye Disease Study: AREDS Report No. 13. *Arch. Ophthalmol.,* 2004; 122(5): 716-726.

[55] Van Leeuwen R, Boekhoorn S, Vingerling JR, Witteman JC, Klaver CC, Hofman A, de Jong PT. Dietary intake of antioxidants and risk of age-related macular degeneration. *JAMA,* 2005; 294 (24): 3101-3107.

[56] Chong EW, Wong TY, Kreis AJ, Simpson JA, Guymer RH. Dietary antioxidants and primary prevention of age related macular degeneration: systematic review and meta-analysis. *BMJ,* 2007; 335 (7623): 755.

[57] Marshall LL, Roach JM. Prevention and treatment of age-related macular degeneration: an update for pharmacists. *Consult. Pharm.,* 2013;28(11):723-37.

[58] Wisniewska A, Subczynski WK. Distribution of macular xanthophylls between domains in a model of photoreceptor outer segment membranes. *Free Radic. Biol. Med.,* 2006; 41 (8): 1257-1265.

[59] Seddon JM, Ajani UA, Sperduto RD, Hiller R, Blair N, Burton TC, Farber MD, Gragoudas ES, Haller J, Miller DT. Dietary carotenoids, vitamins A, C, and E, and advanced age-related macular degeneration. Eye Disease Case-Control Study Group. *JAMA,* 1994; 272(18): 1413-1420. Erratum in*: JAMA,* 1995; 273 (8): 622.

[60] Delcourt C, Carriere I, Delage M, Barberger-Gateau P, Schalch W. Plasma lutein and zeaxanthin and other carotenoids as modifiable risk factors for age-related maculopathy and cataract: the POLA Study. *Invest. Ophthalmol. Vis. Sci.,* 2006; 47 (6): 2329-2335.

[61] Neelam K, Hogg RE, Stevenson MR, Johnston E, Anderson R, Beatty S, Chakravarthy U. Carotenoids and co-antioxidants in age-related maculopathy: design and methods. *Ophthalmic Epidemiol.,* 2008; 15(6): 389-401.

[62] Wang JJ, Buitendijk GH, Rochtchina E, Lee KE, et al. Genetic Susceptibility, Dietary Antioxidants, and Long-term Incidence of Age-related Macular Degeneration in Two Populations. *Ophthalmology,* 2013.

[63] The Age-Related Eye Disease Study 2 (AREDS2) Research Group, Secondary Analyses of the Effects of Lutein/Zeaxanthin on Age-Related Macular Degeneration Progression: AREDS2 Report No. 3. *JAMA Ophthalmol.,* 2013.

[64] Nidhi B, Mamatha BS, Padmaprabhu CA, Pallavi P, Vallikannan B. Dietary and lifestyle risk factors associated with age-related macular degeneration: A hospital based study. *Indian J. Ophthalmol.,* 2013.

[65] Rotstein NP, Politi LE, German OL, Girotti R. Protective effect of docosahexaenoic acid on oxidative stress-induced apoptosis of retina photoreceptors. *Invest. Ophthalmol. Vis. Sci.,* 2003; 44 (5): 2252-9.

[66] Arnarsson A, Sverrisson T, Stefansson E, Sigurdsson H, Sasaki H, Sasaki K, Jonasson F. Risk factors for five-year incident age-related macular degeneration: the Reykjavik Eye Study. *Am. J. Ophthalmol.,* 2006;142 (3): 419-428.

[67] Chua B, Flood V, Rochtchina E, Wang JJ, Smith W, Mitchell P. Dietary fatty acids and the 5-year incidence of age-related maculopathy. *Arch. Ophthalmol.,* 2006; 124 (7): 981-986.

[68] SanGiovanni JP, Chew EY, Clemons TE, Davis MD, Ferris FL, III, Gensler GR, Kurinij N, Lindblad AS, Milton RC, Seddon JM, Sperduto RD. The relationship of dietary lipid intake and age-related macular degeneration in a case-control study: AREDS Report No. 20. *Arch. Ophthalmol.,* 2007; 125 (5): 671-679.

[69] SanGiovanni JP, Chandra SR, Chew EY, Friberg TR, Klein ML, Kurinij N, Seddon JM. Dietary omega-3 long chain polyunsaturared fatty acids and risk for age-related macular degeneration. ARVO. Fort Lauderdale, USA, May 4-9, 2003. *Invest. Ophthalmol. Vis. Sci.,* 2003; 44 (4 Suppl.).

[70] SanGiovanni JP, Chew EY, Clemons TE, Davis MD, Ferris FL, III, Gensler GR, Kurinij N, Lindblad AS, Milton RC, Seddon JM, Sperduto RD. The relationship of dietary lipid intake and age-related macular degeneration in a case-control study: AREDS Report No. 20. *Arch. Ophthalmol.,* 2007; 125 (5): 671-679.

[71] SanGiovanni JP, Chew EY, Agron E, Clemons TE, Ferris FL, III, Gensler G, Lindblad AS, Milton RC, Seddon JM, Klein R, Sperduto RD. The relationship of dietary omega-3 long-chain polyunsaturated fatty acid intake with incident age-related macular degeneration: AREDS Report No. 23. *Arch. Ophthalmol.,* 2008; 126 (9): 1274-1279.

[72] Dawczynski J, Jentsch S, Schweitzer D, Hammer M, Lang GE, Strobel J. Long term effects of lutein, zeaxanthin and omega-3-LCPUFAs supplementation on optical density of macular pigment in AMD patients: the LUTEGA study. *Arch. Clin. Exp. Ophthalmol.,* 2013.

[73] Tan JS, Wang JJ, Flood V, Mitchell P. Dietary fatty acids and the 10-year incidence of age-related macular degeneration: the Blue Mountains Eye Study. *Arch. Ophthalmol.,* 2009; 127 (5): 656-665.

[74] Chong EW, Robman LD, Simpson JA, Hodge AM, Aung KZ, Dolphin TK, English DR, Giles GG, Guymer RH. Fat consumption and its association with age-related macular degeneration. *Arch. Ophthalmol.*, 2009; 127 (5): 674-680.

[75] A randomized, placebo-controlled, clinical trial of high-dose supplementation with vitamins C and E, beta carotene, and zinc for age-related macular degeneration and vision loss: AREDS Report No. 8. *Arch. Ophthalmol.*, 2001; 119 (10): 1417-1436. Erratum in: 2008; 126 (9): 1251.

[76] Sheu SJ, Liu NC, Ou CC, Bee YS, Chen SC, Lin HC, Chan JY. Resveratrol stimulates mitochondrial bioenergetics to protect retinal pigment epithelial cells from oxidative damage. *Invest. Ophthalmol. Vis. Sci.,* 2013 Sep 27;54(9):6426-38.

[77] Seddon JM, Cote J, Rosner B. Progression of age-related macular degeneration: association with dietary fat, transunsaturated fat, nuts, and fish intake. *Arch. Ophthalmol.,* 2003; 121 (12): 1728-37.

In: Oxidative Stress
Editor: Cassidy Croft

ISBN: 978-1-63117-578-7

Chapter 4

Traditional Chinese Medicine Exerts Cardioprotective Effects Against Myocardial Ischemia/Reperfusion Injury

Ru Tie, Wenjuan Xing, Lele Ji and Haifeng Zhang*
Experiment Teaching Center and Department of Physiology,
Fourth Military Medical University, China

Abstract

Myocardial infarction (MI) remains one of the leading causes of death and disability throughout the world. MI and related complications (e.g., heart failure) are great socio-economic burdens to society and healthcare systems. Blood flow restoration through the culprit coronary artery is necessary to save endangered myocardium after acute myocardial infarction. It is well established that early reperfusion limits infarct size and improves clinical outcome of patients with acute MI. The process of restoring blood flow to the ischemic myocardium, however,

* Corresponding author: Haifeng Zhang, M.D., Ph.D., Associate Professor of Medicine and Physiology, Associate Dean, Experiment Teaching Center and Department of Physiology, Fourth Military Medical University, 169 Changlexi Road, Xi'an 710032, China, E-mail: hfzhang@fmmu.edu.cn, Tel: 86-29-84779277, Fax: 86-29-84774764. Supported by the NSFC (No.81270330, 81300190) and Shaanxi Science & Technology Program (No. 2013KJXX-89).

can induce injury, myocardial reperfusion injury, which can paradoxically reduce the beneficial effects of myocardial reperfusion and cause contractile dysfunction and cellular damage. Despite intensive research, therapeutic strategies are limited and there is as yet no routine effective, generally accepted and promising approach for myocardial ischemia/reperfusion (I/R) injury. In recent years, there is a growing interest in the treatment of myocardial I/R-induced cardiac dysfunction with plant-based therapy including traditional Chinese medicine, for which extensive experience has been accumulated over thousands of years. In this review, we propose a systematic approach to the molecular basis of the cardioprotective effects of antioxidant traditional Chinese medicine that could offer a novel therapeutic opportunity against this oxidative tissue damage.

Keywords: Traditional Chinese medicine, myocardial ischemia/reperfusion injury

1. Introduction

According to the WHO, cardiovascular diseases (CVD) are the leading causes of death worldwide. CVD with all its appearances and complications is responsible for approximately 50% of all deaths in the world today. As the population becomes increasingly elderly, almost 23.6 million people will die from CVD by 2030 [1]. The majority of these deaths will be due to coronary heart disease (CHD). Almost 3.8 million men and 3.4 million women dead from CHD per year on average. According to the statistics, Myocardial infarction (MI) or heart failure is the leading causes of death in the future, especially in the elderly of developed and developing nations [2]. Myocardial ischemia refers to a clinical state characterized by low coronary blood flow arising from various causes but resulting in a lack of myocardial oxygen supply which damages myocardial structure and heart function [3, 4]. In most cases MI occurs after rupture, erosion or ulceration of an atherosclerotic plaque in a coronary artery, and this event is rapidly followed by acute thrombosis of these vessels, blocking blood flow. The perfusion imbalance between supply and demand leads to ischemia in the affected myocardium around the thrombotic artery. Necrosis of the cells in the ischemic zone completes 2-4 hours after the onset of decreased perfusion [5]. During MI, cardiomyocytes are subjected to nutrient and oxygen deprivation resulting in acidosis. In most cases, the damaged structure can be repaired and heart function can be restored to its basal condition through ischemia/reperfusion (I/R). However, in some instances, I/R can have the opposite effect, which not only fails to improve heart function but instead exacerbates cardiac function and worsens structural damage. On the basis of the resultant aggravation in myocardial ischemic tissue damage or even irreversible damage after blood flow is increased, this phenomenon is known as myocardial ischemia/reperfusion injury. After reperfusion, when oxidative metabolism restarts, huge ion fluxes are observed, concerted with a burst of reactive oxygen species (ROS). These events trigger the so called reperfusion injury, which finally results in apoptotic and/or necrotic cell death. Therefore, it is necessary for the development of cardioprotective agents to improve myocardial function, limit the total extent of infarction during I/R and decrease the incidence of cardiovascular events [6].

2. Mechanisms of Myocardial Ischemia/ Reperfusion Injury

Myocardial ischemia occurs when the blood supply of the heart is interrupted, generally due to occlusion of coronary arteries. Restoration of blood flow is necessary or myocardium salvage and improves survival after myocardial ischemia. However, the reperfusion of ischemic tissue itself is deleterious and can lead to arrhythmias and contractile dysfunction [7]. Ischemic heart disease does seriously harm to human health, while the most effective clinical measures that restoring blood flow also bring about reperfusion injury [8]. It's a complex and slow process to recovery after I/R injury. It has an important impact factor on myocardial infarction, stroke, organ transplantation and cardiovascular surgery. The I/R injury was mainly occurred in the interaction of the endothelial cells, calcium overload, the reaction of oxygen free radicals, the complement system and so on [9]. I/R injury is inevitable in the treatment for acute myocardial infarction. It is a complicated inflammatory response involved by variety of inflammatory cytokines and cellular pathways, which are involved in oxidative stress, mitochondrial damage and calcium overload [10]. I/R can induce myocardial cell apoptosis, and cell apoptosis is an important link mechanism of myocardial I/R injury [11]. To make the injury minimize, many researchers carried on to explore the specific mechanisms.

2.1. Oxidative Stress

Reactive oxygen species (ROS) plays a crucial role in I/R-induced myocardial damage. Oxidative stress constitutes a unifying mechanism of injury of many types of disease processes; considerable clinical and experimental evidences show that oxidative stress caused by an imbalance between the oxidant and antioxidant systems of the body in favor of the oxidants should be a major apoptotic stimulus in ischemic heart disease (IHD). In the ischemic myocardium, the generation and accumulation of ROS can overwhelm the intrinsic antioxidants and bring about damages to cardiac cells, as a result of peroxidation of lipids, proteins, carbohydrates and DNA. This kind of ROS-induced cardiomyocyte injury plays an important role in the pathogenesis of myocardial I/R injury [12].

ROS is widely recognized as important mediators of cell growth, adhesion, differentiation, senescence, and apoptosis, which are small molecules or molecular ions, initially generated by oxygen reduction, characterized by the presence of unpaired electrons, which are formed during the normal metabolism of oxygen as natural by-products [7, 13]. ROS has both physiological and pathological roles in cellular and tissue adaptation to environmental factors. Normally, low levels of oxygen radicals and oxidants are present in cells and are important in maintaining cellular homeostasis, mitosis, differentiation, and signaling. However, during I/R, ROS formation is markedly increased and cellular injury occurs [14]. In pathophysiological conditions, the main sources of ROS include the mitochondrial respiratory electron transport chain, xanthine oxidase (XO) activation through I/R, the respiratory burst associated with neutrophil activation, and arachidonic acid metabolism [15].

Although mammalian cells express endogenous free radical scavenging enzymes, such as superoxide dismutase (SOD), catalase (CAT), and glutathione peroxidase (GPx), these antioxidative defenses are insufficient during I/R. Oxidative stress during I/R injury contributes to a vicious cycle as it promotes mitochondrial dysfunction, excitotoxicity, lipid peroxidation, and inflammation. Accordingly, successful antioxidant interventions targeted to cleave ROS, which to date has attracted intensive interests from investigators offer insights into delaying or preventing onset of IHD.

2.2. Calcium Overload

Myocardial I/R injury includes intracellular calcium ($[Ca^{2+}]_i$) overload. During ischemia, a reduction in mitochondrial energy production ensues that is accompanied by decreased intracellular pH (pH_i) due to increased lactic acid production consequent to anaerobic glycolysis. The reduction in pH_i, in turn, causes disruption of ionic homeostasis and subsequent $[Ca^{2+}]_i$ overload. This occurs because during ischemia, activation of sarcolemmal Na^+/H^+ exchanger occurs as the cell attempts to restore its pH_i. However, the Na^+ that enters the cell on the Na^+/H^+ exchanger is not pumped out efficiently because a fall in ATP and an increase in phosphate (Pi) inhibit the Na^+/K^+-ATPase [16]. The Na^+/H^+-Na^+/Ca^{2+} exchanger combination, which are important mediators of $[Ca^{2+}]_i$ overload in the ischemic/reperfused heart. Prominent among the diverse consequences of excessive $[Ca^{2+}]_i$ accumulation is the induction of the mitochondrial permeability transition pore, which increases matrix volume by allowing solutes and water to enter the mitochondria [17].

2.3. Inflammation

Increasing evidence indicates that inflammation is involved in the pathophysiology of myocardial I/R injury [18]. During myocardial I/R, the sterile inflammation plays detrimental roles as demonstrated by extensive experimental evidence. Myocardial I/R is characterized by a rapid increase in cytokines and chemokines and an influx of leukocytes into the vulnerable region bordering the infarcted site. This inflammatory response not only results in cardiomyocyte apoptosis during the acute phase, but also results in an adverse myocardial remodeling that further compromises cardiac function. This sterile inflammation is mainly triggered by the interactions between toll-like receptors (TLRs) and their endogenous ligands generated in ischemic and reperfused myocardium, such as apoptotic cell debris, fibrinogen, high mobility group box (HMGB) 1, and heat shock proteins (HSPs). TLR4 has been identified as a mediator of inflammation and organ injury in several models of sterile tissue injury including myocardial I/R. during myocardial I/R, the expression of TLR4 is significantly increased in both the failing myocardium and infiltrated macrophages and thus TLR4 is thought to be a central mediator of inflammation and cardiac injury. A soluble inhibitor of TLR4 was found able to prevent contractile dysfunction in wild-type cells [19]. Another prominent and early mediator for inflammation in I/R injury is interleukin-1β (IL-1β). I/R induces IL-1β expression in the heart and inhibition of IL-1β prevents myocardial injury after I/R, suggesting that the deleterious effects of myocardial I/R are mediated, at least in part, by IL-1β [20]. Therefore, limiting I/R induced myocardial inflammation may not only lower the acute death rate, but also improve long term survival and quality of life.

2.4. Energy Metabolism

In the event of ischemia and hypoxia, myocardial cells can transform rapidly from aerobic to anaerobic glycolysis. Adenosine triphosphate (ATP) generation will significantly reduce the obstacles in the mitochondrial energy synthesis. In the process of the three pathological which the disorders of Ca^{2+} homeostasis and a large number of free radicals producing, energy metabolic dysfunction are likely to be the link in the myocardial I/R injury, which causes the intracellular calcium overload, in order to maintain homeostasis of cytoplasm Ca^{2+}, mitochondria absorb excess Ca^{2+} from cytoplasm, and result in higher Ca^{2+} in the mitochondria, high concentrations of Ca^{2+} can harm the function of mitochondria, change mitochondrial permeability, reduce oxidative phosphorylation efficiency and hinder the ATP synthesis and vicious circle. Energy metabolism dysfunction is the foundation of producing free radicals. Meanwhile, free radical can damage and increase energy metabolic disorders. As a result, mitochondrial damage and energy metabolism disorder is also one of the main reasons in myocardial I/R injury.

2.5. Cell Death

Myocardial I/R leads to the activation of cell death programs, including apoptosis, autophagy and necrosis. Apoptosis characterized by the shrinkage of the cell and its nucleus and persisting plasma membrane integrity, is a major contributor to myocardial I/R injury and left ventricular dysfunction. Caspases are cysteine proteinases that have been shown to be specifically involved in the initiation and execution phases of apoptosis. The balance between apoptotic factors Bcl-2 and Bax has been found altered in cardiomyocytes during ischemia. Autophagy is stimulated by nutrient starvation and growth factor deprivation when cells are unable to take up external nutrients. Autophagy is also activated by decreases in ATP in order for the cell to maintain energy homeostasis and survival. Autophagy may serve primarily to maintain energy production during acute ischemia but switch to clear up damaged organelles during chronic ischemia or reperfusion.

3. Therapeutic Measure

In recent years, emerging research has been shown to possess a remarkable ability to deal with MI/R injury. In conjunction with preventive strategies, major advances in the treatment of acute coronary syndromes and myocardial infarction have occurred over the past 20 years. In particular the ability to rapidly restore blood flow to the myocardium during heart attack, using interventional cardiologic or thrombolytic approaches has been a major step forward [21]. A number of approaches including surgical intervention, traditional pharmacological therapy, physical exercise regimes and evengene-based therapies have been prescribed for the treatment of patients with cardiovascular disease. However, cardiovascular responsiveness to these therapies are not so satisfying in some pathological conditions. The discovery of the major forms of cardioprotective mechanisms has promoted the exploration of new medicine to protect against myocardial I/R injury. Many researches have been conducted to identify strategies and substances that can improve the myocardial response to reperfusion injury. Fortunately, a number of active principles from herbal extracts have been identified for management of cardiovascular diseases including I/R injury.

4. Chinese Medicinal Therapy

In recent years, there is a growing interest in the treatment of myocardial I/R-induced cardiac dysfunction with plant-based therapy including traditional Chinese medicines (TCMs), for which extensive experience has been accumulated over thousands of years. Chinese herbal medicine, especially combined herbal formulations, has been widely used in TCMs for the treatment of myocardial infarction for hundreds of years. Moreover, it has been observed that a lot of TCMs alleviate injury of myocardial reperfusion. A wealth of evidence affirms that TCMs can exert protective effects against myocardial I/R injury by reducing oxidative stress. Some TCMs have been observed to have positive effects of cardioprotection through release of endogenous substances or stimulating endogenous mechanisms. More importantly, as the complementary and alternative medicine, TCMs have shown promising beneficial effects on prevention of cardiovascular disorders partly due to its cell-protection via amelioration of detrimental factors and activation of survival signals. The various actions of TCMs exist in a balance that contributes to cardiovascular homeostasis, suggesting that long-term uptake of TCMs would be effective in prevention and treatment of IHD.

4.1. Anti-Oxidative Stress

Many TCMs, including extracted compounds, single herbs, decoctions, and patent drugs, exert their beneficial effects against I/R injury via their anti-oxidative activity. A number of biomarkers have been used to evaluate the anti-oxidative effects of these TCMs, such as ROS, SOD, GPx, CAT, nitric oxide synthase (NOS), malondialdehyde (MDA), myeloperoxidase (MPO), hemeoxygenase (HO)-1, superoxide anion, GOT, 15-F2t-isoprostane (15-F2t-IsoP), ET-1, cycloxygenase-2 (COX-2), thioredoxin-1 (Trx-1), thioredoxin-related protein-32 (TRP32), redox-sensitive PKC/mKATP pathway, glutathione (GSH), oxidized glutathione (GSSG), glutathione reductase (GRD), CuZn-superoxide dismutase (CuZn-SOD), and Mn-SOD [22].

Normally, low levels of oxygen radicals and oxidants are present in cells and are important in maintaining cellular homeostasis, mitosis, differentiation, and signaling. However, during myocardial I/R, ROS formation is markedly increased and cellular injury occurs. Myocardial ischemia begin to improve when blood flow is restored, but reperfusion injury occurs when blood flow carries ROS, including peroxynitrite, which is derived from reactions between nitric oxide (NO) and superoxide anions, into the affected tissue [12]. Excessive ROS produced by I/R results in increased infarct size and various deleterious events. Moreover, massive ROS release leads to activation of transcription factors, such as nuclear factor κB (NF-κB), which in turn result in augmented expression of adhesion molecules and leukocyte infiltration. Given to the central role of ROS in I/R injury, alleviating the oxidative stress is considered to be a potential option in limiting I/R-induced myocardial injury [23-27].

There are several kinds of TCMs reported to have similar effects. Achyranthes bidentata polypeptides (ABPP) preconditioning for one week significantly improved cardiac function following myocardial I/R, reduced infarct size, plasma creatine kinase (CK)/lactate dehydrogenase (LDH) activities and myocardial apoptosis at the end of reperfusion in rat hearts.

Moreover, ABPP preconditioning significantly inhibited superoxide generation, $gp91^{phox}$ expression, MDA formation and enhanced SOD activity in I/R hearts [28]. Others' studies have showed that a compound Chinese medicine cardiotonic pill (CP) currently used in China for treatment of ischemic angina pectoris, which can attenuate I/R-induced myocardial injury and cardiac microcirculatory disturbance by significantly alleviating the oxidative stress. CP dramatically inhibited I/R-induced nicotinamide adenosine dinucleotide phosphate (NADPH) oxidase subunit $gp91^{phox}$ expression and $p67^{phox}$ and $p47^{phox}$ translocation from cytosol to cell membrane [29]. Song et al. [30] found that Water-soluble polysaccharide (SMP1) was isolated from the roots of Salvia miltiorrhiza. SMP1 has a protective effect against myocardial I/R injury in rats by ameliorating oxidative stress and inhibiting myocardial apoptosis. Panacis japonica rhizoma, also named king of herbs in traditional Tujia and Hmong medicine, is derived from the dried rhizome of Panaxjaponicus (PJ), and belongs to Araliaceae Panax family in the plant kingdom. PJ exerts beneficially cardioprotective effects on myocardial ischemia injury rats, mainly scavenging oxidative stress-triggered overgeneration and accumulation of ROS, alleviating myocardial ischemia injury and cardiac cell death[12]. He H et al. [31] studied that Cortex Dictamni (CD) aqueous extract exerts protective effect against myocardial I/R injury in rats. The possible mechanism may be via the inhibition of peroxidation by increasing the antioxidant enzyme activities. Another study showed that Shenfu injection (SFI) pretreatment had a protective effect on I/R myocardium, which might be associated with anti-oxygen free radical, protecting muscular tissues and suppressing myocardial cells apoptosis [32]. Devi R et al. reported that Clerodendrum colebrookianum Walp (CC) leaf extract protects against oxidative stress and cellular injury associated with I/R injury of rat heart, in which the protective effects of CC extract depend on its antioxidant properties [33]. Li et al. [34] found that Pucrarin's effect of anti-oxidative stress on myocardial I/R rats can reduce the changes of serum CK, thereby reducing myocardial infarct size, and presence of a dose-response relationship.

4.2. Inhibition of Calcium Overload

Wang et al. found that Saponins are prone to alleviate Ca^{2+}overload. Compound acanthopanax senticosus injection (CASI) is of protective effect on myocardial I/R arrhythmia, which may be related to scavenging the oxygen free radicals and Ca^{2+} overload formed during reperfusion [35]. Other study showed that anti-digoxin antiserum has protective and therapeutic effects against I/R injury probably by antagonizing the action of endoxin. The underlying mechanism may be ascribed to restoration of energy metabolism, and attenuation of intracellular Ca^{2+} overload [36]. Li Q et al. found that Anandamide suppresses calcium overload through inhibition of Na^+/Ca^{2+} exchanger current during perfusion with simulated ischemic solution; the effects may be mediated by cannabinoid 2 (CB2) receptor via pertussis toxin (PTX)-sensitive $G_{i/o}$ proteins [37]. It is reported that Motherwort, Astragalus, Salviahave, Rhizomaligustici chuanxiong, extract of ginkgo biloba, Taurine and Ginseng have obvious therapeutic effect against I/R injury and alleviate cell Ca^{2+} overload. In addition, oxymatrine alleviates the membrane lipid peroxidation damage caused by free radicals, reduces myocardial cell membrane permeability and mitochondrial injury caused by Ca^{2+} overload.

4.3 Anti-Inflammation

Ischemia and reperfusion cause sterile inflammation which plays a vital role in myocardial I/R injury. The consequences of myocardial I/R share many phenotypic parallels with activation of a host immune response directed toward invading microorganisms. Gross saponins from Tribulus terrestris had the actions of protecting myocardium from I/R injury, inhibiting the inflammatory damage and decreasing the release of TNF-α and IL-1β [38]. Icariin preconditioning reduces inflammatory responses in the process of myocardial I/R injury in a dose-dependent manner [39]. Wei G et al. [40] found that Protocatechuic aldehyde (PA) could exert great protective effects against myocardial I/R injury in rats and the underlying mechanism might be the suppression of inflammatory response via inhibiting the NF-κB signaling pathway. XuefuZhuyu decoction can protect myocardium from MI/R injury, and the mechanism of action is related to inhibiting inflammatory reaction and reducing arrhythmia and the injury of the myocardial ultrastructure [41]. The other findings found that Guan-Xin-Er-Hao exhibited an anti-inflammatory effect through inhibition of the NF-κB-mediated signaling pathway leading to downregulation of pro-inflammatory cytokine expression and generated cardioprotective effect through reduction of infarct size by mediating lots of endogenous materials via multiple pathways to act on myocardial cells in the treatment of cardiovascular disease [42]. Chronic α-Linolenic acid (ALA) intake confers cardioprotection including inhibiting apoptosis, in part by exerting anti-inflammatory and anti-oxidative stress effects in diabetic rats, which is possibly through PI3K-Akt-dependent mechanism [43]. Vitexin plays a cardioprotection role against myocardial I/R injury in rat via regulating inflammatory cytokines and MAPK pathway [44]. Another previous study found that pretreatment with luteolin play an important role in the cardioprotection against myocardial I/R injury by anti-inflammatory, antioxidant and anti-carcinogenic [45].

4.4. Improving Energy Metabolism

Li et al. reported that energy metabolism is also involved in myocardial I/R. ShuangshenNingxin (SSNX) formula can maintain energy charge in cardiomyocytes and relieve I/R injury by preserving ischemic myocardium ATP [46]. Li et al. [47] found that Shenfu Injection attenuates I/R injury by raising the content of high energy phosphate and SOD activity in myocardium, meanwhile decreasing the content of MDA. Others' study has showed that Danshen dripping pill (DSDP) increases the energy storage of myocardium and protects it by inhibiting the generation of lipid peroxide [48]. Fan et al. showed that Baicalein, Puerarin and Dioscin significantly improve the myocardium energy metabolism in I/R rat [49]. Wen et al. [50] reported that Crocetin protects the myocardial tissues from the I/R injury by boosting ATPase activities associated with energy metabolism.

4.5. Anti-Apoptosis

Zhou et al. [51] revealed that Breviscapine significantly protects myocardial cell against apoptosis induced by hypoxia/reoxygenation which is associated with the increase in Bcl-2 expression, inhibition of CytC release and Casepase-3 activity. Bian et al. [52] reported that Madecassoside (MA), one of the principle terpenoids in Centella asiatica, has shown protect effect on isolated rat hearts and isolated cardiomyocytes against reperfusion injury due to its anti-lipid peroxidation, anti-inflammation and anti-apoptosis function and the enhancement of SOD activity. Others study have showed that Tongxinluo capsule has the effects of resisting oxygen free radical injury, anti-myocardial apoptosis and protecting I/R cardiomyocytes, and with a dose dependence [53]. Du et al. revealed that QDPTP protects myocardium against I/R injury in rats, which might be related with its effects of restoring cardiac function, alleviating oxidative stress and inhibiting apoptosis [54]. Liu et al. reported that 3,5-Dimethoxy-4-(3-(2-carbonyl-ethyldisulfanyl)-propionyl)-benzoic acid 4-guanidino-butyl ester, derived from the Chinese herb Leonurus, inhibited apoptosis by increasing the ratio of Bcl-2/Bax, decreasing the level of cleaved-caspase-3, and enhancing the phosphorylation of Akt [55]. Ling et al. studied the effects of the patent drug, Cardiotonic Pill (CP) combined with the Chinese herb, Salvia miltiorrhiza. They found that CP treatment significantly inhibits TNF-α-induced apoptosis in cardiomyocytes through activating Akt signaling [56]. Others' study has showed that Salvianolic acid A (SAA) possesses marked protective effect on myocardial I/R injury, which is related to its ability to reduce myocardial cell apoptosis and damage induced by oxidative stress [57].

4.6. Other Mechanisms

Angiogenesis limits I/R damage by restoring tissue blood flow. Many TCMs have been used as the targets for angiogenesis promotion to protect cardiomyocytes against I/R. Liu et al. [58] found that the ginsenoside Rb1 have important effect on blood vessel regeneration after ischemia and reperfusion in rats, which can increase capillary density, enhance myocardial angiogenesis and improve left ventricular function. Tanshinone IIA (Tan IIA) promotes angiogenesis and up-regulating VEGF expression in I/R rats due to the enhancement of HIF-1α mRNA expression [59]. Radix et Rhizoma Rhodiolae Kirilowii may promote angiogenesis in myocardium of rats with acute MI through elevating the expressions of HIF-1α, HIF-1β, and VEGF. Salidroside may be one of the effective components in Radix et Rhizoma Rhodiolae Kirilowii [60].

Conclusion

In conclusion, TCMs study of I/R protection is one of the breakthrough point in cooperation of Chinese and western medicine in recent years. Significant progress in prevention and treatment of myocardial I/R injury by TCMs has been proven. More and more research work focused on clarifying the mechanisms of TCMs. TCMs have been proved to serve as promising effective complementary and alternative medicine in treatment myocardial I/R. But much work remains because a large number of TCMs have not been found, developed, researched and clinical applied by now. Most Basic and clinical studies showed limitation of extra value, meanwhile experimental studies have focused mainly on single compounds extracted from Chinese medicines. These studies help us to understand the mechanisms underlying the use of TCMs and formulations for the treatment of myocardial I/R. Establishment of some appropriate methods to define the active components of TCMs and find more effective formulations should be executed to guarantee stable pharmacological and clinical effects. Accordingly, there is a strong likelihood that such ongoing research will lead to novel strategies for the treatment of myocardial I/R injury using TCMs.

References

[1] *Global status report on noncommunicable disaeses 2010.* Geneva, World Health Organization, 2011.

[2] Zhao YL. Research on myocardial ischemia reperfusion injury. *Chinese Circulation Journal.* 2011,26(5):396-398.

[3] Minamino, T. Cardioprotection from ischemia/reperfusion injury: Basic and translational research. *Circ J.* 2012,76(5), 1074-1082.

[4] Moens AL, Claeys MJ, Timmermans JP, Vrints CJ. Myocardial ischemia/reperfusion-injury, a clinical view on a complex pathophysiological process. *Int J Cardiol.* 2005,100(2):179-190.

[5] Dongó E, Hornyák I, Benko Z, Kiss L. The cardioprotective potential of hydrogen sulfide in myocardial ischemia/reperfusion injury. *Acta Physiologica Hungarica.* 2011,98(4):369-381.

[6] Xu T, Li D, Jiang D. Targeting cell signaling and apoptotic pathways by luteolin: cardioprotective role in rat cardiomyocytes following ischemia/reperfusion. *Nutrients.* 2012,4(12):2008-2019.

[7] Braunersreuther V, Jaquet V. Reactive oxygen species in myocardial reperfusion injury: from physiopathology to therapeutic approaches. *Curr Pharm Biotechnol.* 2012,13(1):97-114.

[8] Yun HX. Lu DX. Research Progress of anti-,yocardial ischemia/reperfusion injury and gene expression of tradional Chinese medicine. *Chinese Journal of Experimental Trational Medical Formulae,* 2013, 19(10):360-364

[9] Yang JD, Cui W, Gao GD, Qing H. *The progress of the research on ischemia re-perfusion injury.* 3013,15(165):139-182.

[10] Gao XQ, Xue L. Advances in myocardial ischemia reperfusion injury and its related cytokines and cellular pathways. *Chin J Arterioscler.* 2013, 21(6): 562-566.

[11] Yang Q, Yang K, Li AY, Tan WP. Anti-apoptosis and expression of microRNA-21 in rat myocardium during early ischemia-reperfusion injury. *J Cent South Univ* (Med Sci) 2013, 38(5):483-489.

[12] He H, Xu J, Xu Y, Zhang C, Wang H, He Y, Wang T, Yuan D. Cardioprotective effects of saponins from Panaxjaponicus on acute myocardial ischemia against oxidative stress-triggered damage and cardiac cell death in rat. *J Ethnopharmacol.* 2012, 140(1):73-82.

[13] Ji L, Fu F, Zhang L, Liu W, Cai X, Zhang L, Zheng Q, Zhang H, Gao F. Insulin attenuates myocardial ischemia/reperfusion injury via reducing oxidative/nitrative stress. *Am J Physiol Endocrinol Metab.* 2010,298(4):E871-E880.

[14] Liu Q, Li J, Wang J, Li J, Janicki JS, Fan D. Effects and mechanisms of chinese herbal medicine in ameliorating myocardial ischemia-reperfusion injury. *Evid Based Complement Alternat Med.* 2013:925625.

[15] Rodrigo R, Libuy M, Feliú F, Daniel H. Oxidative stress-related biomarkers in essential hypertension and ischemia-reperfusion myocardial damage. *Dis Markers.* 2013;35(6):773-790.

[16] Mozaffari MS, Liu JY, Abebe W, Baban B. Mechanisms of load dependency of myocardial ischemia reperfusion injury. *Am J Cardiovasc Dis.* 2013, 13(4):180-196.

[17] Mozaffari MS, Patel C, Schaffer SW. Mechanisms underlying afterload-induced exacerbation of myocardial infarct size. Role of T-type Ca^{2+} channel. *Hypertension.* 2006, 47:1-8.

[18] Yellon DM, Hausenloy DJ. Myocardial reperfusion injury. *N Engl J Med.* 2007, 357:1121-1135.

[19] Yu L, Wang L, Chen S. Endogenous toll-like receptor ligands and their biological significance. *Journal of Cellular and Molecular Medicine*, 2010, 14(11):2592-2603.

[20] Kawaguchi M, Takahashi M, Hata T, Kashima Y, Usui F, Morimoto H, Izawa A, Takahashi Y, Masumoto J, Koyama J, Hongo M, Noda T, Nakayama J, Sagara J, Taniguchi S, Ikeda U. Inflammasome activation of cardiac fibroblasts is essential for myocardial ischemia/reperfusion injury. *Circulation.* 2011,123(6):594-604.

[21] Huang C, Cui Y, Ji L, Zhang W, Li R, Ma L, Xing W, Zhou H, Chen B, Yu J, Zhang H. Catalpol decreases peroxynitrite formation and

consequently exerts cardioprotective effects against ischemia/reperfusion insult. *Pharm Biol.* 2013. 51(4):463-473.
[22] Yang XY, Zhao N, Liu YY, Hu BH, Sun K, Chang X, Wei XH, Fan JY, Han JY. Inhibition of NADPH oxidase mediates protective effect of cardiotonic pills against rat heart ischemia/reperfusion injury. *Evid Based Complement Alternat Med.* 2013:728020.
[23] Ambrosio G, Becker LC, Hutchins GM, Weisman HF, Weisfeldt ML. Reduction in experimental infarct size by recombinant human superoxide dismutase: insights into the pathophysiology of reperfusion injury. *Circulation.* 1986, 74(6):1424-1433.
[24] Hamilton KL. Antioxidants and cardioprotection. *Medicine and Science in Sports and Exercise.* 2007, 39(9):1544-1553.
[25] Pagliaro P, Moro F, Tullio F, Perrelli M, Penna C. Cardioprotective pathways during reperfusion: focus on redox signaling and other modalities of cell signaling. *Antioxidants and Redox Signaling.* 2011,14(5):833-850.
[26] Webster KA. Mitochondrial membrane permeabilization and cell death during myocardial infarction: roles of calcium and reactive oxygen species. *Future Cardiology.* 2012, 8(6):863–884.
[27] Tie R, Ji L, Nan Y, Wang W, Liang X, Tian F, Xing W, Zhu M, Li R, Zhang H. Achyranthesbidentata polypeptides reduces oxidative stress and exerts protective effects against myocardial ischemic/reperfusion injury in rats. *Int J Mol Sci.* 2013, 14(10):19792-19804.
[28] Yang XY, Zhao N, Liu YY, Hu BH, Sun K, Chang X, Wei XH, Fan JY, Han JY. Inhibition of NADPH oxidase mediates protective effect of cardiotonic pills against rat heart ischemia/reperfusion injury. *Evid Based Complement Alternat Med.* 2013:728020.
[29] Song M, Huang L, Zhao G, Song Y. Beneficial effects of a polysaccharide from Salvia miltiorrhiza on myocardial ischemia-reperfusion injury in rats. *Carbohydr Polym.* 2013, 6, 98(2):1631-1636.
[30] Xu ML, Wang LL, Li L, Li ZQ, Qin M, Li JM, Xu Y. Protective effects of aqueous extract of Cortex dictamni on myocardial ischemia reperfusion injury in rats. *Acta Laboratorium Animalis Scientia Sinica.* 2013, 21(1):47-52.
[31] Tan B, Xiong Y. Protective Effects of Shenfu Injection pretreatment on myocardial ischemia-reperfusion injury model rats. *China Pharmacy.* 2013,24(27): 2513-2515.

[32] Li J, Huang KX, Wang YC, Shi B. Effect of puerarin on myocardial ischemia-reperfusion injury in rat cardiac enzymes. *Chin J Lab Diagn.* 2013, 17,(2): 244-246.

[33] Devi R, Banerjee SK, Sood S, Dinda AK, Maulik SK. Extract from Clerodendrum colebrookianum Walp protects rat heart against oxidative stress induced by ischemic-reperfusion injury (IRI). *Life Sci.* 2005, 77(24):2999-3009.

[34] Li Q, Cui N, Du Y, Ma H, Zhang Y. Anandamide reduces intracellular Ca^{2+} concentration through suppression of Na^{+}/Ca^{2+} exchanger current in rat cardiac myocytes. *PLoS One.* 2013, 8(5):63386.

[35] Ke YS, Wang DG, Wang HG, Yang SY. Endoxin antagonist lessens myocardial ischemia reperfusion injury. *Cardiovasc Drugs Ther.* 2004, 18(4):289-293.

[36] Wang L, Yu XF, Qu SC, Xu HL, Sui DY. *Effects of CASI on myocardial ischemia-reperfusion arrhythmia in rats.* Zhong Guo Zhong Yao Za Zhi. 2007, 32(20):2174-2177.

[37] Yin HJ, Wang XG, Shi DZ. Effects of GSTT on release of TNF-α and IL-1β in rats with myocardial ischemia/reperfusion injury. *Med J Chin PLA.* 2006,10(31):986-987.

[38] Guo QJ, Wang GM, Zhang XX. Effects of icariin preconditioning on inflammatory responses in myocardial ischemia reperfusion injury. *Chinese Journal of Pathophysiology.* 2013, 29(11): 2034-2038.

[39] Zhang XY, Huang X, Qin F, Ren P. Anti-inflammatory effect of Guan-Xin-Er-Hao via the nuclear factor-kappa B signaling pathway in rats with acute myocardial infarction. *Exp Anim.* 2010, 59(2):207-214.

[40] Tang D, Liu Z, Zhang H, Sun M, Sui Y. Protective effects of Xuefuzhuyu decoction on myocardium ischemia reperfusion injury in rats. *China Journal of Chinese Materia Medica.* 2010, 35(22):3077-3079.

[41] Wei G, Guan Y, Yin Y, Duan J, Zhou D, Zhu Y, Quan W, Xi M, Wen A. Anti-inflammatory effect of protocatechuic aldehyde on myocardial ischemia/reperfusion injury in vivo and in vitro. *Inflammation.* 2013, 36(3):592-602.

[42] Xie N, Zhang W, Li J, Liang H, Zhou H, Duan W, Xu X, Yu S, Zhang H, Yi D. α-linolenic acid intake attenuates myocardial ischemia/reperfusion injury through anti-inflammatory and anti-oxidative stress effects in diabetic but not normal rats. *Arch Med Res.* 2011, 42(3):171-181.

[43] Dong LY, Li S, Zhen YL. Cardioprotection of vitexin on myocardial ischemia/reperfusion injury in rat via regulating inflammatory cytokines and MAPK pathway. *Am J Chin Med.* 2013, 41(6):1251-1266.
[44] Xu T, Li D, Jiang D. Targeting cell signaling and apoptotic pathways by luteolin: cardioprotective role in rat cardiomyocytes following ischemia/reperfusion. *Nutrients.* 2012, 4(12):2008-2019.
[45] Liu XL, Yang Y, Liu X. Effect of ShenfuInjection on myocardial energy metabolism following acute myocardial ischemic reperfusion in rats. *JETCM*, 2009,18 (7):1117-1118.
[46] Li XL, Liu JX,Guo YJ. Effect of shuangshenningxin formula on energy metabolism of myocardial ischemia/reperfusion rats. *China Journal of Chinese Material Medical.* 2013, 38(17):2874-2877.
[47] Zhao YJ, Zhu SJ, Shi CN, Jiang XS, Wang XM, Ma LY. Energy metabolism and lipid peroxidation in rat myocardium with ischemia/reperfusion and protective effect of compound Danshen dripping pills. *Journal of Harbin Medical University.* 2003, 37(4):290-293.
[48] Fan XJ, Jiao JJ, Zhao YQ, Wang W, Kang Y, Lou JS, Zhang Z, Yu L, Gao WZ. Effects of dioscin on adenosine phosphates in rat myocardium with ischemia-reperfusion. *Journal of Tianjin Medical University.* 2008,14(4):409-429.
[49] Wen N, Qian ZY, Rao SY, Shen XC. Effect of crocetin on energy metablism in rats with myocardial ischemia-reperfusion injury. *Chinese Journal of New Drugs* 2005,14(11):1294-1297.
[50] Gao XF, Shi HM, Sun T, Ao H. Effects of Radix et Rhizoma Rhodiolae Kirilowii on expressions of von Willebrand factor, hypoxia-inducible factor 1 and vascular endothelial growth factor in myocardium of rats with acute myocardial infarction. *Journal of Chinese Integrative Medicine*, 2009, 7(5): 434-440.
[51] Zhou XH, Gong MY, Yan FX. Inhibition of breviscapine on apoptosis of cultured myocardial cell of neonatal rat. *Chinese Traditional Patent Medicine.* 2009, 31(12):1823-1827.
[52] Bian GX, Li GG, Yang Y, Liu RT, Ren JP, Wen LQ, Guo SM, Lu QJ. Madecassoside reduces ischemia-reperfusion injury on regional ischemia induced heart infarction in rat. *Biol Pharm Bull.* 2008, 31(3):458-463.
[53] Qin J, Zhang WJ, Jin MH, Wu GZ, Liu HJ, Zhang Y. Effect of tongxinluo capsule on reperfusion myocardial apoptosis. *Rehabilitation of Traditional Chinese Medicine.* 2005,9(31):228-230.

[54] Du J, Lian H, Zhang X. Protective Effects of QDPTP against myocardial ischemia reperfusion injury in rats. *Acta Med Univ Sci Technol Huazhong*. 2006,35(5):576-579.

[55] Liu C, Guo W, Maerz S, Gu X, Zhu Y. 3, 5-Dimethoxy-4-(3-(2-carbonyl-ethyldisulfanyl)-propionyl)-benzoic acid 4-guanidino-butyl ester: a novel twin drug that prevents primary cardiac myocytes from hypoxia-induced apoptosis. *European Journal of Pharmacology*. 2013, 118-126.

[56] Ling S, Luo R, Dai A, Guo Z, Guo R, and Komesaroff PA. A pharmaceutical preparation of Salvia miltiorrhiza protects cardiac myocytes from tumor necrosis factor-induced apoptosis and reduces angiotensin II-stimulated collagen synthesis in fibroblasts. *Phytomedicine*. 2009, 16(1): 56-64.

[57] Fan H, Yang L, Fu F, Xu H, Meng Q, Zhu H, Teng L, Yang M, Zhang L, Zhang Z, Liu K. Cardioprotective effects of salvianolic acid a on myocardial ischemia-reperfusion injury in vivo and in vitro. *Evid Based Complement Alternat Med*. 2012:508938.

[58] Liu YF, Liu SW, Liu ZX. Effects of Ginsenoside Rb1 on Blood Vessel Regeneration after ischemia and Reperfusion Rats. *Chinese Journal of Histochemistry and Cytochemistry*. 2008,17(1): 39-43.

[59] Xu W, Yang J, Wu LM. Cardioprotective effects of tanshinone IIA on myocardial ischemia injury in rats. *Pharmazie*. 2009, 64(5): 332-336.

[60] Gao XF, Shi HM, Sun T, Ao H. Effects of Radix et Rhizoma Rhodiolae Kirilowii on expressions of von Willebrand factor, hypoxia-inducible factor 1 and vascular endothelial growth factor in myocardium of rats with acute myocardial infarction, *Journal of Chinese Integrative Medicine*. 2009, 7(5): 434-440.

In: Oxidative Stress
Editor: Cassidy Croft

ISBN: 978-1-63117-578-7

Chapter 5

Controlling Oxidative Stress in Non-Alcoholic Steatohepatitis (NASH)

***Akinobu Takaki*[*], *Daisuke Kawai*[†] and *Kazuhide Yamamoto*[‡]**
Department of Gastroenterology and Hepatology, Okayama University
Graduate School of Medicine, Dentistry and Pharmaceutical Sciences
Okayama City, Okayama, Japan

Abstract

Non-alcoholic steatohepatitis (NASH) is a severe form of non-alcoholic fatty liver disease (NAFLD), in which most patients exhibit non-progressive non-alcoholic fatty liver (NAFL) representing simple steatosis of the liver. Multiple hits, including genetic differences, fat accumulation, insulin resistance and intestinal microbiota changes, account for the progression NASH. NAFLD is strongly associated with obesity, which induces adipokine secretion, endoplasmic reticulum (ER) and oxidative stress at the cellular level, and induces hepatic steatosis, inflammation and fibrosis. Among these factors, oxidative stress is

[*] Corresponding author: Akinobu Takaki; E-mail: akitaka@md.okayama-u.ac.jp; Tel.: +81-86-235-7219; Fax: +81-86-225-5991.
[†] daicawai@yahoo.co.jp.
[‡] kazuhide@md.okayama-u.ac.jp.

considered a key contributor to the progression from NAFL to NASH. Although several clinical trials have shown that anti-oxidative therapy with vitamin E can effectively control the effects of hepatitis in the short term, the long-term effects remains obscure. Several trials of long-term anti-oxidant protocols aimed at treating cerebrovascular diseases or cancer development have failed to demonstrate benefits. This might be attributed to the non-selective anti-oxidant properties or excessive anti-oxidative effects of these drugs. Molecular hydrogen has recently been identified as an effective antioxidant that specifically reduces cytotoxic reactive oxygen species (ROS). Several diseases associated with oxidative stress, such as ischemia reperfusion injury of brain or heart, Parkinson's disease, post-chemotherapeutic renal injury, or transplant rejection, are responsive to hydrogen. The progress of NASH and transition of NASH to hepatocellular carcinoma can be controlled using hydrogen-rich water in mouse models. Long-term clinical intervention is required to control this complex lifestyle-related disease.

Keywords: Non-alcoholic steatohepatitis, oxidative stress

1. Introduction

Non-alcoholic fatty liver disease (NAFLD) is a common cause of chronic liver disease and a major indicator of the increasingly prevalent metabolic syndrome [1]. Most patients with NAFLD exhibit non-progressive simple fatty liver, namely non-alcoholic fatty liver (NAFL). Non-alcoholic steatohepatitis (NASH) is a more severe form of NAFLD that is broadly defined by the presence of steatosis with inflammation and progressive fibrosis [2, 3], ultimately leading to cirrhosis and hepatocellular carcinoma (HCC) [4-7]. A subset of patients with NAFLD develops NASH through poorly understood mechanisms.

The development of NASH has been considered a "two hit" process [8]. The first hit is the development of hepatic steatosis and the second hit includes cellular stresses such as oxidative stress, apoptosis and gut-derived stimulation. However, a "multiple hit" process has recently been advocated due to inflammation being able to induce steatosis and the discovery that genetic background is correlated with disease progression (Figure 1). A recent genome wide association study (GWAS) revealed patatin-like phospholipase 3 (PNPLA3) as a key gene in the development of NASH. Although NAFL is usually non-progressive, it can progress in patients harboring the risk allele of the PNPLA3 gene.

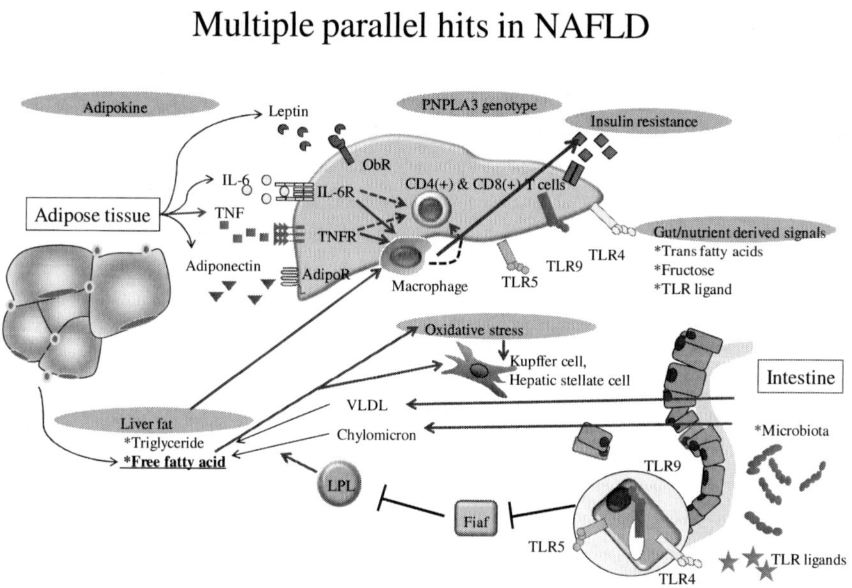

Figure 1. Multiple parallel hits in NAFLD. Genome-wide association studies have confirmed the importance of a patatin-like phospholipase 3 (PNPLA3) gene polymorphism in NAFLD. This genetic polymorphism can differentiate simple steatosis, with or without minimal inflammation, and fibrosis progressing to NASH. In some instances, inflammation can precede steatosis, and anti-tumor necrosis factor (TNF)-α antibody therapy improves steatosis in ob/ob mice. Obesity and diabetes induce insulin resistance, adipocyte proliferation and changes in intestinal flora. Macrophages have an important role in the induction of inflammation and insulin resistance. CD4(+) and CD8(+) T cells are found after NASH development. Adipokines produced by adipocytes, such as IL-6 and TNF-α, affect hepatocyte fat content and the liver inflammatory environment. Gut-derived signals can be affected by ingested trans fatty acids, fructose, or TLR ligands resulting in hepatic inflammation. Ingested free fatty acids and free cholesterol induce ER stress and oxidative stress resulting in hepatic inflammation and fibrogenesis.

Many sources of cellular stresses, including oxidative stress, apoptosis and gut-derived LPS, trigger an inflammatory response and progressive liver damage [9]. Oxidative stress appears to be responsible for initiating necroinflammation. Reactive oxygen species (ROS) generated during free fatty acid metabolism in microsomes, peroxisomes, and mitochondria, comprise an established source of oxidative stress [10]. Mitochondria are the most important cellular source of ROS, and mitochondrial dysfunction might therefore play a central role in the pathological mechanisms of NASH. Although the mechanisms of mitochondrial dysfunction are not clearly understood, emerging data suggest that ROS, lipid peroxidation products, and tumor necrosis factor-α (TNF-α) are involved in the second hit, which induces the progression of simple steatosis to NASH. Furthermore, ROS induces the directional migration of resident hepatic pro-fibrogenic cells, resulting in liver fibrosis [11].

Several studies have suggested that antioxidants such as vitamin E along with 1-aminobenzotriazole (ABT) and thiazolidinediones (insulin sensitizers) confer benefits to patients with NAFLD or NASH [12-15]. Because NASH pathogenesis includes insulin resistance and oxidative stress, insulin sensitizers appear to be promising as therapeutics. The thiazolidinedione pioglitazone improves insulin sensitivity, steatosis, and inflammation. However, the improvement is not clear from a histological perspective and vitamin E might be a better candidate [12]. The American Association for the Study of Liver Disease (AASLD) recommends the use of high dose vitamin E for NASH. However, most clinical studies of atherosclerotic diseases with dietary antioxidants have not generated clear results, partly because of the non-selective effects of these anti-oxidative drugs and difficulties associated with cytosolic distribution [16].

Molecular hydrogen has therapeutic value as an antioxidant through its ability to specifically reduce the cytotoxic ROS hydroxyl radicals, but not superoxide, hydrogen peroxide, or nitric oxide. Hydrogen freely diffuses into the cytosol without the need for specific receptors or hydrophilicity [17]. Inhaled hydrogen gas (~4% H_2 in air) can reduce infarct size in rat models of focal cerebral and myocardial ischemia-reperfusion injury [18]. Drinking water containing therapeutic doses of hydrogen (hydrogen-rich water; HW) represents an alternative model for delivering molecular hydrogen to treat ROS-induced pathologies [19]. We recently showed that HW counteracts oxidative stress in mouse models of NASH.

Here, we review the importance of oxidative stress in the pathogenesis of NASH and the effect of anti-oxidants including HW.

2. General Characteristics of NAFLD

NAFLD is diagnosed with the following findings; alcohol intake < 20 g / day (30 g / day for men), fatty liver diagnosed by imaging or histology, exclusion of other liver disease. The clinical characteristics of NAFLD are correlated with obesity and related general disorders. The two-hit theory indicates that the first hit is hepatic steatosis, and obesity induced NAFL is the defining feature of NAFLD [20]. However, as inflammation can occasionally precede steatosis and anti- TNF α antibody treatment improves steatosis in ob/ob mice, hepatic steatosis is now regarded to be one of the many factors contributing to the development of NAFLD [21, 22]. Genetic background, visceral obesity, insulin resistance, and steatosis are the features of NASH, however, diagnosis is still performed according to liver histology and requires a liver biopsy. Liver biopsies are expensive, time consuming, and involve a degree of morbidity as well as a very rare mortality risk, and therefore should be performed only on patients with progressive disease risk [23]. Serological markers are required to enable the differentiation of NAFL and NASH. Measurement of CK-18 fragments has been reported in different populations and found to be a reliable non-invasive NAFLD diagnostic marker [24].

2.1. Genetic Background

Genome-wide association studies (GWAS) have uncovered many disease- or treatment-susceptible genes. Several GWAS of various races have confirmed the importance of PNPLA3 gene polymorphisms in NAFLD [25]. This genetic polymorphism differentiates between simple steatosis with or without minimal inflammation and fibrosis that progresses to NASH [26, 27]. Patients with the NASH-sensitive single nucleotide polymorphism (SNP) rs738409 G/G genotype might progress to simple steatosis as well as to NASH, probably under the same metabolic conditions. The function of PNPLA3 is not well known since mice deficient in PNPLA3 develop neither fatty liver nor liver injury. However, the overexpression of sterol-regulated binding protein 1c (SREBP-1c) results in its binding to the transcription start site of the mouse PNPLA3 gene and additional PNPLA3 knockdown can decrease intracellular triglyceride content in primary hepatocytes [28]. Thus, PNPLA3 might function as a downstream target gene of SREBP-1c to mediate SREBP-1c stimulation of lipid accumulation. This genetic characteristic might be the "first hit" and subsequent hits might affect disease progression.

2.2. Visceral Obesity

Obesity is a growing global epidemic among adults and children and is associated with many diseases such as hypertension, diabetes mellitus, hyperlipidemia, and NAFLD. Obesity, hypertriglyceridemia, and hypertension are predictive risk factors for NAFLD [29]. Visceral fat accumulation in obesity correlates with various organ pathologies including cerebrovascular diseases, cancer, and NASH. Visceral fat accumulation is regarded as a significant risk factor for the development of NAFLD and NASH. A study from Japan has found that the severity of hepatic steatosis determined by ultrasound positively correlates with visceral fat accumulation and insulin resistance in both obese and non-obese individuals, suggesting that hepatic steatosis is influenced by visceral fat accumulation regardless of obesity [30]. Over the past decade, visceral obesity has become quite common world-wide, even among children, due to a shift towards Western style diets that are high in calories, fat, and fructose [31].

2.3. Insulin Resistance

Insulin resistance is an independent risk factor for NAFLD severity [30]. Adipose and hepatic insulin resistance progressively increases across NAFLD stages, even in non-obese, non-diabetic, and normolipidemic patients. The oral glucose tolerant test (OGTT) shows impaired pancreatic β-cell function in patients with NASH but not in those with simple steatosis [32]. Furthermore, a more atherogenic postprandial lipoprotein profile indicates systemic insulin resistance and hepatic free fatty acid (FFA) accumulation.

2.4. Hepatic Steatosis

Triglycerides are the main types of lipids stored in the liver of patients with NAFLD. The toxic lipids in NASH and the non-toxic lipids in NAFL (simple steatosis) might be different [33]. Diacylglycerol acyltransferase 2 (DGAT2) catalyzes the final step in hepatocyte triglyceride biosynthesis. The induction of hepatic steatosis and elevated plasma triglyceride content in a model of obese simple fatty liver are reduced by DGAT2 antisense oligonucleotides in a manner that does not correlate with changes in body weight, adiposity or insulin sensitivity [34]. However, in mice fed with a methionine choline-deficient (MCD) diet that generates inflammation and fibrosis with hepatic steatosis, DGAT2 antisense oligonucleotides increased levels of hepatic free fatty acids, lipid oxidant stress, lobular necroinflammation and fibrosis, whereas hepatic triglyceride content decreased [33]. These results suggest that the pathogenesis and treatment of steatosis in simple fatty liver and in NASH are different. An analysis of the effect of human genetic variability on lifestyle intervention has shown that the DGAT2 gene polymorphism is related to a decrease in liver fat, while changes in insulin resistance do not correlate [35]. Since insulin resistance is the key marker for NASH, the DGAT2 gene polymorphism might only be associated with non-progressive fatty liver.

2.5. Differential Diagnosis of NAFL and NASH

Fatty liver is the basic feature of NAFLD and NASH that can be diagnosed with abdominal ultrasound characterized by the detection of bright, fat-deposited liver. The differential diagnosis of NAFL and NASH is still based on liver histology. The histological features of NASH include the presence of macrovesicular steatosis, the ballooning degeneration of hepatocytes, and lobular inflammation. In addition, Mallory hyaline bodies and pericellular fibrosis are observed surrounding the central veins. In 1999, Matteoni *et al.* reported a classification system that categorized NAFLD into four stages, type 1: steatosis alone, type 2: steatosis with lobular inflammation, type 3: steatosis with hepatocyte ballooning, type 4: type 3 plus either Mallory hyaline bodies or fibrosis (Figure 2) [2]. They found that type 1 and 2 are non-progressive and are now regarded as NAFL, while type 3 and 4 are progressive and are now regarded as NASH. From this result, hepatocyte degeneration is the key feature of progressive NAFLD. Recently, Younossi *et al.* reported the histological features indicative of long-term (median 146 months) liver-related mortality in 209 NAFLD patients [36]. They concluded that only fibrosis is an independent predictor of liver-related mortality. Patients with advanced fibrosis were predicted to succumb to liver related deaths in 12 years, however, an early diagnostic feature of later progression NASH remains to be identified. Although it is not statistically significant, the frequent existence of hepatocellular ballooning was found in 72% of the patients who died of liver related diseases by using multivariate analysis. Longer follow-up of these patients is required to determine the life-long natural course of this "modern disease".

Many scoring systems for the differentiation of NAFL and NASH have been reported, such as the FIB-4 score (age x AST / platelet x √ALT), AST to ALT ratio, BARD score (BMI > 28, AST / ALT > 0.8, diabetes), APRI score (AST to platelet ratio), Fibro test (includes total bilirubin, gamma GTP, alpha 2 macroglobulin, apolipoprotein A1, haptoglobulin), cytokeratin 18 (CK-18) fragments, hyaluronic acid, soluble Fas and Fas ligand, C-reactive protein, fibroblast growth factor-21, adiponectin, and desmosterol [37, 38]. Of these, measurement of CK-18 fragments have been found to be reliable with more than ten reports from different populations [24].

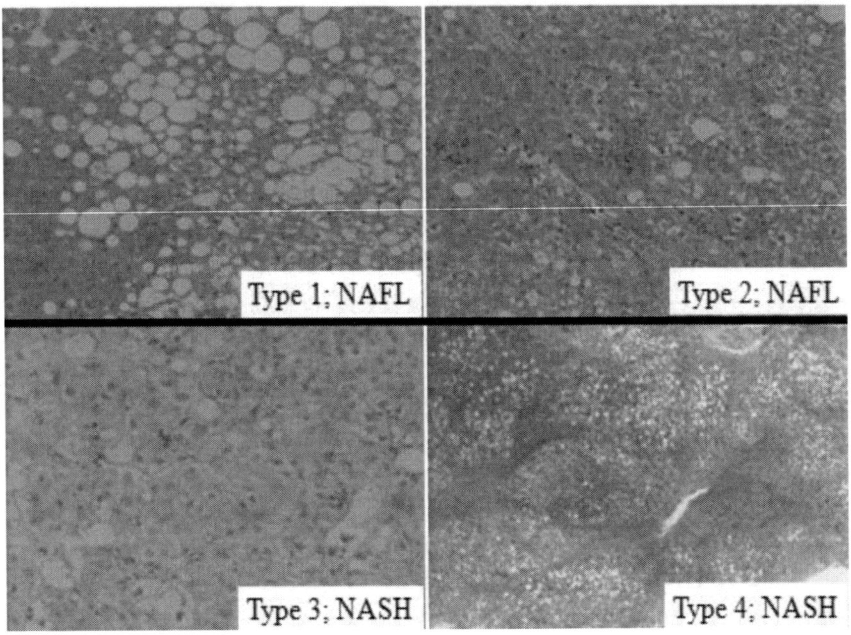

Figure 2. Histological findings of NAFLD. Liver biopsy specimens of NAFLD patients are shown. Images representative of the four classes of NAFLD reported by Matteoni *et al.* are shown. Type 1: steatosis alone (x100, H&E staining), Type 2: steatosis with lobular inflammation (x100, H&E staining), Type 3: steatosis with hepatocyte ballooning (x200, H&E staining), Type 4: type 3 plus either Mallory-Denk bodies or fibrosis (x40, Azan staining).

3. Pathogenesis of NAFLD

As the importance of superficially similar fat droplets observed in simple fatty liver and NASH hepatocytes differs in DGAT2 knockdown experiments, analyzing the molecular pathogenesis of NASH at the cellular level is quite important (Table 1).

Table 1. Molecular characteristics of NAFL and NASH

NAFL	Characteristics	NASH
Triglyceride	Hepatic lipid content	Free fatty acid
Mild	Insulin resistance	Severe
Macrophage	Infiltrating cells	Macrophage
CD8(+) T cell		CD4(+) T cell
		CD8(+) T cell
CCL-2	Chemokine, Cytokine	IL-6, IL-8

3.1. Adipokines

Adipokines are multifunctional secreted factors thought to be primarily derived from adipose tissue. The function of adipose tissue has been traditionally regarded simply as a location for storing energy, whereas it is now considered to be a complex organ that is involved in the control of many processes including metabolic, immunological, and inflammatory responses. Adiponectin is the most abundant adipose tissue-specific adipokine. Mature adipocytes mainly produce adiponectin in white adipose tissue and the levels of expression and secretion increase during adipocyte differentiation. Levels of adiponectin are significantly higher in females than in males, in whom serum androgens become more evident during puberty [39]. Adiponectin levels inversely correlate with visceral obesity and insulin resistance, while weight loss is an inducer of adiponectin synthesis. Proinflammatory adipokines such as TNF-α or IL-6 suppress adiponectin, which has anti-inflammatory, anti-atherogenic, and anti-diabetic properties [40]. Adipose tissue is also the main source of the adipokine leptin, the levels of which directly correlate with body fat mass and adipocyte size [41]. Leptin production is mainly regulated by food intake, and hormones related to eating, such as insulin, increase leptin secretion and vice versa. Leptin is also regulated by sex hormones, with testosterone inhibiting leptin production and ovarian sex steroids increasing production, resulting in higher levels in females. Proinflammatory endotoxin, IL-1, and TNF-α increase the secretion of leptin, which has central and peripheral effects. Leptin acts on hypothalamic cells, inhibits anabolic pathways, activates catabolic pathways, inhibits appetite, and stimulates energy expenditure. Peripheral leptin increases basal metabolism, regulates pancreatic cell function and insulin secretion, affects T cell generation, and the differentiation of T helper 1 cells in lymph nodes. Leptin-deficient (ob/ob) mice and leptin receptor-deficient (db/db) mice are severely obese and have increased pituitary and adrenal hormone production, hyperglycemia, elevated insulin, and decreased immune function.

Several groups have produced conflicting information on serum adiponectin levels, with reports of either unchanged or lower levels in NAFLD than in NASH [42-45]. A meta-analysis of 27 studies of 698 controls and 1545 patients with NAFLD found that serum adiponectin levels are low in NAFLD and very low in NASH [40]. Since adiponectin and leptin exert antagonistic effects on liver fibrogenesis and inflammation, the ratio of adiponectin to leptin might be a better marker with which to distinguish NASH from NAFLD. Levels of adiponectin receptor II are decreased in human liver biopsy specimens and in mouse models of NASH [46, 47]. However, since contradictory results have suggested that lower serum adiponectin levels induce a high expression of hepatic adiponectin receptor II as a compensatory response, the function of these novel adipokines and receptors requires further investigation [48, 49].

3.2. Endotoxin and Gut Derived Signals

Gut microbiota play many roles in NAFLD and NASH, hepatocellular carcinoma, cardiac function, vascular atherosclerosis, diabetes, and other conditions. Endotoxin or LPS produced by gut microbiota could be delivered to the liver via the portal vein, which raises the question of why such toxic materials flow into the portal vein through the intestinal barrier. Patients with biopsy-proven NAFLD have increased intestinal permeability with disrupted intercellular tight junctions in the intestine [50]. These abnormalities are related to increased bacterial overgrowth in the small intestine. Murine NAFLD models of bacterial overgrowth develop compositional changes and increased intestinal permeability with a concurrent reduction in the expression of tight junction proteins [51]. Plasma endotoxin levels are significantly higher in patients with NAFLD and in murine NASH models [50, 52]. High-fat diets are capable of increasing LPS concentrations two- to three-fold [53]. Proinflammatory inflammasomes induce inflammation in the liver of patients with NAFLD, but an inflammasome-deficient mouse model developed exacerbated hepatic steatosis and inflammation through the influx of TLR4 and TLR9 agonists into the portal vein [54]. The microbiota of these inflammasome-deficient mice differed from those of wild-type mice with NASH. Furthermore, co-housing inflammasome-deficient and wild-type mice resulted in intestinal inflammation and exacerbated hepatic steatosis in the wild-type mice. This finding suggests that altered microbiota in inflammasome-deficient mice could be transferred to healthy mice resulting in intestinal inflammation, increased permeability, and NAFLD. Gut and oral periodontal status correlates with the progression of liver disease [55]. Treating periodontitis could improve elevation of transaminases in NAFLD and, in fact, several probiotics that control gut microbiota improve NAFLD [56, 57, 58]. Studies using models of hepatocarcinogenesis have found that a high-fat diet increases levels of deoxycholic acid, a gut bacterial metabolite that damages DNA and exacerbates hepatocarcinogenesis [59]. Antibiotics could abrogate these effects. Therefore, gut microbiota are an important factor affecting not only NAFLD, but also obesity-related hepatocarcinogenesis.

3.3. Immune Mechanisms

It is accepted that immune responses and inflammation are involved in metabolic diseases such as diabetes mellitus, atherosclerosis, and NASH. Many obese people do not progress to metabolic abnormalities, and most patients with mild metabolic abnormalities do not progress to metabolic syndrome or further overt diabetes. Adipose tissue derived cytokines are accepted as promoters of metabolic disease progression. In obesity, excessive numbers of proinflammatory, M1-like macrophages accumulate in adipose tissue and liver [60]. Even in simple fatty liver, macrophage infiltration and the expression of the macrophage attractant chemokine CCL2 are significantly increased compared to controls [61]. Such inflammatory macrophages induce insulin resistance. Inflammatory pathways in macrophages are under the strict control of several transcription factors, such as NF-kB, AP1, the peroxisome proliferator-activated receptor (PPAR) family, LXR, and associated coactivating and coregulatory molecules. The major corepressor, nuclear receptor corepressor (NCoR) has an important role in metabolic processes. In the basal state, NCoR is resident on a number of inflammatory pathway genes maintaining them in the repressed state, while upon inflammatory pathway activation, NCoR dissociates from the promoter complex following activation of proinflammatory transcription factors such as NF-kB and AP1 [62]. However, macrophage and neutrophil specific NCoR knockout mice display an anti-inflammatory and insulin sensitive phenotype. This apparent opposite phenotype is due to derepression of LXR, which leads to the induction of the lipogenic pathway and increased biosynthesis of palmitoleic acid (POA) and omega 3 fatty acids, which exert local anti-inflammatory effects and insulin sensitization [63]. Macrophages are an important mediator of inflammation and insulin resistance, which are common characteristics of NAFLD. Neutrophils are also frequently found in NASH liver specimens and thought to have important pathological roles. Neutrophils secrete several proteases, including neutrophil elastase. Treatment of hepatocytes with neutrophil elastase causes cellular insulin resistance, while the deletion of neutrophil elastase improves insulin resistance and tissue inflammation [64]. In advanced NASH, CD4(+) and CD8(+) T cell infiltration, and inflammatory cytokines, such as IL-6 or IL-8, have been observed to increase [61]. Adaptive immune response linked CD8(+) T cells usually respond after innate immune cell reactions, however, obese adipose tissue could recruit CD8(+) T cells prior to macrophage accumulation [65]. Therefore, numerous types of inflammatory cells could gather in obesity and, accompanied by increased adipose tissue quantity, result in inflammation and insulin resistance.

Toll-like receptors are sensors of microbial and endogenous danger signals, and are expressed and activated in innate immune cells and liver parenchymal cells; furthermore, these receptors also contribute to the progression of NASH. Gut microbiota can release pathogen- or damage-associated molecular pattern molecules (PAMPs or DAMPs), which are TLR ligands, following the activation of downstream signals. Among the 10 TLRs (TLR1-10) identified in humans and 13 (TLR1-9, 11-13) identified in mammals, TLR2, TLR4, and TLR9 appear to be involved in the pathogenesis of NASH. TLR2 is a receptor for multiple bacterial glycolipids or lipoproteins adhering to the cell surface of monocytes, myeloid dendritic cells or mast cells. TLR4 recognizes LPS and is located on the surfaces of monocytes, myeloid dendritic cells, mast cells, B cells, and intestinal epithelium. The activation of this receptor by representative pathogens of gut microbiota has been studied in detail. Levels of free cholesterol (but not cholesterol ester) are increased in hepatic stellate cells (HSC) in NAFLD, resulting in increased TLR4 protein levels and fibrogenic HSC [66]. Kupffer cells phagocytize various cellular, viral, or bacterial components and are sources of hepatic pro-inflammatory and pro-fibrogenic cytokines. Cholesterol phagocytized by Kupffer cells can induce their activation along with TLR4 up-regulation [67]. TLR9 is located on the endoplasmic reticulum (ER) or endosomes of plasmacytoid dendritic cells or B cells and is regarded as a ligand for unmethylated CpG DNA particles released from bacteria. These molecules have been analyzed in several NAFLD and NASH models. Free cholesterol can accumulate in fibrogenic hepatic stellate cells, resulting in an increase in TLR4 through suppression of the endosomal-lysosomal degradation pathway of TLR4. The increased expression of TLR4 sensitizes cells to TGF-β-induced activation [66]. There is a notable amount of variation in the results of TLR studies in different NASH models. Currently, mouse models of NASH can reproduce only a portion of the pathogenesis. For example, the choline-deficient amino acid-defined (CDAA) diet mouse model develops steatosis with relatively mild hepatitis or fibrosis with obesity, whereas the methionine and choline deficient (MCD) diet mouse model develops steatosis with severe hepatitis and fibrosis without obesity. The CDAA diet improves NASH outcomes, whereas the MCDD diet worsens NASH outcomes in TLR2 knockout mice [68, 69]. This discrepancy might be valid, as NASH itself is heterogeneous and complex. TLR4 and TLR9 agonists might flow into the portal veins of inflammasome-deficient MCDD mice and thus exacerbate NASH [54]. Inflammasomes are multiprotein complexes composed of a nucleotide-binding domain and leucine-rich repeat protein 3 (NLRP3), apoptosis-associated speck-like protein containing CARD (ASC), and procaspase 1, and are DAMP or PAMP sensors. Inflammasome activation leads to the processing and secretion of proinflammatory cytokines IL1β and IL-18, whereas knockdown results in MCD NASH exacerbation. These perplexing findings indicate that the intestinal DAMP or PAMP barrier function that is disrupted in inflammasome knockout mice overcomes the anti-inflammatory effect in the liver and that TLR4 and TLR9 ligands flow into the portal vein where they stimulate NASH progression. TLR5 is the receptor for microbial flagellin. Mice that are deficient in TLR5 develop spontaneous colitis, profound metabolic syndrome with hyperphagia, hypertension and insulin resistance, as a result of intestinal microbiota transport [70, 71]. However, another study found no such pathologies in TLR5-deficient mice [72]. The authors concluded that this discrepancy might have been due to conditions in their animal facilities, an indication that environmental factors might be an important consideration for all such molecular functions.

3.4. Endoplasmic Reticulum (ER) Stress

Toxic lipids, such as free fatty acids, diacylglyceride, phospholipids, and free cholesterol, activate several cellular stress pathways [73]. One epicenter for this stress response is the ER, a membranous network that functions in the synthesis and assembly of secretory and membrane proteins to achieve their proper conformation. Proteins that are related to lipid metabolism are enriched, whereas protein synthesis and transport functions are down-regulated in obese hepatic ER [74]. The maintenance of ER function requires high concentrations of intra-ER Ca^{2+}, which is actively controlled by sarco(endo)plasmic reticulum Ca^{2+}-ATPase (SERCA). Free cholesterol accumulation triggers ER stress by altering the critical free cholesterol-to-phospholipid ratio of the ER membrane, which is needed to maintain its fluidity. Among the ER enzymes, SERCA ATPase is particularly sensitive to ER membrane cholesterol content, which can inhibit SERCA conformational changes and activity. Such changes induce a decrease in physiologically high intra-ER Ca^{2+} concentrations and results in impaired ER function and induction of ER stress. ER stress is one of the most important factors for disease progression in NASH, along with hepatocyte apoptosis and hepatic stellate cell (HSC) or Kupffer cell activation.

The chaperone response is blunted in obese mice as a result of dysfunctional X-Box binding protein 1 (XBP1), which is a master regulator of ER folding capacity [75].

Levels of liver-specific SERCA2b are reduced in obese mice with increased ER stress. Increasing SERCA2b levels reduces ER stress in the liver and increases glucose tolerance [76]. The SERCA inhibitor thapsigargin induces an increase in cytosolic calcium content accompanied by a decrease in ER calcium resulting in mitochondrial cytochrome C release and apoptosis in cultured primary rat hepatocytes [77]. Kupffer cells function as antigen presenting cells by displaying major histocompatibility complex (MHC) peptides on the cell surface. These peptides are processed by proteasomal degradation in the cytosol with subsequent translocation to the ER, where they undergo N-terminal trimming and loading onto MHC for export to the cell surface.

The ER also contains inflammatory cytokine-inducible factors, such as stimulator of interferon genes (STING), that induce type I interferon genes upon release [78]. ER stress induces the activation of such MHC-related and non-related pro-inflammatory responses. These results suggest that diseases could be treated with anti-ER stress agents as noted in the above mouse models. However, ER stress also sensitizes activated, but not quiescent, HSCs to apoptosis, resulting in the resolution of fibrosis [79]. Non-selective anti-ER stress treatment might be ineffective and treatment targeted towards ER stress should be designed to focus on the specific status of ER conditions.

3.5. Oxidative Stress

3.5.1. Oxidative Stress IN Hepatocytes

Oxidative stress is involved in the mechanisms of aging, carcinogenesis and atherosclerotic progression. Excessive oxidative stress induced by mitochondrial, peroxisomal and microsomal ROS in NASH results in apoptosis as well as damage to nuclear and mitochondrial DNA. Limited antioxidant defenses contribute to the processes of both NASH and hepatocarcinogenesis [80, 81]. Physiologically low levels of ROS are involved in necessary vital cellular processes, indicating that the balance of oxidative anti-oxidative responses is important [82]. An imbalance in the mitochondrial respiratory chain is the main source of ROS, superoxide ($O_2\cdot^-$), hydrogen peroxide (H_2O_2), and hydroxyl radicals ($\cdot OH$). Acute oxidative stress can be induced by several types of organ stress such as inflammation, organ infarction, shock and reperfusion injury. Oxidative reactions such as β-oxidation, tricarboxylic acid (TCA) cycle turn oxidized (NAD+ and FAD) into reduced (NADH and FADH2) cofactors (Figure 3). Subsequent oxidation of these reduced cofactors results in the delivery of electrons to the final acceptor, molecular oxygen, through the mitochondrial respiratory chain, namely the electron transport chain (ETC; complexes I, III, and IV). Under physiological conditions, most reactive, incompletely reduced forms of oxygen, such as superoxide ($O_2\cdot^-$), are detoxified into water by various anti-oxidant defenses and repair enzymes to maintain a relatively low steady state of oxidants.

The mitochondrial capacity to control the oxidative balance will collapse under continuous oxidative stress. Excess superoxide ($O_2\cdot^-$) could be generated within injured mitochondria through electron leakage and the resulting excess of superoxide ($O_2\cdot^-$) would be converted to hydrogen peroxide (H_2O_2) by superoxide dismutase (SOD). Glutathione peroxidase (GPx) or catalase can metabolize hydrogen peroxide (H_2O_2) to non-toxic H_2O, but the Fenton and/or Haber-Weiss reactions generate highly reactive toxic ROS, hydroxyl radical ($\cdot OH$). Oxidative stress produced by Fenton reactions is mediated by iron. Although its role in NASH is not fully understood, levels of iron are elevated in NASH, which is an inducer of oxidative stress, and reduced iron levels result in fair outcomes for patients with chronic liver diseases [83]. Elevated plasma citrate levels in NAFLD promote iron mediated hydroxyl radical formation *in vitro* [84]. Excess fatty acids and glucose result in the elevation of pyruvate and acetyl-CoA, which subsequently increase the formation of citrate and induces iron related oxidative stress. The reactivity of ROS dictates toxicity and high reactivity results in a short half-life and limited diffusion (half-life: $O_2\cdot^-$ and $\cdot OH$ 10^{-6} and 10^{-9} seconds, respectively) [82].

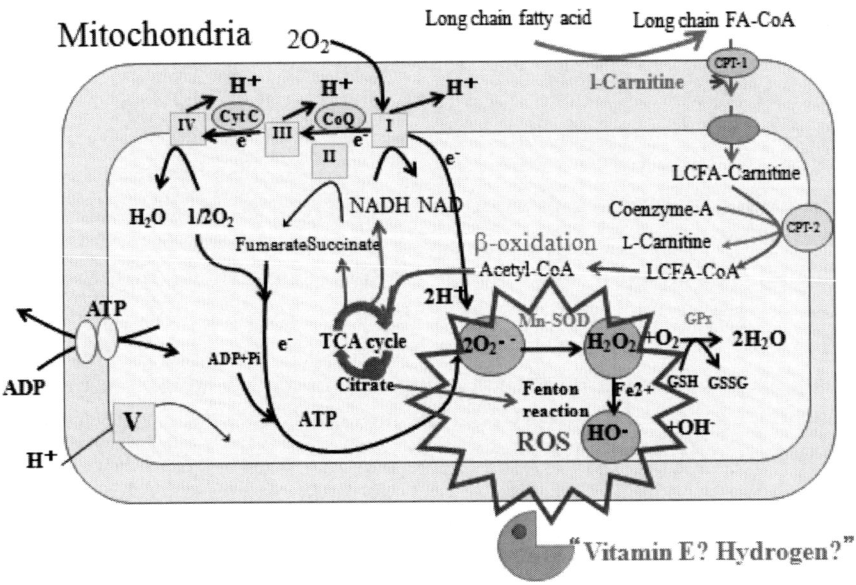

Figure 3. Oxidative stress production and treatment targets in mitochondria. High levels of plasma free fatty acids increase levels of hepatic free fatty acids. Long-chain fatty acids taken up by the mitochondria as complexes with L-carnitine are subsequently metabolized in the β-oxidation pathway. Under conditions of oxidative stress, oxidative reactions convert oxidized cofactors (NAD+ and FAD) into reduced cofactors (NADH and FADH2) and deliver electrons to the respiratory chain. An imbalance between increased delivery of electrons to the respiratory chain and decreased outflow from the respiratory chain causes the accumulation of electrons and ROS products. Anti-oxidant defenses, such as superoxide dismutase (SOD), glutathione peroxidase (GPx) or catalase, can metabolize hydrogen peroxide (H_2O_2) to non-toxic H_2O. However, the Fenton and/or Haber-Weiss reactions generate the highly reactive toxic ROS, hydroxyl radical ($\cdot OH$). The ROS scavenger vitamin E, the selective cytotoxic ROS scavenger hydrogen, and L-carnitine, which is a factor that supports mitochondrial function, might be good candidates for controlling mitochondrial oxidative stress.

However, ROS can attack polyunsaturated fatty acids (PUFA) and initiate lipid peroxidation resulting in the formation of aldehyde by-products such as 4-hydroxy-2-nonenal (4-HNE) or malondialdehyde (MDA) [85]. 4-HNE and MDA have longer half-lives than ROS and can diffuse into other sites and thus spread oxidative stress. Mitochondrial free fatty acid oxidation is not inhibited until respiration is severely impaired, resulting in accelerated ROS production until mitochondrial function is lost. Thus, mitochondria comprise the main source of oxidative stress, while ER stress can induce superoxide ($O_2\cdot^-$) and hydrogen peroxide (H_2O_2) with monooxygenases, such as cytochrome P450, and peroxisomes can induce cytosolic hydrogen peroxide (H_2O_2) associated with fatty acid oxidation [86, 87].

Mitochondrial antioxidant defenses are not powerful enough to control continuous oxidative stress, such as that imposed by long chain free fatty acids, thereby resulting in oxidative damage to the ETC complexes and mitochondrial DNA [88, 89]. The production of ROS in the inner mitochondrial membrane readily attacks proximal mitochondrial DNA. However, DNA repair mechanisms are thought to play a central role in preventing the accumulation of DNA mutations and in the maintenance of DNA stability [90]. Although both nuclear and mitochondrial DNA repair pathways exist, mitochondria are deficient in several of these [90]. Interestingly, estrogen can salvage one mitochondrial DNA repair pathway, namely the base excision repair (BER) pathway that becomes impaired in aged female rats, indicating that estrogen confers benefits to DNA pathways in females [91]. Because of these mitochondrial DNA deficiencies guarding against stress reactions, mitochondrial DNA are susceptible to oxidative stress-induced damage or mutation [92]. The accumulation of mitochondrial DNA mutations and damage results in ETC dysfunction and leads to increased ROS as well as further DNA damage. These oxidative stress chain reactions produce large amounts of ROS that affect other mitochondria or organelles and ultimately induce cellular apoptosis.

The mitochondrial proliferation and differentiation program might be impaired in NASH. The most important regulator of mitochondrial biogenesis is the transcription coactivator PPAR-γ-coactivator-1α (PGC-1α) [93], which coordinates the large number of genes required for mitochondrial biogenesis. The activity of PGC-1α is impaired in the fatty liver, which results in a decrease in mitochondrial biogenesis [94]. Decreases in mitochondrial DNA and mitochondrial DNA-encoded polypeptides are representative findings in NASH, whereas mitochondrial DNA content is increased in simple fatty liver [95]. The compensatory activation of mitochondrial DNA in simple fatty liver might help to protect the liver from inflammation and fibrosis, whereas a decrease in NASH induces progressive inflammation and fibrosis.

3.5.2. Oxidative Stress Affects Non-Hepatocyte Liver Cells

Among the non-parenchymal cells that comprise almost 40% of all liver cells, Kupffer cells and HSC play significant roles in the progression of chronic liver inflammation and fibrosis progression [85]. Excess fatty acid accumulation in hepatocytes induces oxidative stress in mitochondria as well as peroxisomes or microsomes. These cytotoxic ROS and lipid peroxidation products can diffuse into the extracellular space and affect Kupffer cells and HSCs. The cellular oxidative stress from hepatocytes and the direct uptake of free fatty acids or free cholesterol by Kupffer cells induce the activation of nuclear-factor κB, which induces the synthesis of TNF-α and several proinflammatory cytokines, including IL-6 or IL-8 [96]. Kupffer cells in patients with NASH produce TGF-β resulting in HSCs acquiring a fibrogenic myofibroblast-like phenotype.

Exposing primary HSC or HSC cell lines to hydrogen peroxide (H_2O_2) leads to an increase in the gene expression of ER chaperone BIP binding transmembrane proteins, such as inositol, requiring enzyme 1 (IRE1a), or activating transcription factor 4 (ATF4). ER stress in HSCs results in increased autophagy and HSC activation to fibrogenic status [97]. Among the most characteristic features of HSC activation is the loss of cytoplasmic lipid droplets, which are composed of retinyl esters and triglycerides [98]. Autophagy is present in all cell types and is up-regulated as an adaptive response under cellular stress to generate intracellular nutrients and energy. Autophagy is up-regulated in activated HSCs of mice with liver damage. However, cytoplasmic lipid droplets are maintained and remain quiescent in autophagy-defective HSCs, indicating that oxidative stress-induced ER stress and autophagy are key events in HSC activation [99].

4. Treatments for NASH

4.1. General Aspects

Since NAFLD and NASH have emerged as lifestyle-associated diseases, lifestyle intervention is an important approach to their treatment. Healthy and Western-style diets differentiate the risk for NAFLD progression [100]. It has been demonstrated that a one-year intensive lifestyle intervention comprised of dietary modifications and physical activity improved waist circumference, visceral abdominal fat, blood pressure, insulin resistance and hepatic fat content in obese patients [101]. Western-style diets, especially those that are rich in trans-fatty acids, are powerful inducers of obesity and NAFLD and need to be avoided [102]. However, it is mentally challenging to maintain compliance with therapeutic measures involving restrained food consumption and the relapse rate is high [103]. Patients that struggle to comply with dietary interventions may require pharmacological therapies.

4.2. Antioxidant Supplementation As a Standard Treatment for NASH

Vitamin E supplementation, the prototypical antioxidant drug treatment, has become a standard treatment for NASH [23]. Administration of vitamin E improves non-alcoholic fatty liver disease activity scores (NAS) for clinical and histological activity within two years, but also increases insulin resistance and plasma triglyceride levels [12]. However, recovery of fibrosis progression was not demonstrated [104]. Antioxidants do not affect body weight, waist circumference, and cholesterol metabolism.

Controversy surrounds antioxidant therapies because ROS have essential functions in living organisms. Balancing oxidative stress is the key issue, and bioavailability and bioaccessibility are needed to elicit an effective response to drugs. Antioxidants have effective chemical activities *in vitro*, however, demonstrating efficacy *in vivo* has resulted in many failures [105]. Many cerebrovascular studies have investigated the effects of vitamin E. A meta-analysis of the effect of vitamin E on stroke revealed a 10% reduction in ischemic stroke accompanied by a 22% increase in hemorrhagic stroke. Furthermore, antioxidants are likely to cause the progression of cancer [106]. Stem cell-like cancer cells have powerful antioxidative properties that confer protection against oxidative stress and are thus anti-apoptotic [107]. Oxidative stress in normal cells can induce the transition to cancer cells that are highly resistant to further oxidative stress. Inducing oxidative stress under these conditions is an approach that is being used in several cancer treatment trials [108]. However, this approach is likely to kill normal cells and induce new cancer development from normal cells. Thus, clinical circumstances must be considered when attempting to control oxidative stress. The clinical results of antioxidant therapies have not always been favorable [109]. It is not clear whether antioxidant therapies are too strong and result in destruction of necessary oxidative stress, or too weak, or have inappropriate distribution resulting in no favorable effects [110].

4.3. Second Line Treatment Options for NASH

Because obesity and insulin resistance are general characteristics of NASH, anti-insulin resistance treatment is commonly employed. From this viewpoint, the ability of insulin sensitizing anti-diabetic drugs to treat NASH has been analyzed. Among these treatments, use of the PPAR-α agonist pioglitazone and the biguanide metformin have produced clinical improvements in NASH. However, neither of these drugs improved liver histology. Metformin induced weight loss, whereas pioglitazone induced weight gain. Metformin has brought about histological improvements in the non-diabetic NASH mouse model [112], whereas human trials are usually too short to generate histological improvements. These anti-diabetic insulin-sensitizing drugs also have anti-oxidative effects. Glucagon like peptide-1 (GLP-1) and gastric inhibitory polypeptide (GIP) are both incretins, which are a group of gastrointestinal hormones that cause increased insulin release from pancreatic beta cells, and might be good targets for treating NASH. A GLP-1 receptor agonist analogue improved metabolic, biochemical and histopathological indices of NASH in mice via restoring hepatic lipid oxidation [113]. A GLP-1 receptor agonist in type 2 diabetic patients with NAFLD caused a reduction in intrahepatic lipid content that correlated with diabetic control [114]. Dipeptidylpeptidase-IV (DPP-IV) degrades GLP-1 and GIP and thus the inhibition of DPP-IV extends the half-life of endogenous GLP-1 and GIP and results in diabetic control. The long-term administration of a DPP-IV inhibitor has reduced liver fat content in animals with diet-induced hepatic steatosis and insulin resistance [115].

Pentoxifylline is a methylxanthine derivative that increases red blood cell flexibility, reduces blood viscosity and decreases platelet aggregation. In addition, pentoxifylline suppresses TNF-α gene expression and is a hydroxyl and peroxyl radical scavenger that produces anti-oxidative effects. A randomized controlled trial (RCT) has proven that pentoxifylline decreases free-radical-mediated lipid oxidation and improves clinical and histological NASH [116, 117].

Lipid-lowering drugs, such as statins, can also improve ALT and radiological steatosis in hyperlipidemic patients with NAFLD, but histological improvements are not evident [118]. Ezetimibe is a Niemann-Pick C1-like protein inhibitor that can reduce intestinal accumulation of free cholesterol. Ezetimibe has reduced histological NAS in mice and in 10 patients with NASH, indicating a need for larger RCT [119, 120].

Ursodeoxycholic acid (UDCA) is also reportedly effective in some instances. Several RCTs have found improvements in ALT, but not in liver histology even at high doses [121]. Combinations of UDCA and vitamin E have improved ALT and histological NAS scores [122].

Tumor necrosis factor (TNF)-α is one of the main cytokines involved in adipocyte-related inflammation. Powerful anti-TNF-α agents, such as infliximab (a chimeric monoclonal antibody), adalimumab (a human monoclonal antibody), and etanercept (a fusion protein), have severe side effects, including tuberculosis, that render them unacceptable as therapies for NAFLD [123]. The anti-oxidative agent pentoxifylline, described above, also has an anti-TNF-α function that is partially involved in the favorable effects on NASH.

A pro-inflammatory intestinal microbiome has been identified in mice and in patients with NASH. Probiotics, such as butyrate-producing agents, reduce hepatic triglyceride contents and induce anti-oxidative enzymes that help to prevent the progression of NASH to hepatocellular carcinoma [57].

4.4. Emerging Treatment Candidates for NASH

4.4.1. Hydrogen As an Antioxidant

Ohsawa *et al.* have found that molecular hydrogen has powerful antioxidant effects with unique features [18]. In cultured cells, H_2 scavenges hydroxyl radicals (·OH) but not superoxide ($O_2\cdot^-$) or hydrogen peroxide (H_2O_2) and nitric oxide (NO). Levels of intracellular superoxide are increased in cells cultured with the mitochondrial respiratory complex III inhibitor antimycin A, which are rapidly converted to hydrogen peroxide and hydroxyl radicals. Cultures with H_2 exhibit decreased cellular levels of hydroxyl radicals, but not superoxide, hydrogen peroxide or steady-state levels of NO. Furthermore, nuclear levels of hydroxyl radicals are notably decreased. As a result, H_2 prevents a decline in the mitochondrial membrane potential and decreases in cellular ATP synthesis, an effect that is consistent with effective antioxidants.

To defend cells against bacterial invasion, hydrogen peroxide is converted to hypochlorous acid by myeloperoxidase, indicating that oxidative stress is important for microbial defense [124]. Additionally, NO functions as a neurotransmitter that is essential for blood vessel dilation and protects against endothelial cell activation, suggesting that oxidative stress is important for vascular function [125]. Since treatment with H_2 specifically reduces levels of hydroxyl radicals, it does not interfere with the physiological roles of superoxide and hydrogen peroxide in cell survival.

Most hydrophilic compounds are retained at membranes and do not reach the cytoplasm, whereas hydrophobic compounds, such as vitamin E, cannot penetrate biomembranes in the absence of specific carriers or receptors. In contrast, H_2 can diffuse into cytoplasm and intracellular organelles, including the mitochondria, ER, and nucleus.

High concentrations of H_2 are not cytotoxic. Indeed, inhalation of high concentrations of H_2 in gas has been used to treat decompression sickness and arterial gas thrombosis after deep diving [126].

Several disease models have been utilized to determine the effects of molecular hydrogen (Table 2) [19, 80, 127-139]. Hydrogen can be ingested by gas inhalation or drinking HW. Hydrogen can be inhaled via hydrogen gas delivered through a ventilator with a facemask. Arterial blood H_2 levels increase depending on the concentration of inhaled H_2 gas. The diffusion of H_2 gas has been monitored in the rat myocardium [128] and H_2 concentration reportedly increased by two thirds in the ischemic compared to the non-ischemic myocardium. Furthermore, H_2-treated (inhalation) rats exhibited decreased ischemic volume one day after middle cerebral artery occlusion in a cerebral infarction model, with a greater volume difference observed one week after injury, indicating improvements in chronic ischemic stress [18]. The inhalation of H_2 reduces inflammatory responses associated with ventilator-induced lung injury at local and systemic levels via its antioxidant, anti-inflammatory and anti-apoptotic effects [140].

Drinking HW is a simple and facile method for daily administration at outpatient clinics, because up to 0.8 mM H_2 (1.6 ppm, wt/vol) can be dissolved in water under atmospheric pressure. Glass or plastic containers are unsuitable for conserving H_2 since it can rapidly penetrate these containers, whereas aluminum bags retain H_2 for long periods [110]. HW can be prepared by dissolving hydrogen gas in water under high pressure or by reacting magnesium metal with water. The detection of H_2 at μM levels in the liver and the fact that the H_2 concentration peaks five minutes after HW reaches the stomach suggests that the liver is a good H_2 target [132].

The effects of hydrogen on chemically-induced (by diethylnitrosamine (DEN), GalN/LPS, and CCl_4) liver damage have been studied in mouse models [135]. Hydrogen was given intraperitoneally every three hours after the administration of the chemicals. Serum levels of TNF-α and IL-6 and transaminase levels decreased in mice with GalN/LPS-induced acute liver injury after H_2 administration. Hepatic fibrogenesis markers such as collagen-α1 or α-smooth muscle actin (SMA) were reduced in mice with CCl_4-induced liver cirrhosis; while proliferative activities of hepatocytes were reduced in mice with DEN induced hepatic tumorigenesis.

Table 2. Effectiveness of hydrogen [Consider the alternative "Hydrogen therapy studies"]

	Hydrogen administration	Reference number
Disease model		
Cerebral ischemia reperfusion injury	Gas	[18]
Liver ischemia reperfusion injury	Gas	[127]
Myocardial ischemia reperfusion injury	Gas	[128]
Lung ischemia reperfusion injury	Gas	[129]
Parkinson's disease	Drinking water	[130]
Atherosclerosis	Drinking water	[131]
Obese diabetes	Drinking water	[132]
Type1 diabetes	Drinking water and intraperitoneal injection	[133]
Diabetic retinopathy	Intraperitoneal injection	[134]
Chemically-induced liver injury	Intraperitoneal injection	[135]
NASH	Drinking water	[80]
Cisplatin-induced renal injury	Gas and drinking water	[136]
Post renal transplant rejection	Drinking water	[19]
Intestinal transplant rejection	Graft storage in hydrogen bubbled preservative	[137]
Clinical trial		
Glucose and lipid metabolism type 2 diabetes	Drinking water	[138]
Metabolic syndrome	Drinking water	[139]

Kawai *et al.* have reported that drinking HW has favorable effects in NASH models [80]. Plasma transaminase levels, histological NAS, hepatic TNF-α, IL-6, fatty acid synthesis-related gene expression, and the oxidative stress biomarker 8-OHdG were decreased in the livers of MCD diet-induced NASH mice administered either HW or the anti-oxidant pioglitazone. Although the decrease in hepatic cholesterol was smaller in the group given HW, serum oxidative stress was reduced and antioxidant function was higher than that in the pioglitazone group. Another NASH mouse model was constructed to determine whether hydrogen affects hepatocarcinogenesis. The Stellic Research Institute created a mouse model of streptozotocin-induced NASH (STAM) that produces hepatocarcinogenesis within 16 weeks [141].

HW reduced the number and size of hepatocellular carcinoma lesions in this model compared with controls.

The consumption of HW might be effective in treating NASH through the reduction of hepatic oxidative stress, inflammation, and hepatocarcinogenesis. We emphasize that because the results of many investigations into the effects of antioxidants on diseases associated with oxidative stress have been disappointing, the effects of hydrogen may ultimately prove to be similar to the previously discouraging agents. More basic and clinical information on the potential benefits of this novel treatment option is required.

4.4.2. L-Carnitine As a Mitochondrial Function Modifier

L-carnitine is a substrate of carnitine-palmitoyltransferase 1 (CPT-1), the rate-limiting enzyme for mitochondrial β-oxidation that affects mitochondrial function. Any deficiency in the mitochondrial carnitine-dependent transport system results in curtailed fatty acid oxidation. L-carnitine supplementation reduces TNF-α, liver function parameters, plasma glucose levels and histological scores [111]. This is not an oxidative stress scavenger but it may stimulate mitochondrial function and the effect would be different from the antioxidants usually used. Additional data is needed to confirm the clinical effect.

4.4.3. Adiponectin Receptor Agonist

An adiponectin receptor agonist AdipoRon has been reported as a new treatment candidate for type 2 diabetes [142]. By screening small molecules in a chemical library, AdipoRon was found to bind both adiponectin receptors 1 and 2 (AdipoR 1 and AdipoR 2) and increase AMPK activation, PGC-1α expression and mitochondrial biogenesis. Administration of AdipoRon induced phosphorylation of AMPK in the muscle and liver of wild-type mice, but not in $Adipor1^{-/-}Adipor2^{-/-}$ mice, indicating that this small molecule activates AMPK in skeletal muscle and liver via AdipoR1 and AdipoR2. Orally administered AdipoRon resulted in significant reductions in fasting plasma glucose and insulin levels as well as glucose and insulin responses to an oral glucose tolerance test. Plasma concentrations of triglycerides and free fatty acids (FFA) were also reduced following AdipoRon administration. In skeletal muscles, AdipoRon increased the expression of genes involved in mitochondrial biogenesis and increased mitochondrial DNA content. In the liver, AdipoRon reduced triglyceride content, oxidative stress, and inflammatory cytokine expression, indicating that this therapy is likely to be effective in treating NASH.

Conclusion

Multiple parallel hits associated with current lifestyle factors are now believed to cause NASH. While the pathogenesis of cellular damage is heterogeneous, oxidative stress appears to be a key factor affecting the progression of NASH. Several approaches to control this complex process are often unsuccessful, because oxidative stress is also essential for life. However, new approaches that target mitochondria, such as L-carnitine, pentoxifylline, or molecular hydrogen, have produced favorable effects. Optimal treatment protocols and combinations of these therapies should be further investigated.

Conflict of Interest

The authors declare no conflict of interest.

References

[1] Pacifico L, Anania C, Martino F, Poggiogalle E, Chiarelli F, Arca M, et al. Management of metabolic syndrome in children and adolescents. *Nutr Metab Cardiovasc Dis.* 2011;21(6):455-66.

[2] Matteoni CA, Younossi ZM, Gramlich T, Boparai N, Liu YC, McCullough AJ. Nonalcoholic fatty liver disease: a spectrum of clinical and pathological severity. *Gastroenterology.* 1999;116(6):1413-9.

[3] Brunt EM, Kleiner DE, Wilson LA, Unalp A, Behling CE, Lavine JE, et al. Portal chronic inflammation in nonalcoholic fatty liver disease (NAFLD): a histologic marker of advanced NAFLD-Clinicopathologic correlations from the nonalcoholic steatohepatitis clinical research network. *Hepatology.* 2009;49(3):809-20.

[4] Yatsuji S, Hashimoto E, Tobari M, Taniai M, Tokushige K, Shiratori K. Clinical features and outcomes of cirrhosis due to non-alcoholic steatohepatitis compared with cirrhosis caused by chronic hepatitis C. *J Gastroenterol Hepatol.* 2009;24(2):248-54.

[5] Hatanaka K, Kudo M, Fukunaga T, Ueshima K, Chung H, Minami Y, et al. Clinical characteristics of NonBNonC- HCC: Comparison with HBV and HCV related HCC. *Intervirology.* 2007;50(1):24-31.

[6] Fassio E, Alvarez E, Dominguez N, Landeira G, Longo C. Natural history of nonalcoholic steatohepatitis: a longitudinal study of repeat liver biopsies. *Hepatology*. 2004;40(4):820-6.

[7] Ono M, Saibara T. Clinical features of nonalcoholic steatohepatitis in Japan: Evidence from the literature. J Gastroenterol. 2006;41(8):725-32.

[8] Gentile CL, Pagliassotti MJ. The role of fatty acids in the development and progression of nonalcoholic fatty liver disease. *J Nutr Biochem.* 2008;19(9):567-76.

[9] Csak T, Ganz M, Pespisa J, Kodys K, Dolganiuc A, Szabo G. Fatty acids and endotoxin activate inflammasome in hepatocytes which release danger signals to activate immune cells in steatohepatitis. *Hepatology*. 2011.

[10] Pessayre D. Role of mitochondria in non-alcoholic fatty liver disease. *J Gastroenterol Hepatol.* 2007;22 Suppl 1:S20-7.

[11] Novo E, Busletta C, Bonzo LV, Povero D, Paternostro C, Mareschi K, et al. Intracellular reactive oxygen species are required for directional migration of resident and bone marrow-derived hepatic pro-fibrogenic cells. *J Hepatol.* 2011;54(5):964-74.

[12] Sanyal AJ, Chalasani N, Kowdley KV, McCullough A, Diehl AM, Bass NM, et al. Pioglitazone, vitamin E, or placebo for nonalcoholic steatohepatitis. *N Engl J Med.* 2010;362(18):1675-85.

[13] Nan YM, Wu WJ, Fu N, Liang BL, Wang RQ, Li LX, et al. Antioxidants vitamin E and 1-aminobenzotriazole prevent experimental non-alcoholic steatohepatitis in mice. *Scand J Gastroenterol.* 2009;44(9):1121-31.

[14] Bugianesi E, Gentilcore E, Manini R, Natale S, Vanni E, Villanova N, et al. A randomized controlled trial of metformin versus vitamin E or prescriptive diet in nonalcoholic fatty liver disease. *Am J Gastroenterol.* 2005;100(5):1082-90.

[15] Musso G, Gambino R, Cassader M, Pagano G. A meta-analysis of randomized trials for the treatment of nonalcoholic fatty liver disease. *Hepatology*. 2010;52(1):79-104.

[16] Steinhubl SR. Why have antioxidants failed in clinical trials? *Am J Cardiol.* 2008;101(10A):14D-9D.

[17] Ohta S. Molecular hydrogen is a novel antioxidant to efficiently reduce oxidative stress with potential for the improvement of mitochondrial diseases. *Biochim Biophys Acta.* 2011.

[18] Ohsawa I, Ishikawa M, Takahashi K, Watanabe M, Nishimaki K, Yamagata K, et al. Hydrogen acts as a therapeutic antioxidant by

selectively reducing cytotoxic oxygen radicals. *Nature Medicine.* 2007;13(6):688-94.

[19] Cardinal JS, Zhan J, Wang Y, Sugimoto R, Tsung A, McCurry KR, et al. Oral hydrogen water prevents chronic allograft nephropathy in rats. *Kidney Int.* 2010;77(2):101-9.

[20] Day CP, James OF. Steatohepatitis: a tale of two "hits"? *Gastroenterology.* 1998;114(4):842-5.

[21] Li Z, Yang S, Lin H, Huang J, Watkins PA, Moser AB, et al. Probiotics and antibodies to TNF inhibit inflammatory activity and improve nonalcoholic fatty liver disease. *Hepatology.* 2003;37(2):343-50.

[22] Tiniakos DG, Vos MB, Brunt EM. Nonalcoholic fatty liver disease: pathology and pathogenesis. *Annu Rev Pathol.* 2010;5:145-71.

[23] Chalasani N, Younossi Z, Lavine JE, Diehl AM, Brunt EM, Cusi K, et al. The diagnosis and management of non-alcoholic fatty liver disease: practice guideline by the American Gastroenterological Association, American Association for the Study of Liver Diseases, and American College of Gastroenterology. *Gastroenterology.* 2012;142(7):1592-609.

[24] Machado MV, Cortez-Pinto H. Non-invasive diagnosis of non-alcoholic fatty liver disease. A critical appraisal. *J Hepatol.* 2013;58(5):1007-19.

[25] Romeo S, Kozlitina J, Xing C, Pertsemlidis A, Cox D, Pennacchio LA, et al. Genetic variation in PNPLA3 confers susceptibility to nonalcoholic fatty liver disease. *Nat Genet.* 2008;40(12):1461-5.

[26] Valenti L, Alisi A, Galmozzi E, Bartuli A, Del Menico B, Alterio A, et al. I148M patatin-like phospholipase domain-containing 3 gene variant and severity of pediatric nonalcoholic fatty liver disease. *Hepatology.* 2010;52(4):1274-80.

[27] Kawaguchi T, Sumida Y, Umemura A, Matsuo K, Takahashi M, Takamura T, et al. Genetic polymorphisms of the human PNPLA3 gene are strongly associated with severity of non-alcoholic fatty liver disease in Japanese. *PLoS One.* 2012;7(6):e38322.

[28] Qiao A, Liang J, Ke Y, Li C, Cui Y, Shen L, et al. Mouse patatin-like phospholipase domain-containing 3 influences systemic lipid and glucose homeostasis. *Hepatology.* 2011;54(2):509-21.

[29] Tsuneto A, Hida A, Sera N, Imaizumi M, Ichimaru S, Nakashima E, et al. Fatty liver incidence and predictive variables. *Hypertens Res.* 2010;33(6):638-43.

[30] Eguchi Y, Eguchi T, Mizuta T, Ide Y, Yasutake T, Iwakiri R, et al. Visceral fat accumulation and insulin resistance are important factors in nonalcoholic fatty liver disease. *J Gastroenterol.* 2006;41(5):462-9.

[31] Nobili V, Svegliati-Baroni G, Alisi A, Miele L, Valenti L, Vajro P. A 360-degree overview of paediatric NAFLD: Recent insights. *J Hepatol.* 2013;58(6):1218-29.
[32] Musso G, Cassader M, De Michieli F, Rosina F, Orlandi F, Gambino R. Nonalcoholic steatohepatitis versus steatosis: adipose tissue insulin resistance and dysfunctional response to fat ingestion predict liver injury and altered glucose and lipoprotein metabolism. *Hepatology.* 2012;56(3):933-42.
[33] Yamaguchi K, Yang L, McCall S, Huang J, Yu XX, Pandey SK, et al. Inhibiting triglyceride synthesis improves hepatic steatosis but exacerbates liver damage and fibrosis in obese mice with nonalcoholic steatohepatitis. *Hepatology.* 2007;45(6):1366-74.
[34] Yu XX, Murray SF, Pandey SK, Booten SL, Bao D, Song XZ, et al. Antisense oligonucleotide reduction of DGAT2 expression improves hepatic steatosis and hyperlipidemia in obese mice. *Hepatology.* 2005;42(2):362-71.
[35] Kantartzis K, Machicao F, Machann J, Schick F, Fritsche A, Haring HU, et al. The DGAT2 gene is a candidate for the dissociation between fatty liver and insulin resistance in humans. *Clin Sci* (Lond). 2009;116(6):531-7.
[36] Younossi ZM, Stepanova M, Rafiq N, Makhlouf H, Younoszai Z, Agrawal R, et al. Pathologic criteria for nonalcoholic steatohepatitis: interprotocol agreement and ability to predict liver-related mortality. *Hepatology.* 2011;53(6):1874-82.
[37] McPherson S, Stewart SF, Henderson E, Burt AD, Day CP. Simple non-invasive fibrosis scoring systems can reliably exclude advanced fibrosis in patients with non-alcoholic fatty liver disease. *Gut.* 2010;59(9):1265-9.
[38] Ratziu V, Massard J, Charlotte F, Messous D, Imbert-Bismut F, Bonyhay L, et al. Diagnostic value of biochemical markers (FibroTest-FibroSURE) for the prediction of liver fibrosis in patients with non-alcoholic fatty liver disease. *BMC Gastroenterol.* 2006;6:6.
[39] Corbetta S, Bulfamante G, Cortelazzi D, Barresi V, Cetin I, Mantovani G, et al. Adiponectin expression in human fetal tissues during mid- and late gestation. *J Clin Endocrinol Metab.* 2005;90(4):2397-402.
[40] Polyzos SA, Toulis KA, Goulis DG, Zavos C, Kountouras J. Serum total adiponectin in nonalcoholic fatty liver disease: a systematic review and meta-analysis. *Metabolism.* 2011;60(3):313-26.

[41] Carbone F, La Rocca C, Matarese G. Immunological functions of leptin and adiponectin. *Biochimie.* 2012;94(10):2082-8.

[42] Shimada M, Kawahara H, Ozaki K, Fukura M, Yano H, Tsuchishima M, et al. Usefulness of a combined evaluation of the serum adiponectin level, HOMA-IR, and serum type IV collagen 7S level to predict the early stage of nonalcoholic steatohepatitis. *Am J Gastroenterol.* 2007;102(9):1931-8.

[43] Younossi ZM, Jarrar M, Nugent C, Randhawa M, Afendy M, Stepanova M, et al. A novel diagnostic biomarker panel for obesity-related nonalcoholic steatohepatitis (NASH). *Obes Surg.* 2008;18(11):1430-7.

[44] Argentou M, Tiniakos DG, Karanikolas M, Melachrinou M, Makri MG, Kittas C, et al. Adipokine serum levels are related to liver histology in severely obese patients undergoing bariatric surgery. *Obes Surg.* 2009;19(9):1313-23.

[45] Lemoine M, Ratziu V, Kim M, Maachi M, Wendum D, Paye F, et al. Serum adipokine levels predictive of liver injury in non-alcoholic fatty liver disease. *Liver Int.* 2009;29(9):1431-8.

[46] Kaser S, Moschen A, Cayon A, Kaser A, Crespo J, Pons-Romero F, et al. Adiponectin and its receptors in non-alcoholic steatohepatitis. *Gut.* 2005;54(1):117-21.

[47] Matsunami T, Sato Y, Ariga S, Sato T, Shimomura T, Kashimura H, et al. Regulation of synthesis and oxidation of fatty acids by adiponectin receptors (AdipoR1/R2) and insulin receptor substrate isoforms (IRS-1/-2) of the liver in a nonalcoholic steatohepatitis animal model. *Metabolism.* 2011;60(6):805-14.

[48] Nannipieri M, Cecchetti F, Anselmino M, Mancini E, Marchetti G, Bonotti A, et al. Pattern of expression of adiponectin receptors in human liver and its relation to nonalcoholic steatohepatitis. *Obes Surg.* 2009;19(4):467-74.

[49] Ma H, Gomez V, Lu L, Yang X, Wu X, Xiao SY. Expression of adiponectin and its receptors in livers of morbidly obese patients with non-alcoholic fatty liver disease. *J Gastroenterol Hepatol.* 2009;24(2):233-7.

[50] Miele L, Valenza V, La Torre G, Montalto M, Cammarota G, Ricci R, et al. Increased intestinal permeability and tight junction alterations in nonalcoholic fatty liver disease. *Hepatology.* 2009;49(6):1877-87.

[51] Brun P, Castagliuolo I, Di Leo V, Buda A, Pinzani M, Palu G, et al. Increased intestinal permeability in obese mice: new evidence in the

pathogenesis of nonalcoholic steatohepatitis. *Am J Physiol Gastrointest Liver Physiol.* 2007;292(2):G518-25.

[52] Cani PD, Bibiloni R, Knauf C, Waget A, Neyrinck AM, Delzenne NM, et al. Changes in gut microbiota control metabolic endotoxemia-induced inflammation in high-fat diet-induced obesity and diabetes in mice. *Diabetes.* 2008;57(6):1470-81.

[53] Cani PD, Amar J, Iglesias MA, Poggi M, Knauf C, Bastelica D, et al. Metabolic endotoxemia initiates obesity and insulin resistance. *Diabetes.* 2007;56(7):1761-72.

[54] Henao-Mejia J, Elinav E, Jin C, Hao L, Mehal WZ, Strowig T, et al. Inflammasome-mediated dysbiosis regulates progression of NAFLD and obesity. *Nature.* 2012;482(7384):179-85.

[55] Tamaki N, Takaki A, Tomofuji T, Endo Y, Kasuyama K, Ekuni D, et al. Stage of hepatocellular carcinoma is associated with periodontitis. *J Clin Periodontol.* 2011;38(11):1015-20.

[56] Yoneda M, Naka S, Nakano K, Wada K, Endo H, Mawatari H, et al. Involvement of a periodontal pathogen, Porphyromonas gingivalis on the pathogenesis of non-alcoholic fatty liver disease. *BMC Gastroenterol.* 2012;12:16.

[57] Endo H, Niioka M, Kobayashi N, Tanaka M, Watanabe T. Butyrate-producing probiotics reduce nonalcoholic Fatty liver disease progression in rats: new insight into the probiotics for the gut-liver axis. *PLoS One.* 2013;8(5):e63388.

[58] Xu RY, Wan YP, Fang QY, Lu W, Cai W. Supplementation with probiotics modifies gut flora and attenuates liver fat accumulation in rat nonalcoholic fatty liver disease model. *J Clin Biochem Nutr.* 2012;50(1):72-7.

[59] Yoshimoto S, Loo TM, Atarashi K, Kanda H, Sato S, Oyadomari S, et al. Obesity-induced gut microbial metabolite promotes liver cancer through senescence secretome. *Nature.* 2013;499(7456):97-101.

[60] Lanthier N, Molendi-Coste O, Horsmans Y, van Rooijen N, Cani PD, Leclercq IA. Kupffer cell activation is a causal factor for hepatic insulin resistance. *Am J Physiol Gastrointest Liver Physiol.* 2010;298(1):G107-16.

[61] Gadd VL, Skoien R, Powell EE, Fagan KJ, Winterford C, Horsfall L, et al. The portal inflammatory infiltrate and ductular reaction in human non-alcoholic fatty liver disease. *Hepatology.* 2013.

[62] Glass CK, Saijo K. Nuclear receptor transrepression pathways that regulate inflammation in macrophages and T cells. *Nat Rev Immunol.* 2010;10(5):365-76.

[63] Li P, Spann NJ, Kaikkonen MU, Lu M, Oh da Y, Fox JN, et al. NCoR repression of LXRs restricts macrophage biosynthesis of insulin-sensitizing omega 3 fatty acids. *Cell.* 2013;155(1):200-14.

[64] Talukdar S, Oh da Y, Bandyopadhyay G, Li D, Xu J, McNelis J, et al. Neutrophils mediate insulin resistance in mice fed a high-fat diet through secreted elastase. *Nat Med.* 2012;18(9):1407-12.

[65] Nishimura S, Manabe I, Nagasaki M, Eto K, Yamashita H, Ohsugi M, et al. CD8+ effector T cells contribute to macrophage recruitment and adipose tissue inflammation in obesity. *Nat Med.* 2009;15(8):914-20.

[66] Tomita K, Teratani T, Suzuki T, Shimizu M, Sato H, Narimatsu K, et al. Free cholesterol accumulation in hepatic stellate cells: Mechanism of liver fibrosis aggravation in nonalcoholic steatohepatitis in mice. *Hepatology.* 2013.

[67] Leroux A, Ferrere G, Godie V, Cailleux F, Renoud ML, Gaudin F, et al. Toxic lipids stored by Kupffer cells correlates with their pro-inflammatory phenotype at an early stage of steatohepatitis. *J Hepatol.* 2012;57(1):141-9.

[68] Miura K, Yang L, van Rooijen N, Brenner DA, Ohnishi H, Seki E. Toll-like receptor 2 and palmitic acid cooperatively contribute to the development of nonalcoholic steatohepatitis through inflammasome activation in mice. *Hepatology.* 2013;57(2):577-89.

[69] Rivera CA, Gaskin L, Allman M, Pang J, Brady K, Adegboyega P, et al. Toll-like receptor-2 deficiency enhances non-alcoholic steatohepatitis. *BMC Gastroenterol.* 2010;10:52.

[70] Vijay-Kumar M, Sanders CJ, Taylor RT, Kumar A, Aitken JD, Sitaraman SV, et al. Deletion of TLR5 results in spontaneous colitis in mice. *J Clin Invest.* 2007;117(12):3909-21.

[71] Vijay-Kumar M, Aitken JD, Carvalho FA, Cullender TC, Mwangi S, Srinivasan S, et al. Metabolic syndrome and altered gut microbiota in mice lacking Toll-like receptor 5. *Science.* 2010;328(5975):228-31.

[72] Letran SE, Lee SJ, Atif SM, Flores-Langarica A, Uematsu S, Akira S, et al. TLR5-deficient mice lack basal inflammatory and metabolic defects but exhibit impaired CD4 T cell responses to a flagellated pathogen. *J Immunol.* 2011;186(9):5406-12.

[73] Musso G, Gambino R, Cassader M. Cholesterol metabolism and the pathogenesis of non-alcoholic steatohepatitis. *Prog Lipid Res.* 2013;52(1):175-91.

[74] Fu S, Yang L, Li P, Hofmann O, Dicker L, Hide W, et al. Aberrant lipid metabolism disrupts calcium homeostasis causing liver endoplasmic reticulum stress in obesity. *Nature.* 2011;473(7348):528-31.

[75] Park SW, Zhou Y, Lee J, Lu A, Sun C, Chung J, et al. The regulatory subunits of PI3K, p85alpha and p85beta, interact with XBP-1 and increase its nuclear translocation. *Nat Med.* 2010;16(4):429-37.

[76] Park SW, Zhou Y, Lee J, Ozcan U. Sarco(endo)plasmic reticulum Ca2+-ATPase 2b is a major regulator of endoplasmic reticulum stress and glucose homeostasis in obesity. *Proc Natl Acad Sci U S A.* 2010;107(45):19320-5.

[77] Canova NK, Kmonickova E, Martinek J, Zidek Z, Farghali H. Thapsigargin, a selective inhibitor of sarco-endoplasmic reticulum Ca2+ -ATPases, modulates nitric oxide production and cell death of primary rat hepatocytes in culture. *Cell Biol Toxicol.* 2007;23(5):337-54.

[78] Barker JR, Koestler BJ, Carpenter VK, Burdette DL, Waters CM, Vance RE, et al. STING-dependent recognition of cyclic di-AMP mediates type I interferon responses during Chlamydia trachomatis infection. *MBio.* 2013;4(3):e00018-13.

[79] De Minicis S, Candelaresi C, Agostinelli L, Taffetani S, Saccomanno S, Rychlicki C, et al. Endoplasmic Reticulum stress induces hepatic stellate cell apoptosis and contributes to fibrosis resolution. *Liver Int.* 2012;32(10):1574-84.

[80] Kawai D, Takaki A, Nakatsuka A, Wada J, Tamaki N, Yasunaka T, et al. Hydrogen-rich water prevents progression of nonalcoholic steatohepatitis and accompanying hepatocarcinogenesis in mice. *Hepatology.* 2012;56(3):912-21.

[81] Bugianesi E. Non-alcoholic steatohepatitis and cancer. *Clin Liver Dis.* 2007;11(1):191-207, x-xi.

[82] Mittler R, Vanderauwera S, Suzuki N, Miller G, Tognetti VB, Vandepoele K, et al. ROS signaling: the new wave? *Trends Plant Sci.* 2011;16(6):300-9.

[83] Nelson JE, Wilson L, Brunt EM, Yeh MM, Kleiner DE, Unalp-Arida A, et al. Relationship between the pattern of hepatic iron deposition and histological severity in nonalcoholic fatty liver disease. *Hepatology.* 2011;53(2):448-57.

[84] van de Wier B, Balk JM, Haenen GR, Giamouridis D, Bakker JA, Bast BC, et al. Elevated citrate levels in non-alcoholic fatty liver disease: the potential of citrate to promote radical production. *FEBS Lett.* 2013;587(15):2461-6.
[85] Rolo AP, Teodoro JS, Palmeira CM. Role of oxidative stress in the pathogenesis of nonalcoholic steatohepatitis. *Free Radic Biol Med.* 2012;52(1):59-69.
[86] Fritz R, Bol J, Hebling U, Angermuller S, Volkl A, Fahimi HD, et al. Compartment-dependent management of H(2)O(2) by peroxisomes. Free *Radic Biol Med.* 2007;42(7):1119-29.
[87] Zangar RC, Davydov DR, Verma S. Mechanisms that regulate production of reactive oxygen species by cytochrome P450. *Toxicol Appl Pharmacol.* 2004;199(3):316-31.
[88] Rachek LI, Yuzefovych LV, Ledoux SP, Julie NL, Wilson GL. Troglitazone, but not rosiglitazone, damages mitochondrial DNA and induces mitochondrial dysfunction and cell death in human hepatocytes. *Toxicol Appl Pharmacol.* 2009;240(3):348-54.
[89] Ricci C, Pastukh V, Leonard J, Turrens J, Wilson G, Schaffer D, et al. Mitochondrial DNA damage triggers mitochondrial-superoxide generation and apoptosis. *Am J Physiol Cell Physiol.* 2008;294(2):C413-22.
[90] Gredilla R, Bohr VA, Stevnsner T. Mitochondrial DNA repair and association with aging--an update. *Exp Gerontol.* 2010;45(7-8):478-88.
[91] Leclere R, Torregrosa-Munumer R, Kireev R, Garcia C, Vara E, Tresguerres JA, et al. Effect of estrogens on base excision repair in brain and liver mitochondria of aged female rats. *Biogerontology.* 2013.
[92] Murphy MP. How mitochondria produce reactive oxygen species. *Biochem J.* 2009;417(1):1-13.
[93] Scarpulla RC. Metabolic control of mitochondrial biogenesis through the PGC-1 family regulatory network. *Biochim Biophys Acta.* 2011;1813(7):1269-78.
[94] Aharoni-Simon M, Hann-Obercyger M, Pen S, Madar Z, Tirosh O. Fatty liver is associated with impaired activity of PPARgamma-coactivator 1alpha (PGC1alpha) and mitochondrial biogenesis in mice. *Lab Invest.* 2011;91(7):1018-28.
[95] Chiappini F, Barrier A, Saffroy R, Domart MC, Dagues N, Azoulay D, et al. Exploration of global gene expression in human liver steatosis by high-density oligonucleotide microarray. *Lab Invest.* 2006;86(2):154-65.

[96] Hui JM, Hodge A, Farrell GC, Kench JG, Kriketos A, George J. Beyond insulin resistance in NASH: TNF-alpha or adiponectin? *Hepatology.* 2004;40(1):46-54.

[97] Hernandez-Gea V, Hilscher M, Rozenfeld R, Lim MP, Nieto N, Werner S, et al. Endoplasmic reticulum stress induces fibrogenic activity in hepatic stellate cells through autophagy. *J Hepatol.* 2013;59(1):98-104.

[98] Blaner WS, O'Byrne SM, Wongsiriroj N, Kluwe J, D'Ambrosio DM, Jiang H, et al. Hepatic stellate cell lipid droplets: a specialized lipid droplet for retinoid storage. *Biochim Biophys Acta.* 2009;1791(6):467-73.

[99] Hernandez-Gea V, Ghiassi-Nejad Z, Rozenfeld R, Gordon R, Fiel MI, Yue Z, et al. Autophagy releases lipid that promotes fibrogenesis by activated hepatic stellate cells in mice and in human tissues. *Gastroenterology.* 2012;142(4):938-46.

[100] Oddy WH, Herbison CE, Jacoby P, Ambrosini GL, O'Sullivan TA, Ayonrinde OT, et al. The Western dietary pattern is prospectively associated with nonalcoholic fatty liver disease in adolescence. *Am J Gastroenterol.* 2013;108(5):778-85.

[101] Goodpaster BH, Delany JP, Otto AD, Kuller L, Vockley J, South-Paul JE, et al. Effects of diet and physical activity interventions on weight loss and cardiometabolic risk factors in severely obese adults: a randomized trial. *JAMA.* 2010;304(16):1795-802.

[102] Neuschwander-Tetri BA, Ford DA, Acharya S, Gilkey G, Basaranoglu M, Tetri LH, et al. Dietary trans-fatty acid induced NASH is normalized following loss of trans-fatty acids from hepatic lipid pools. *Lipids.* 2012;47(10):941-50.

[103] Soetens B, Braet C, Moens E. Thought suppression in obese and non-obese restrained eaters: piece of cake or forbidden fruit? *Eur Eat Disord Rev.* 2008;16(1):67-76.

[104] Hoofnagle JH, Van Natta ML, Kleiner DE, Clark JM, Kowdley KV, Loomba R, et al. Vitamin E and changes in serum alanine aminotransferase levels in patients with non-alcoholic steatohepatitis. *Aliment Pharmacol Ther.* 2013;38(2):134-43.

[105] Bast A, Haenen GR. Ten misconceptions about antioxidants. *Trends Pharmacol Sci.* 2013;34(8):430-6.

[106] Watson J. Oxidants, antioxidants and the current incurability of metastatic cancers. *Open Biol.* 2013;3(1):120144.

[107] Yae T, Tsuchihashi K, Ishimoto T, Motohara T, Yoshikawa M, Yoshida GJ, et al. Alternative splicing of CD44 mRNA by ESRP1 enhances lung colonization of metastatic cancer cell. *Nat Commun.* 2012;3:883.

[108] Trachootham D, Alexandre J, Huang P. Targeting cancer cells by ROS-mediated mechanisms: a radical therapeutic approach? *Nat Rev Drug Discov.* 2009;8(7):579-91.

[109] Hackam DG. Review: antioxidant supplements for primary and secondary prevention do not decrease mortality. *ACP J Club.* 2007;147(1):4.

[110] Ohta S. Recent progress toward hydrogen medicine: potential of molecular hydrogen for preventive and therapeutic applications. *Curr Pharm Des.* 2011;17(22):2241-52.

[111] Malaguarnera M, Gargante MP, Russo C, Antic T, Vacante M, Avitabile T, et al. L-carnitine supplementation to diet: a new tool in treatment of nonalcoholic steatohepatitis--a randomized and controlled clinical trial. *Am J Gastroenterol. 2010*;105(6):1338-45.

[112] Musso G, Cassader M, Rosina F, Gambino R. Impact of current treatments on liver disease, glucose metabolism and cardiovascular risk in non-alcoholic fatty liver disease (NAFLD): a systematic review and meta-analysis of randomised trials. *Diabetologia.* 2012;55(4):885-904.

[113] Svegliati-Baroni G, Saccomanno S, Rychlicki C, Agostinelli L, De Minicis S, Candelaresi C, et al. Glucagon-like peptide-1 receptor activation stimulates hepatic lipid oxidation and restores hepatic signalling alteration induced by a high-fat diet in nonalcoholic steatohepatitis. *Liver Int.* 2011;31(9):1285-97.

[114] Cuthbertson DJ, Irwin A, Gardner CJ, Daousi C, Purewal T, Furlong N, et al. Improved glycaemia correlates with liver fat reduction in obese, type 2 diabetes, patients given glucagon-like peptide-1 (GLP-1) receptor agonists. *PLoS One.* 2012;7(12):e50117.

[115] Kern M, Kloting N, Niessen HG, Thomas L, Stiller D, Mark M, et al. Linagliptin improves insulin sensitivity and hepatic steatosis in diet-induced obesity. *PLoS One.* 2012;7(6):e38744.

[116] Zein CO, Lopez R, Fu X, Kirwan JP, Yerian LM, McCullough AJ, et al. Pentoxifylline decreases oxidized lipid products in nonalcoholic steatohepatitis: new evidence on the potential therapeutic mechanism. *Hepatology.* 2012;56(4):1291-9.

[117] Zein CO, Yerian LM, Gogate P, Lopez R, Kirwan JP, Feldstein AE, et al. Pentoxifylline improves nonalcoholic steatohepatitis: a randomized placebo-controlled trial. *Hepatology.* 2011;54(5):1610-9.

[118] Nelson A, Torres DM, Morgan AE, Fincke C, Harrison SA. A pilot study using simvastatin in the treatment of nonalcoholic steatohepatitis: A randomized placebo-controlled trial. *J Clin Gastroenterol.* 2009;43(10):990-4.

[119] Deushi M, Nomura M, Kawakami A, Haraguchi M, Ito M, Okazaki M, et al. Ezetimibe improves liver steatosis and insulin resistance in obese rat model of metabolic syndrome. *FEBS Lett.* 2007;581(29):5664-70.

[120] Yoneda M, Fujita K, Nozaki Y, Endo H, Takahashi H, Hosono K, et al. Efficacy of ezetimibe for the treatment of non-alcoholic steatohepatitis: An open-label, pilot study. *Hepatol Res.* 2010;40(6):613-21.

[121] Leuschner UF, Lindenthal B, Herrmann G, Arnold JC, Rossle M, Cordes HJ, et al. High-dose ursodeoxycholic acid therapy for nonalcoholic steatohepatitis: a double-blind, randomized, placebo-controlled trial. *Hepatology.* 2010;52(2):472-9.

[122] Pietu F, Guillaud O, Walter T, Vallin M, Hervieu V, Scoazec JY, et al. Ursodeoxycholic acid with vitamin E in patients with nonalcoholic steatohepatitis: long-term results. *Clin Res Hepatol Gastroenterol.* 2012;36(2):146-55.

[123] Ford AC, Peyrin-Biroulet L. Opportunistic Infections With Anti-Tumor Necrosis Factor-alpha Therapy in Inflammatory Bowel Disease: Meta-Analysis of Randomized Controlled Trials. *Am J Gastroenterol.* 2013.

[124] Winterbourn CC. Biological reactivity and biomarkers of the neutrophil oxidant, hypochlorous acid. *Toxicology.* 2002;181-182:223-7.

[125] Liao JK. Linking endothelial dysfunction with endothelial cell activation. *J Clin Invest.* 2013;123(2):540-1.

[126] Fontanari P, Badier M, Guillot C, Tomei C, Burnet H, Gardette B, et al. Changes in maximal performance of inspiratory and skeletal muscles during and after the 7.1-MPa Hydra 10 record human dive. *Eur J Appl Physiol.* 2000;81(4):325-8.

[127] Fukuda KI, Asoh S, Ishikawa M, Yamamoto Y, Ohsawa I, Ohta S. Inhalation of hydrogen gas suppresses hepatic injury caused by ischemia/reperfusion through reducing oxidative stress. *Biochem Bioph Res Co.* 2007;361(3):670-4.

[128] Hayashida K, Sano M, Ohsawa I, Shinmura K, Tamaki K, Kimura K, et al. Inhalation of hydrogen gas reduces infarct size in the rat model of myocardial ischemia-reperfusion injury. *Biochem Biophys Res Commun.* 2008;373(1):30-5.

[129] Kawamura T, Huang CS, Tochigi N, Lee S, Shigemura N, Billiar TR, et al. Inhaled hydrogen gas therapy for prevention of lung transplant-

induced ischemia/reperfusion injury in rats. *Transplantation.* 2010;90(12):1344-51.
[130] Fu Y, Ito M, Fujita Y, Ichihara M, Masuda A, Suzuki Y, et al. Molecular hydrogen is protective against 6-hydroxydopamine-induced nigrostriatal degeneration in a rat model of Parkinson's disease. *Neurosci Lett.* 2009;453(2):81-5.
[131] Ohsawa I, Nishimaki K, Yamagata K, Ishikawa M, Ohta S. Consumption of hydrogen water prevents atherosclerosis in apolipoprotein E knockout mice. *Biochem Biophys Res Commun.* 2008;377(4):1195-8.
[132] Kamimura N, Nishimaki K, Ohsawa I, Ohta S. Molecular hydrogen improves obesity and diabetes by inducing hepatic FGF21 and stimulating energy metabolism in db/db mice. *Obesity* (Silver Spring). 2011;19(7):1396-403.
[133] Amitani H, Asakawa A, Cheng K, Amitani M, Kaimoto K, Nakano M, et al. Hydrogen improves glycemic control in type1 diabetic animal model by promoting glucose uptake into skeletal muscle. *PLoS One.* 2013;8(1):e53913.
[134] Feng Y, Wang R, Xu J, Sun J, Xu T, Gu Q, et al. Hydrogen-rich saline prevents early neurovascular dysfunction resulting from inhibition of oxidative stress in STZ-diabetic rats. *Curr Eye Res.* 2013;38(3):396-404.
[135] Sun H, Chen L, Zhou W, Hu L, Li L, Tu Q, et al. The protective role of hydrogen-rich saline in experimental liver injury in mice. *J Hepatol.* 2011;54(3):471-80.
[136] Nakashima-Kamimura N, Mori T, Ohsawa I, Asoh S, Ohta S. Molecular hydrogen alleviates nephrotoxicity induced by an anti-cancer drug cisplatin without compromising anti-tumor activity in mice. *Cancer Chemother Pharmacol.* 2009;64(4):753-61.
[137] Buchholz BM, Kaczorowski DJ, Sugimoto R, Yang R, Wang Y, Billiar TR, et al. Hydrogen inhalation ameliorates oxidative stress in transplantation induced intestinal graft injury. *Am J Transplant.* 2008;8(10):2015-24.
[138] Kajiyama S, Hasegawa G, Asano M, Hosoda H, Fukui M, Nakamura N, et al. Supplementation of hydrogen-rich water improves lipid and glucose metabolism in patients with type 2 diabetes or impaired glucose tolerance. *Nutr Res.* 2008;28(3):137-43.
[139] Nakao A, Toyoda Y, Sharma P, Evans M, Guthrie N. Effectiveness of hydrogen rich water on antioxidant status of subjects with potential

metabolic syndrome - an open label pilot study. *J Clin Biochem Nutr.* 2010;46(2):140-9.

[140] Huang CS, Kawamura T, Lee S, Tochigi N, Shigemura N, Buchholz BM, et al. Hydrogen inhalation ameliorates ventilator-induced lung injury. *Crit Care.* 2010;14(6):R234.

[141] Fujii M, Shibazaki Y, Wakamatsu K, Honda Y, Kawauchi Y, Suzuki K, et al. A murine model for non-alcoholic steatohepatitis showing evidence of association between diabetes and hepatocellular carcinoma. *Med Mol Morphol.* 2013.

[142] Okada-Iwabu M, Yamauchi T, Iwabu M, Honma T, Hamagami K, Matsuda K, et al. A small-molecule AdipoR agonist for type 2 diabetes and short life in obesity. *Nature.* 2013;503(7477):493-9.

In: Oxidative Stress
Editor: Cassidy Croft

ISBN: 978-1-63117-578-7

Chapter 6

Current Approaches to Redox Therapies in Multiple Sclerosis

Elżbieta Miller[1, 2], Jarosław Jakubik[3] and B. Wachowicz[4]
[1]Department of Physical Medicine, Medical University of Lodz, Poland
[2]Neurorehabilitation Ward, III General Hospital in Lodz, Lodz, Poland
[3]Department of Surgical Oncology Medical University of Lodz, Poland
[4]Faculty of Biology and Environmental Protection,
Department of General Biochemistry, University of Lodz,
Lodz, Poland

Abstract

Multiple sclerosis (MS) is a heterogeneous disease with the different and unpredictable clinical courses. Investigations of MS are very wide due to its complex pathogenesis that involves several components: autoimmune, inflammatory, demyelinisation, neurodegeneration and oxidative stress. The development of effective antioxidative therapy for MS patients is intricated by the heterogenity of pathophysiological mechanisms involved. There is a strong need for further research in this field especially in progressive subtypes of MS that have no effective pharmacological treatment. In this review we try to focus on the oxidative stress not only as a specific biochemical process of this complex disease but also as a potential target of the therapies in MS, therefore some exogenous compounds have been proposed as such approach to MS treatment.

The redox therapeutic approach can target: degenerative, inflammatory/autoimmune and neurodegenerative components. Redox therapy should not be applied uniformly, and must be developed to target specific mechanisms. The results of redox studies could lead to new therapies in MS, as well as to knowledge about life style adjustments that would contribute to well being of the MS patients.

Introduction

Multiple sclerosis (MS) is a heterogenous disease of the central nervous system (CNS) and results in variety of clinical presentation. The main histopathological feature of MS is the focal demyelinisation of CNS [1]. The course of the disease is unpredictable and characterized by recurrent neurological relapses and/or progression. The prevalence of MS is 1 per 1000 (1.5 female to 1 man) [2]. The early phase of MS is characterized by immune-mediated responses with microglial activation and massive cellular infiltration connected mainly with inflammation of white matter in patches named plaques (destruction of myelin) [1, 3, 4]. There is a wide range of clinical symptoms in MS different at the early and progressive stage. Early MS symptoms are vision impaired due to optic neuritis connected with inflammation of optic nerve and sensation deficits such as burning or prickling [2]. The progressive form of MS presents paresis/paralysis (mainly lower extremities), spasticy, ataxia, fatigue and incontinence, tremor, difficulty of speaking, loss of bladder control and constipation) depending on where in CNS the demyelinisation and axonal loss have occurred [1, 2]. Cognitive impairment is very characteristic for MS, first of all memory and concentration difficulties. Clinical symptoms are the basis for diagnosis. The emergence of neurological symptoms is named relapse [2]. It must be more than one neurological exacerbation (relapse) with dissemination in time and space to diagnosed MS [5]. Other diagnostic methods including computerized tomography scan (CTS), magnetic resonance imaging (MRI), cerebrospinal fluid analyses for immunoglobulin and oligoclonal banding only confirm clinical observations. Four subtypes of MS exist: relapsing-remitting (RRMS), secondary progressive (SPMS) and primary progressive (PPMS) disorders [6].

The most usual subtype is relapsing-remitting course (RRMS) with frequent intervals of exacerbations with complete or partial recovery followed by periods of remission. RRMS is characterized mainly by multifocal inflammation. The brain-blood barrier damage is a cardinal feature of active MS allowing to the influx of inflammatory cells [2].

At the age of about 40 years (about 10-20 disease duration) MS takes secondary progressive course (SPMS) characterized by accumulation of irreversible neurological deficits with no relapses and new “plaques” in MRI. SPMS is dominated by neuronal and axonal degeneration and CNS atrophy with slow progression of neurological symptoms [4].

About 20% of MS patients have primary progressive form of disease (PPMS) with less inflammation and earlier axonal loss. Progressive forms of MS (PPMS; SPMS) are mainly dominated by neuroaxonal degeneration that correlate with neurological deficits and CNS atrophy. CNS atrophy is a progressive phenomenon that worsens with increasing disease duration and worsening disease course [5]. A number of studies have established an association between brain atrophy and cognitive impairment in MS patients. Less favourable prognosis is in patients with higher number of relapses at the early stage of disease. Numerous drugs targeting the immune system slow down the progression of the disease were introduced [3].

In spite of MS investigation many elements of complex pathogenesis of MS are still unknown [3]. Oxidative stress appears to provide a critical link between environmental factors and genetic risk factors. The presence of four different patterns in MS lesion is showed in table 1. Patterns I and II are involved in autoimmunity and resemble experimental *autoimmune encephalomyelitis* (EAE), while patterns III and IV are not connected with autoimmunity even in the early stages of lesion development. Pattern III lesions are situated near the venules and veins. They are characterized by demyelination and increased activities of antioxidative enzymes. Pattern IV has been found in autopsy samples of PPMS patients and is related to degenerative processes [5].

Various therapies, designed to affect immune response directed against the CNS, are applied, recently addressing the various involvements of redox alterations in MS initiation and progression, but they only slow down and/or reduce severity of the clinical course of MS. This disappointing fact outlines the importance of therapy directed against other components in MS pathology [3]. A large number of studies performed mainly in the past decade indicate a critical role of redox processes in all stages of MS, particularly in the first - the initiation and the last - the neurodegeneration [4].

Table 1. Histopathological patterns of multiple sclerosis (MS)

Pattern I	Macrophage madiated	Radial expression of the lessions, activated by inflammatory compased microglia degenerating myelin
Pattern II	Antibody mediated	Pattern I and deposition of immunoglobin and activated complement in active myelin degeneration
Pattern III	Distal oligodendropathy	Oligodendrocenyt death mediated by inflammmation processes
Pattern IV	Primary oligodendrocyte injury and secondary demyeliniation	Mainly oligodendrocytes degeneration in small rim of periplaque white matter followed by pattern I –like processes

CNS Cells Involved in MS

Oligodendrocytes (ODC)

The oligodendrocyt is a cell that can modulate processes of 50 axons. The most important role of ODC in CNS is producing myelin sheaths that are approximately 1 μm thick and consist of lipids (80%) and proteins (20%) (Figure 1) [5]. Myelin proteins are the crucial molecular targets in immunological activity in MS and its EAE models include myelin oligodendrocyte glycoprotein, proteolipid protein and myelin basic protein (MBP) [12-14]. Moreover, oligodendrocytes have an important role in brain blood-barrier (BBB) integrity (Table 2).

Astrocytes

Astrocytes are the cells available in large quantities and constitute about 90% of the CNS. They are main macroglial cells providing main neuronal support in homeostasis, blood–brain barrierintegrity, myelination, neurotransmitter regulation and synapse function (Figure 1). The widespread of astrocytes throughout the both white and grey matter and their connection with CNS blood vessels involving in most of immunity-related actions create astrocytes as major cells in neuroinflammatory disorders, such as MS [2, 16]. They play a crucial role in supporting neurons function and BBB regulation. During inflammation interleukin (IL)-6, tumor necrosis factor (TNF) – α, IL-

1β is released by astrocytes and the increase of BBB permeability takes place [5, 17]. The ability of astrocytes to modulate BBB permeability has significant implications during inflammation by the effect on the influx of immune cells, ions and toxic molecules into the CNS. Astrocytes play an important role in the reactivation of autoreactive T cells in MS [2, 5] (Table 2).

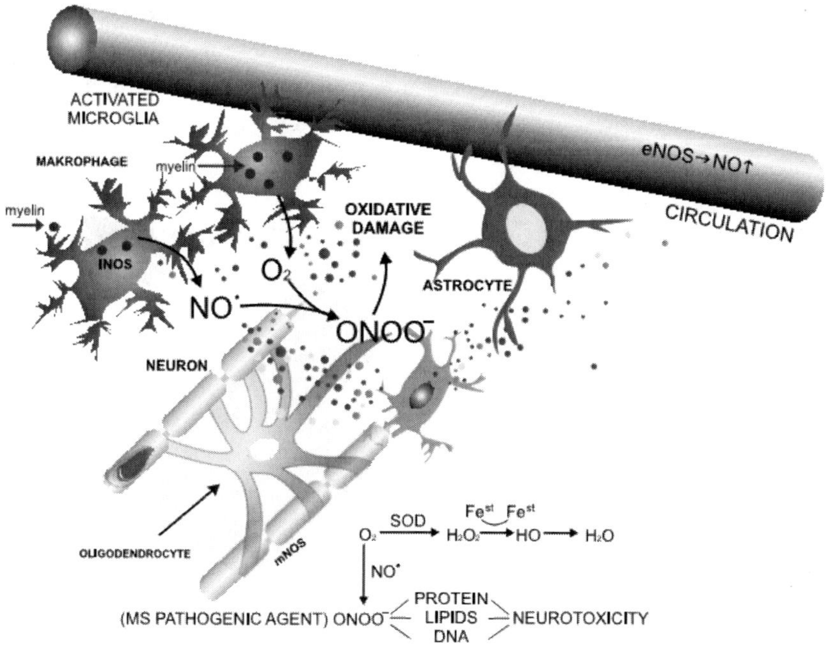

Figure 1. Brain structures involved in MS pathogenesis. The formation of powerful oxidant peroxynitrite ($ONOO^-$).

Microglial Cells

Microglial cells are resident macrophages of the CNS (Figure 1). Their main role is the elimination of cell debris and infected cells after their activation; microglial cells may become classical phagocytic cells [5]. Microglial cells produce inflammatory mediators and effectors (cytokines, prostaglandins, reactive oxygen and nitrogen species (ROS and RNS) and can up regulate major histocompatibility complex (MHC) molecules [2]. Their main function is protection of CNS homeostasis, particularly under pathological conditions such as neurodegenerative processes [5, 18].

Macrophages are phagocytic cells that have important function in innation and adaptation of brain immunity. They are able to eliminate microbes and infected cells, but also are responsible for autoimmunity (Table 2) [18].

There are meningeal, perivascular and choroid plexus macrophages. The dendritic cells (DC) are professional antigen presenting cells (APC). They have the key role in the initiation of the autoimmunity in MS. Generally, it is accepted that there are no DC in the healthy CNS [5]. Neutrophils are absent in the CNS, unlike T and B cells that are present in low numbers. Endothelial cells and pericytes that are constituents of small blood vessels within the CNS have important functions in CNS- immunity relation, especially BBB function.

Nitric Oxide As a Molecule Modulating Neural Activity

Nitric oxide (NO) is an omnipresent multifunctional intercellular molecule that can modulate blood flow, thrombosis and neural activity (Figure 2). NO is produced by all brain cells including neurons, endothelial and glial cells (astrocytes, oligodendrocytes and microglia) by Ca2+/calmodulin-dependent nitric oxide synthases (NOS) isoforms. It is essential for the control of cerebral blood flow and neurotransmission, synaptic plasticity modulation of neuroendocrine functions memory formation and behavioral activity. NO plays an important role in amplifying toxity in the CNS. Under various pathological conditions associated with inflammation large amount of NO is produced as a result of the inducibleNOS (iNOS) in glial cells. The crucial role of NO in physiology and patology is the NO reaction with superoxide and formation the powerful oxidant peroxyntrite $ONOO^-$ [18, 19]. Superoxide is rapidly removed by high concentrations of main antioxidative enzyme superoxide dismutase (SOD) (Figure 1) which izoenzymes are located in cytoplasm, mitochondria, and extracellular compartments. The biological half-life of NO in vivo is less than a second whereas the concentrations of NO relevant for cellular signaling can persist in phosphate-buffered saline for an hour. There is no enzyme to be able to catalyze any reaction as fast as it is required to form peroxynitrite from NO and superoxide [20]. Moreover, even slight higher level of superoxide and NO (10-fold greater rate) can increase peroxynitrite formation by 100-fold. Therefore, brain microglia activation stimulates superoxide and NO production and 1000-fold higher production makes cause the formation of peroxynitrite by a 1000000-fold [21]. Although peroxynitrite is a strong oxidant, it reacts at a relatively slow rate with most biological molecules and can diffuse quite far on cellular scale [20]. Peroxynitrite is able to traverse cell membranes in part through anion channels.

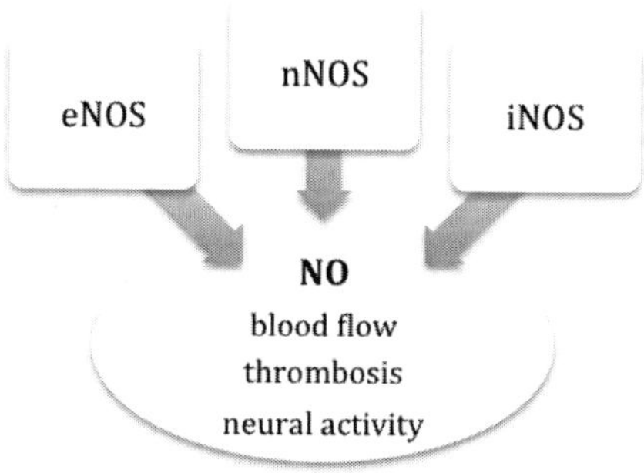

Figure 2. The nitric oxide (NO) role in humans. The NO syntethases (NOS): (eNOS-endothelial; nNOS-neuronal; iNOS-inducible).

Table 2. Central nervous system (CNS) cells involved in multiple sclerosis (MS)

CNS cell	Physiological function	Role in MS
Neuron	Transmit information by electrical and chemical signaling	loss of myelin sheath and next axonal loss; slowing down or blockade of impulses transmission
Oligodendrocyte	Support and insulation for axons by forming the myelin sheath (80%lipids; 20%protein).	myelin proteins (basic protein (MBP), myelin oligodendrocyte glycoprotein (MOG) and proteolipid protein (PLP) are immune targets
Astrocytes	Optimal physical and metabolic environment for neuronal activities	Neuronal redox homeostasis
Microglial - Macrophages	Optimal homeostasis for neural activities	Upregulate major histocompatibility complex (MHC) produce inflammatory mediators
Microglial - Dendritic cell	Professional antigen presenting cells	Initiation of immune response

The brain proved to be rich source of NO synthesis and allowed the first NO synthase (NOS) to be cloned and purified. There are three NOS: nNOS (neuronal NOS) or NOS1; iNOS (inducible NOS) or NOS2 and eNOS (endothelial NOS) or NOS3 (Figure 1) [21, 22]. The iNOS (NOS2) was isolated from macrophages and it is readily induced in many tissues by proinflammatory cytokines. NOS2 is not regulated by changes in intracellular calcium and is often called a high-output source of NO [23]. There is also eNOS synthase that is found not only in endothelium but also in other tissues like neurons. The main feature of eNOS is it relation to calcium increasing. NO (gas) is a small hydrophobic molecule that crosses cell membranes without channels or receptors like oxygen and carbon dioxide, so that there is no barrier to NO. The diffusion coefficient of NO in water at 37*C is slightly faster than oxygen and carbon dioxide [24, 25]. Therefore it can transmit information over short distances very fast. The lifespan of NO is relatively long compared with the firing of nerve or even activation of a neural network and thus help to integrate neuronal activity in small volumes of the brain [26].

The production of oxidants is a crucial mechanism for neutrophils and macrophages to damage or destroy microorganisms. In physiology the production of oxidant such as peroxynitrite is very low. Moderate persistent flux of peroxinitrite results in substantial oxidation and potential destruction of whole cellular components, leading to the cell death through both apoptosis and necrosis. The half-life of peroxinitrite is short (about 10-20ms), but sufficient to cross biological membranes, diffuse one to two cell diameters. In MS with persistent inflammation processes peroxynitrite may play a key role by initiating peroxidation of myelin lipids, leading to demyelination. ONOO can damage DNA by introducing oxidative modification in both nucleobases and sugar-phosphate backbone. The most reactive with peroxynitrite is guanine. In proteins tyrosine nitration caused by peroxynitrite may contribute to the blood-brain barrier damage. Peroxynitrite scavengers such as mercaptoethylguanidine or guanidinoethyldisulphide protected only against the induction phase of EAE but did not prevent disease progression. The main inhibitor of tyrosine nitration is uric acid that protects the brain-blood barrier to the entry of inflammatory cells into the CNS. Plasma uric acid level is proposed as biomarker for monitoring disease activity in MS [27-29].

Increased levels of nitrate, nitrite and free nitrotirosine have been found to be present in cerebral spinal fluid (CSF) and CSF level of these compounds is proposed as a marker of neurodegeneration. iNOS expression decreases in demyelinated plaques from MS patients when inflammation is reduced [30-33].

MS is an immune-mediated, inflammatory disease causing focal damage to the white matter attacking different regions of the CNS apparently random. The ability of neurons to conduct impulses becomes compromised throughout the loss of their myelin sheath and next axonal loss.

MS Traditional Treatment

Currently, most of the drugs and therapies are focused on early phase of MS, especially in relapsing-remitting (RRMS) clinical form. The most effective form of relapses treatment is still using the high doses of corticosteroids due to their strong anti-inflammmatory effects. Current first-line pharmacological treatments of RRMS are disease-modifying drugs (DMD) including interferon (IFN) (1b, 1a) and Glatiramer acetate that represent the gold standard in the modifying the course of MS. The aim of these treatments is reducing the rate of relapses (about 30%) [12]. The first line DMD for MS treatment have good safety profiles. DMD immune response in MS patients is changed due to immunomodulatory and/or immunosuppressive effects. The main problem in treatment MS patients' is heterogeneity of response to DMD [1]. Currently there is also the second-line of treatment for MS including monoclonal antibodies such as Natalizumab and Cladribine or others. Second-line generations of therapies such as Natalizumab, or the most recent Fingolimod (oral drug) are characterized with higher level of effectiveness of reducing the rate of relapses (about 70%). On the other hand, they have a risk of rare but serious complications such as the development of progressive multifocal leukoencephalopathy (Natalizumab) or cardiotoxicity (Fingolimod) [24]. So, they are used in more severe non-IFN-responder cases. Therefore, the therapeutic potential of antioxidative therapies in MS, especially in progressive form of disease is still very needed.

Therapeutic Potential of Antioxidative Therapies in MS

Antioxidants prevent oxidative stress that is the crucial factor both initiation and progression of MS. Therefore, redox therapy can be a useful therapeutic agent in oxidative stress-related disease including MS [34-42]. It is wide range of biochemical molecules (such as uric acid and large like albumin) that are antioxidants. The effectiveness of antioxidant depends on its quick reaction with the ROS at the low concentrations and the product of the oxidation is a stable chemical or molecule that can be easily recycled back to an active antioxidant. There are endogenous antioxidants synthesized in the human body and exogenous compounds (plants, vitamins, minerals) [45, 46].

Accumulating data from epidemiological studies have shown that higher intake of exogenous antioxidants is associated with lower risks of heart disease, some neurodegenerative diseases [31-36] and cancers [37-39].

Expression of the most antioxidant enzymes is regulated through the transcription factor nuclear factor-E2 related factor (Nrf2) and antioxidant response elements (ARE) in the genes encoding enzymatic antioxidants and is induced by oxidative stress. In neurons of MS patients, higher expression of Nrf2/ARE-regulated antioxidants is in relation with the occurrence of oxidative stress in these lesions [47, 48]. Currently, over 200 Nrf2-driven genes connected with antioxidant defense have been identified, including superoxide dismutases (SOD), glutathione peroxidases (GPx), catalase (CAT), peoxiredoxins and NAD(P)H: quinone oxidoreductase. Therefore, antioxidative therapies might be an attractive therapy to limit oxidative tissue injury. However, most antioxidative compunds are not able to cross easily the BBB and have narrow therapeutic window. Nrf2/ARE regulated antioxidant enzymes are up-regulated as an endogenous compensatory system to decrease ROS-induced damage. Using variety of antioxidative therapies is very popular in MS [55]. Schwarz et al. analyzed on the group of 1573 MS patients wide range of complementary and alternative medicine using by them: diet modification (41%), omega-3 fatty acids (37%), vitamin D (28%), Vitamin E (28%) and vitamin C (28%) homeopathy (26%) and selenium (24%). Moreover, majority of respondents (69%) were satisfied with the effects of complementary treatment. Compared with conventional therapy complementary and alternative therapies rarely showed side-effects (9%vs59%) [49, 50].

In active demyelinating MS lesions SOD1 staining was detected in foamy macrophages and astrocytes. Dismutation of superoxide by SODs results in the formation of hydrogen peroxide, which is subsequently converted by catalase, glutathione peroxidases and peroxiredoxins. CAT is low expressed in CNS and is mainly located in peroxisomes. Peroxiredoxins are antioxidant enzymes which are expressed in different CNS cell types (neurons, astrocytes, endothelial cells).

Melatonin

Melatonin (N-acetyl-5-methoxytryptamine) is an indoleamide (indoleamine) secreted by the pineal gland. Endogenous melatonin is directly released into the cerebrospinal fluid (CSF) of the third ventricle of the brain in addition to being discharged into the perfuse capillary bed that permeates the gland [54-55]. Therefore, melatonin could quickly diffuse into the neural tissue to protect against ROS/RNS. Moreover, it can eliminate superoxide anion, NO, ONOO–, can inhibit activity of NO synthases (iNOS, nNOS) and reduces levels of proinflammatory cytokines: IL- 6, IL- 12, TNF-α, IFN [50]. Many studies reported neuroprotective function of melatonin [54-61]. Moreover, melatonin is responsible for higher activation of main antioxidative enzymes and their effectiveness as scavengers. It is suggested that low level of melatonin can have an important role in fatigue, mood disorder fluctuation of symptoms [54, 58], and triglyceride level in MS [58].

Melatonin easily crosses the BBB and reacts with ROS/RNS due to its anti-inflammatory and antioxidative properties [5]. It is suggested that melatonin have an influence on immune system cells via melatonin receptors. Our recent studies showed that 10 mg daily/30 day's melatonin supplementation caused statistically significant increase of SOD, GPx and decrease of MDA in erythrocytes of SPMS patients [61].

Sandyk et al., [62] show an association nocturnal melatonin secretion with duration of clinical symptoms of MS patients. Therefore, the activity of the pineal gland may decline with progression of the disease. However, the other studies did not find this association [60].

Cannabinoids

Cannabinoids are the variety of chemical compounds that activate cannabinoid receptors. There are endocannabinoids (produced in the body), the phytocannabinoids (cannabis and some other plant compounds), and synthetic cannabinoids (produced chemically). Major psychoactive compound of cannabis is the phytocannabinoid Δ9-tetrahydrocannabinol (THC). The brain canabinoid receptor was described by Devane et al. in 1980s. Cannabinoids are used mainly to ameliorate muscle spasticity and pain in MS patients. Their anti-inflammatory properties received experimental support in inflammation models *in vitro* and *in vivo* [63].

There are two cannabinoid receptors named CB_1 and CB_2. The CB_1 receptors are related to all psychotropic and motor impairing effects of cannabis due to their expressed in CNS areas connected with the control of pain [64]. Synthetic THC (dronabinol) and its derivative nabilone are therapeutic agents with antiemetic and analgesic properties (Marinol® and Cesamet®, respectively) [64, 65]. CB_1 receptors are found mainly at the terminals of central and peripheral neurons, where they usually modulate the release of excitatory and inhibitory neurotransmitter [66].

The CB_2 receptors are expressed not only in immune cells but also in CNS, particularly in spinal cord and dorsal root ganglia. In the CNS expresion of CB_2 receptors depend on microglia activation. In healthy CNS, there is no expresion of CB_2. However, CB_2 expression on CNS neurons is still controversial, although its presence in peripheral nociceptive neurons is responsible for modulating many types of pain 1 [67, 68]. The CB_2 cannabinoids receptors, may not only reduce the production of tumor necrosis factor TNF-α, interleukin IL-1β and the p40 subunit of IL-12 and IL-23 by microglia and macrophages but also may play major role in migration cells including neutrophils, macrophages, NK and B cells [66]. Moreover, cannabinoids are able to decrease IL-2 production and T cells proliferation and may change the cytokine profile [65].

Currently, cannabinoid medicine is focused on alleviate neuropathic pain, spasticity, overactive bladder, and other symptoms associated with MS.

Vitamin D

The active form of vitamin D is 1, 25-dihydroxyvitamin D (1, 25(OH)2D). Hypovitaminosis D is key environmental risk factor in MS and also may have a immunomodulatory role in the brain [2, 4]. Moreover, vitamin D, can alter the T- cell into a more anti-inflammatory and regulated state, with inhibition of Th1 and Th17 cells and promotion of Th2 and Treg cells [69]. Treatment with vitamin D has a positive effect on MS patients also as a preventive factor after high dose of sterydotherapy [69, 70]. It is the lower incidence of MS in the region near the equator where sunlight is relatively higher. Furthermore, right level of vitamin D in childhood and adolescence is connected with a low risk of MS [2].

Fumaric Acid Esters (FAE)

Fumaric acid esters (FAE) have been used in psoriasis treatment for over 30 years and are available as health supplements for natural therapy to treat psoriasis. This drug has been involved in altering response to oxidative stress via nuclear-related factor E2-related factor 2 (Nrf2). The Nrf2 pathway increases expression of antioxidative proteins and in this way provides neuroprotection and homeostasis of immune system.

Fumaric acid esters are investigated as an oral therapy for RRMS` and as a neuroprotectants [71-73]. The results of randomized, placebo-controlled phase II study that have been published lately indicate significant positive effects of FAE on diverse MRI parameters in MS patients with relapsing-remitting MS. It has been shown in clinical studies in psoriasis that FAE caused a decrease of peripheral CD4+ and CD8+ T-lymphocytes by stimulation of apoptotic processes [71, 73]. *In vitro* studies showed dimethylfumarate ester's inhibitory effect in human endothelial cells on nuclear factor kappa B (NF-B)-dependent transcription of tumor necrosis factor-alpha (TNF-α) induced genes [71]. Experimental studies of EAE demyelinated central nervous system showed distinct myelin and axonal density protection in the plaque. Molecular reports showed that these processes are dependent on the antioxidative mechanism thorough transcription factor Nrf-2 stimulation. A phase II clinical trial in RRMS patients with dimethylfumarate presented a substantial decrease in the number of gadolinium advancing lesions after 24 weeks [84, 85]. This positive effect of immunomodulation seems to be similar to first line of DMD that are basic treatment of RRMS in the early phase. Many years of treatment in psoriasis showed safety profile of dimethyl- furmate (DMF) formula BG12. Currently, the phase III clinical trials are being conducted to present the longitudal efficiency in patients with RRMS [73].

Cryostimulation

Accumulating clinical studies show that hypothermia is promising neuroprotective therapy [74-77]. Low temperatures were used in late 60s in brain injury and results showed a decrease of metabolism indicators [78]. The clinical studies suggest that even slight fluctuations of brain tissue temperature can alter excitotoxicity, calcium dependent intercellular signaling, hemodynamic, apoptosis, inflammation and oedema and also biochemical makers [78]. The main effect of hypothermia is the cell protection against hypoxia by delaying the pace of damage of cells caused by formation of free radicals, tissue oedema and chemical metabolites [79]. Low temperature therapy was used in neonates hypoxic-ischemic encephalopathy [75] depression [80], brain injury [75], multiple sclerosis [77], and cerebral ischemia [76]. The whole body exposure to cryogenic temperatures (–130°C) was firstly used in late 70s in Japan by Thosiro Yamauchi (Yamauchi 1989) who used it in rheumatism treatment [77]. Whole body cryotherapy is also called cryostimulation. It is an exposure of whole human body to extremely low temperatures (–130° C) in a cryogenic chamber. In the cryogenic chamber there are two rooms: the vestibule where temperature is about –60°C and the main chamber with proper therapeutic temperature (–130°C). The length of one session is 3 minutes per day. Cryostimulation is the therapy that can be used as additional treatment in inflammatory diseases, rheumatic diseases, sport medicine or degenerative joint, spine diseases as well as psychiatric disorders especially for anxiety- depressive syndrome [77]. The main feature of low temperature is less demand of oxygen and the decrease of cell metabolism. Therefore the production of free radicals and ROS leading to oxidative damages are reduced. Membrane lipid peroxidation became slower and belays ischemic cell membranes by stabilizing potassium efflux [78]. Our clinical studies indicate the reduction of TAS (total antioxidant status) in depressive MS patients compared with non- depressive MS patients [79]. After 10 sessions of cryostimulation we observed higher level of TAS in plasma of depressive MS patients. They reached the values of healthy controls. It is still unknown how cryostimulation might have an effect on oxidative stress and futher studies in this area are needed. Results of Miller et al. demonstrate that ten exposures of cryostimulation can not only increase the level of TAS but also uric acid that is the main human antioxidant in MS patients [81]. Moreover, it seems that the lower level of TAS observed in plasma of MS patients is dependent on the low concentrations of endogenous antioxidants, mainly uric acid. Therefore the cryostimulation migth be the effective factor that can suppress oxidative stress and ROS production especially in MS. The longitudal measurement of uric acid level in plasma of MS patients after completion ten sessions of cryostimulation showed an increase of uric acid concentration even 3 months after therapy [81]. Therefore, cryostimulation seems to be a potent adjuvant antioxidative therapy in MS.

Conclusion

The potential protective effects of redox therapies are necessary to be continued to understand cellular immunology of MS neurodegeneration. [87]. It is essential to improve our knowledge about the patomechanisms of this disorder. Moreover, it also helps to establish new aims in innovative methods for treatment of MS.

Conflict of Interest

The author(s) confirm that this article content has no conflicts of interest.

Acknowledgments

Declared none.

References

[1] Van Horssen, J; Witte ME; Schreibelt, G; de Viries HE. (2011) Radical changes in multiple sclerosis pathogenesis. *Biochim. Bioph. Acta,* 1812, 141-50.

[2] Miller, E. (2012). Multiple sclerosis. *Adv. Exp. Med. Biol*, 724, 222-238.

[3] Ortiz, GG; Pacheco-Moises, FP; Bitzer-Quintero, OK; Ramirez-Anguiano AC; Flores-Alvarado, LJ; Ramirez-Ramirez, VR; Macias-Islas MA; Torres-Sanchez ED. (2013) *Immunology and oxidative stress in multiple sclerosis: Clinical Basic Approach.* Clinical and Developmental Immunology, ID708659, 14 pages.

[4] Miller, E; Wachowicz, B; Majsterek, I. (2013) Advances in antioxidative therapy of multiple sclerosis. 20, 1-11.

[5] Milijković, D; Spasojević, I. (2013) Multiple sclerosis: Molecular Mechanisms and Therapeutic Opportunities. *Antioxidants & redox signaling.* 19, 2286-2334.

[6] Bielekova, B; Martin, R. (2004) Development of biomarkers in multiple sclerosis. *Brain,* 127, 1463-1478.

[7] Miller, E; Mrowicka, M; Saluk-Juszczak, J; Majsterek, I. 2011The level of isoprostanes as a non-invasive marker for in vivo lipid peroxidation in secondary progressive multiple sclerosis. *Neurochem. Res.,* 36, 1012-1016.

[8] Miller, E; Walczak, A; Saluk-Juszczak, J; Majsterek, I. Oxidative modification of patient's plasma proteins and its role in pathogenesis of multiple sclerosis. *Clin. Biochem.*, 2012, 45, 26-30.

[9] Witherick, J; Wilkins, A; Scolding, N. Mechanisms of oxidative damage in multiple sclerosis and a cell therapy approach to treatment. *Autoimmune Dis*, 2011, ID 164608: 11.

[10] Gonsette, R. Oxidative stress and excitotoxicity: a therapeutic issue in multiple sclerosis? *Mult. Scler*, 2008, 14, 22-34.

[11] Choi, IY; Lee, SP; Denny, DR.; Lynch LA. Lower levels of gluthatione in the brains of secondary progressive multiple sclero- sis patients measured by 1H magnetic resonance chemical shift imaging at 35. *Mult Scler,* 2011, 17(3), 289-296.

[12] Lerday, E; Yaouanq, J; Le Page, E; Constans, M; Lapland, D; Oger, J; Edan, G. (2010) Evidence for a two-stages multiple sclerosis. *Brain,* 133(7), 1900-1913.

[13] Bradl, M; Lassman, H.(2010) Oligodendrocytes: biology and pathology *Acta Neuropatol.*, 119, 37-53.

[14] Bauman, N; Pham-Dinh, D. (2001) Biology of oligodendrocytes and myelin in the mammalian central nervous system. *Physiol. Rev.*, 81, 871-927.

[15] Watzlawik, J; Warrington, AE; Rodriguez, M. Importance of oligodendrocyte protection BBB. (2010) *Expert Rev. Neurother,* 2010, 10(3), 441-57.

[16] Nair, A; Frederick, TJ; Miller, SD. (2008) Astrocytes in multiple sclerosis: A product of environment. *Cell Mol. Life Sci*, 65, 2702-20.

[17] Abott, NJ; Ronnback, L; Hansson E. (2006) Astrocyte-endothelial interactions at the blood-brain barier. *Nat. Rev. Neurosci.*, 7, 41-53.

[18] Block, ML; Hong, JS. (2005) Microglia and inflammation-mediated neurodegeneration: multiple triggers with a common mechanism. *Prog. Neurobiol.* 76(2), 77–98.

[19] Pacher, P; Backman, JS; Liaudet L.(2007). Nitric Oxide and peroxynitrite in heath and disease. *Physiol. Rev.*, 87, 315-424.

[20] Lancaster, JR.(1994) Simulation of the diffusion and reaction of endogenously produced nitric oxide. *Proc. Natl. Acad. Sci. USA*, 91, 8137-41.

[21] Denicola A;Souza, JM; Radi, R. (1998) Diffusion of peroxynitrite across erythrocute membranes. *Proc. Natl. Acad. Sci. USA*, 95, 3566-3571.

[22] Liu, X; Miller, MJ; Joshi, MS; Thomas, DD; Lancaster, JR; (1998) Accelerated reaction of nitric oxide with O2 within the hydrophobic interior of biological membranes. *Proc. Natl. Acad. Sci. USA*, 95, 2175-2179.

[23] Bredt, DS; Hwang, PM; Snyder, SH. (1990) Localization of nitric oxide synthase indicating a neural role for nitric oxide. *Nature* 347, 768-70.

[24] Calabrese, V; Cornelius, C; Rizzarelli, E. (2009) Nitric oxide in cell survival: a jams molecule. *Antioxid Redox Signal*, 11, 2717-39.

[25] Guix, FX; Uribesalgo, I; Coma, M; Munoz, FJ. (2005) The physiology and pathology of nitric oxide in the brain. *Prog. Neurobiol.*, 76, 126-52.

[26] Moncada, S; Bolanos, JP.(2006) Nitric xide, cell bioenergetics and neurodegeneration. *J. Neurochem.*, 97, 1676-89.

[27] Hooper, DC; Spitsin, S; Kean, RB. (1998) Uric acid, a natural scavenger of peroxynitrite, in experimental allergic encephalomyelitis and multiple sclerosis. *Proc. Natl. Acad. Sci. USA,* 95, 675-80.

[28] Guerrero, AL; Gutierrez, F; Iglesias, F. (2011) Serum uric acid levels in multiple sclerosis patients inversely correlate with disability. *Neurol. Sci.,* 32, 347-50.

[29] Rentzos, M; Nikolaou, C; Anagnostouli, M. (2006) Serum uric acid and multiple sclerosis. *Ciln. Neurol. Neurosurg.*, 108, 527-31.

[30] Onufriev, MV. (2010) Nitrosative stress in the brain: autoantibodies to nitrotyrosine in liquor as a potential marker. *Neurochem. Journal*, 4, 228-234.

[31] Wachowicz, B; Rywaniak, JZ; Nowak, P. (2008) Apoptic matkers in human blood platelets treated with peroxynitrite. *Platelets,* 19, 624-635.

[32] Liu, JS; Zhao, ML; Brosnan, CF; Lee, SC. (2001) Expression of inducible nitric oxide synthetase and nitrityrosine in multiple sclerosis lessions. *Am. J. Pathol.*, 158, 2057-66.

[33] Brown, GC. (2010) Nitric oxide and neuronal death. *Nitric. Oxide,* 23, 153–165.

[34] Devasagayam, TP; Tilak, JC; Boloor, KK; Sane, KS; Ghaskadbi, SS; Lele, RD.(2004) Free radicals and antioxidants in human health: current status and future prospects. *J. Assoc. Physicians India*, 52, 794-804.

[35] Ma, Q. (2010) Transcriptional responses to oxidative stress: pathological and toxicological implications. *Pharmacol. Ther*, 125, 376-93.

[36] Smith, KJ; Kapoor, R; Felts, PA.(1999) Demyelination: the role of reactive oxygen and nitrogen species. *Brain Pathol.*, 9, 69-92.

[37] Cross, AH; Manning, PT; Keeling, RM; Schmidt, RE; Misko, TP. (1998) Peroxynitrite formation within the central nervous system in active multiple sclerosis, *J. Neuroimmunol.*, 88, 45.

[38] Bizzozero, OA; De Jesus, G; Bixler, HA; Pastuszyn, A. (2005) Evidence of nitrosative damage in the brain white matter of patients with multiple sclerosis. *Neurochem. Res.*, 30, 139.

[39] Andrews, HE; Nichols, PP; Bates, D; Turnbull, DM. (2005) Mitochondrial dysfunction plays a key role in progressive axonal loss in Multiple Sclerosis. *Med. Hypotheses*, 64, 669.

[40] Mahad, DJ; Ziabreva, I; Campbell, G; Lax, N; White, K; Hanson, PS; Lassmann, H; Turnbull, D.M. (2009) Mitochondrial changes within axons in multiple sclerosis, *Brain.*

[41] Forman, HJ; Torres, M. (2001) Redox signaling in macrophages, *Mol. Aspects Med.*, 22, 189.

[42] Dutta, R; McDonough, J; Yin, X; Peterson, J; Chang, A; Torres, T; Gudz, T; Macklin, WB; Lewis, DA; Fox, RJ; Rudick, R; Mirnics, K; Trapp, B.D.(2006) Mitochondrial dysfunction as a cause of axonal degeneration in multiple sclerosis patients. *Ann. Neurol.*, 59, 478.

[43] Kalman, B; Laitinen, K; Komoly, S. (2007) The involvement of mitochondria in the pathogenesis of multiple sclerosis, *J. Neuroimmunol,* 188, 1.

[44] Ferguson, B; Matyszak, MK; Esiri, MM; Perry, VH. (1997) Axonal damage in acute multiple sclerosis lesions. *Brain,* 120, 393.

[45] Van Horssen, J; Schreibelt, G; Drexhage, J. Hazes, T; Dijkstra, C.D; Van der Valk P; de Vries, H.E. (2008) Severe oxidative damage in multiple sclerosis lesions coincides with enhanced antioxidant enzyme expression, *Free Radic. Biol. Med.* 45, 1729.

[46] Carlson, NG; Rose, JW. (2006) Antioxidants in multiple sclerosis: do they have a role in therapy? CNS. *Drugs*, 20, 433.

[47] Itoh, K; Tong, KI;Yamamoto, M. (2004) Molecular mechanism activating Nrf2-Keap1 pathway in regulation of adaptive response to electrophiles, *Free Radic. Biol. Med.*, 36, 1208.

[48] Motohashi, H; Yamamoto, M. (2004) Nrf2-Keap1 defines a physiologically important stress response mechanism, *Trends Mol. Med.*, 10, 549.

[49] Kensler, TW;Wakabayashi, N;Biswal, S. (2007) Cell survival responses to environmen- tal stresses via the Keap1-Nrf2-ARE pathway, *Annu. Rev. Pharmacol. Toxicol.*, 47, 89.

[50] Thimmulappa, RK;Mai, KH;Srisuma, S;Kensler, TW; Yamamoto, M; Biswal, S. (2002) Identification of Nrf2-regulated genes induced by the chemopreventive agent sulforaphane by oligonucleotide microarray, *Cancer Res,* 62, 5196.

[51] Weiner, HL.(2009) The challenge of multiple sclerosis: how do we cure a chronic heterogeneous disease? *Annals of Neurology*, 65, 239–248.

[52] Smith, KJ; Kapoor, R; Felts, P. A. (1999) Demyelination: the role of reactive oxygen and nitrogen species, " *Brain Pathology*, 9, 69–92.

[53] Fitzner, D; Simons, M. (2010). Chronic progressive multiple sclerosis-pathogenesis of neurodegeneration and therapeutic strategies. *Curr. Neuropharmac.*, 8, 305-15.

[54] Esposito, E; Cuzzocrea, S.(2010) Antiinflammatory activity of melatonin in central nervous system. *Curr. Neuropharmacol.*, 8, 228-42.

[55] Galano, A; Tan, DX; Reiter RJ. (2011) Melatonin as a natural ally against oxidative stress: a physicochemical examination. *J. Pineal Res,* 51, 1-16.

[56] Melamud, L; Golan, D; Luboshitzky, R; Lavi, I; Miller, A.(2012) Melatonin deregulation, sleep disturbances and fatigue in MS. *J. Neurol.* Sci., 314, 37-40.

[57] Natarajan, R; Einarsdottir, E; Riutta, A; Hagman, S; Raunio, M; Mononen, N; Lehtimäki, T; Elovaara, I. (2012) Melatonin pathway genes are associated with progressive subtypes and disability status in multiple sclerosis among Finnish patients. *J. Neuroimmunol.*, 250, 106-10.

[58] Ghorbani, A; Salari, M; Shaygannejad, V; Norouzi, R. (2013) The role of melatonin in the pathogenesis of multiple sclerosis: a case-control study. *Int. J. Prev. Med.*, 4, 180-184.

[59] Reiter, RJ; Tan, DX; Fuentes-Broto, L. (2010) Melatonin: a multitasking molecule. *Prog. Brain Res.*, 181, 128-151.

[60] Srinivasan, V. (2002) Melatonin oxidative stress and neurodegenerative diseases. *Indian J. Exp. Biol.*, 40, 668-79.

[61] Miller, E; Walczak, A; Majsterek, I; Kędziora, J. (2013) Melatonin reduces oxidative stress in the erythrocytes of multiple sclerosis patients with secondary progressive clinical course. 257, 97-101.

[62] Sandyk, R; Awerbuch, GI. (1992) Nocturnal plasma melatonin and alpha-melanocyte stimulating hormone levels during exacerbation of multiple sclerosis. *Int. J. Neurosci.* 67, 173–86.

[63] Zajicek, J; Ball, S; Wright, D; Nunn, A; Miller, D; Cano, MG; McManus, D; Mallik, S; Hobart, J. (2013) Effect of dronabinol on

progression in progressive multiple sclerosis (CUPID): a randomised, placebo-controlled trial. *Lancet Neurol.*, 12, 857-865.

[64] De Lago, E; Moreno-Martet, M; Cabranes, A; Ramos, JA; Fernandez-Ruiz, J. (2012) Cannabinoids ameliorate disease progression in a model of multiple sclerosis in mice, acting preferentially through CB1 receptor-mediated anti-inflammatory effects. *Neuropharmacology*, 62, 2299-308.

[65] Kozela, E; Nirit, L; Kaushansky, N; Eilam, R; Rimmerman, N; Levy, R; Ben-Nun, A; Juknat, A; Vogel, Z. (2011) Cannabidiol inhibits pathogenic T cells, decreases spinal microglial activation and ameliorates multiple sclerosis-like disease in C57BL/6. *Br. J. Pharmacol.*, 163, 1507-1519.

[66] Saito, VM; Rezende, RM; Teixeira, AL. (2012) Cannabinoid modulation of neuroinflammatory disorders. *Curr. Neuropharmacol.*, 10(2), 159–166.

[67] Walker, JM; Huang, SM. (2002) Cannabinoid analgesia. *Pharmacol. Ther*, 95(2), 127–35.

[68] Zhornitsky, S; Potvin, S. (2012) Cannabidiol in humans-the quest for therapeutic targets. *Pharmaceuticals,* 5, 529-52.

[69] Pedersen, L. B.; Nashold, F. E.; Spach, K. M.; Hayes, C. E. 1, 25-dihydroxyvitamin D3 reverses experimental autoimmune encephalomyelitis by inhibiting chemokine synthesis and monocyte traf- ficking. *J. Neurosci. Res.,* 2007, 85, 2480-2490.

[70] Spach, KM; Hayes, CE. (2005) Vitamin D3 confers protection from autoimmune encephalomyelitis only in female mice. *J Immunol.*, 2005, 175, 4119-4126.

[71] Moharregh-Khiabani, D; Linker, RA; Gold, R; Stangel, M. (2009) Fumaric acid and its esters: an emerging treatment for multiple sclerosis. *Curr. Neuropharmacol.*, 2009, 7(1), 60-64.

[72] Gold, R; Linker, RA; Stangel, M. (2012) Fumaric acid and its esters: an emerging treatment for multiple sclerosis with antioxidative mechanism of action. *Clin. Immunol.*, 2012, 142(1), 44-48.

[73] Killestein, J; Rudick, RA; Polman, CH. (2011) Oral treatment for multiple sclerosis. *Lancet. Neurol.*, 2011, 10(11), 1026-1034.

[74] Duqué, B; Smolander, J; Westerlund, T. (2005) Acute and long-term effects of winter swimming and whole-body cryotherapy on plasma antioxidative capacity in healthy women. *Scand. J. Clin. Lab. Invest,* 65, 395-402.

[75] Jorgensen, SL. (2008) Hypothermia: a cool intervention for hypoxic-ischemic encephalopathy. *JAAPA,* 21, 44-7.

[76] Katz, LM; Young, AS; Frank, JE et al. (2004) Regulated hypothermia reduces brain oxidative stress after hypoxic-ischemia. *Brain Res.,* 1017, 85-91.
[77] Miller, E; Mrowicka, M; Malinowska, K et al. (2010) Effects of whole body cryotherapy on total antioxidative status and activities of antioxidative enzymes in blood of patients with multiple sclerosis. *J. Med. Invest,* 57, 168-173.
[78] Miller, E; Mrowicka, M; Malinowska, K et al. (2010) Effects of whole body cryotherapy on oxidative stress in multiple sclerosis patients *J. Therm. Biol.*, 35, 406-410.
[79] Miller, E; Mrowicka, M; Malinowska, K et al. (2011) Effects of whole body cryotherapy on a total antioxidative status and activity of antioxidant enzymes in blood of depressive multiple sclerosis patients *World J. biol. Psychiatry*, 12.223-7.
[80] Rymaszewska, J; Ramsey, D; Chladzinska-Kiejna, S. (2008) Whole body cryotherapy as adjunct treatment of depressive and anxiety disorders. *Arch. Immun. Therap Exp.*, 56, 63 – 68.
[81] Miller, E; Saluk, J; Morel, A; Wachowicz, B. (2013) Long-term effects of whole body cryostimulation on uric acid concentration in plasma of secondary progressive multiple sclerosis patients. *Scand. J. Med. Invest.*, 73, 635-40.

In: Oxidative Stress
Editor: Cassidy Croft
ISBN: 978-1-63117-578-7

Chapter 7

The Role of Nitric Oxide Toxicity and Oxidative Stress in Graft vs. Host Disease

Osnat Almogi-Hazan[1], Reut Shainer[1], Eytan R. Barnea[2,3] and Reuven Or[1]
[1]Department of Bone Marrow Transplantation,
Hadassah-Hebrew University Medical Center, Jerusalem, Israel
[2]SIEP- The Society for the Investigation of Early Pregnancy,
Cherry Hill, NJ, US
[3]BioIncept LLC (PIF* Proprietary)

Abstract

Allogeneic Hematopoietic Stem Cell Transplantation (HSCT) is widely used for treatment of malignant and non-malignant hematological diseases. Allogeneic transplantation is associated with the beneficial Graft vs. Leukemia/lymphoma (GVL) effect that prevents disease relapse. Often though, allogeneic HSCT leads to graft-versus-host disease (GVHD) which remains a major cause of morbidity and mortality in allogeneic HSCT patients. Clinically, GVHD manifestations present acute and/or chronic form. Acute GVHD is characterized by multi-organ damage targeting mainly skin, liver and gastrointestinal tract, while chronic GVHD can target many organ systems, including acute GVHD target organs as well as connective tissue and exocrine glands.

Monocytes/Macrophages are phagocytic cells that serve as a first-line defense against invading pathogens through the generation of reactive oxygen species (ROS), reactive nitrogen species (RNS, e.g., nitric oxide, NO•), and production of inflammatory cytokines. In pathological inflammatory conditions, overproduction of ROS/RNS coupled with deficiency in enzymatic and non-enzymatic antioxidants can be harmful. In allogeneic HSCT and GVHD, the ROS/RNS balance is disturbed.

Here we review the cumulative knowledge from the past two decades, on the effect of allogeneic HSCT on blood markers for free radicals' toxicity in patients. The role of RNS in the patho-etiology of GVHD, as it emerges from studies in experimental models is presented. In addition, the issue whether drug intervention in ROS/RNS pathways could improve the clinical results after allogeneic HSCT is addressed. We describe the PreImplantation Factor and its projected therapeutic role in reducing GVHD by modulating inflammation and reducing NO production. Evidence suggests that restored free radicals balance is an efficient way to improve clinical GVHD manifestations.

Introduction

Allogeneic Hematopoietic Stem Cell Transplantation (HSCT) is a well-established treatment modality for malignant and non-malignant hematological diseases. The first unrelated-donor HSCT for leukemia patients was carried out in 1980, and currently it is performed in tens of thousands of patients each year. HSCT has been shown to induce Graft vs. Leukemia/lymphoma (GVL) effect, which can prevent relapse of disease [1-4].

Mature donor T-cells within the stem cell graft are the main mediators of these beneficial immune effects, but are also responsible for the induction of graft-versus-host disease (GVHD), which still remained a major cause of morbidity and mortality in the HSCT patients [5, 6]. GVHD occurs when transplanted donor-derived T cells recognize proteins expressed by recipient antigen presenting cells as foreign. Consequently, this recognition induces donor T-cell activation, proliferation and differentiation, leading to a cellular and inflammatory attack on recipient's organs or tissues. Acute GVHD occurs within a 100-day period post-transplant and generally is manifested as dermatitis, enteritis and hepatitis. Chronic GVHD develops after 100 days post-transplant and manifests as an immune mediated disease directed at multiple organs.

GVHD development is a long term threat for patients following HSCT, unless a perfect match is found, and even then immunosuppression is in general the rule. As such, long-term therapy is required, using several immunosuppressive agents, frequently in combination. In addition, prior to HSCT, recipients undergo a conditioning regimen that is myelosuppressive and immunosuppressive (to deplete host stem cells and make space for donor stem cell engraftment and to reduce graft rejection mediated by host immune cells, respectively). The toxicity and suppressive effects of this regimen can cause tissue damage and induce inflammation in the host.

Oxygen free radicals, at low/moderate concentrations, have physiological roles in cellular responses. They are involved in a number of cellular signaling pathways and have a role in defense against infectious agents. Nitric oxide (NO•), at low concentrations, is an intercellular messenger, which modulates blood flow, coagulation, and neural activity. At high concentrations, reactive nitrogen and oxygen species have toxic effects (nitrosative/oxidative stress) and may damage cells and tissues [7-9].

Oxidative stress is a byproduct of most conditioning protocols and nitrosative stress is associated with inflammation during GVHD following allogeneic HSCT, thereby these procedures are associated with severe disturbance of free radicals balance in the host [10-12] The present review provides an update on the effect of allogeneic HSCT on blood markers for free radicals' toxicity in patients, the role of RNS in the patho-etiology of GVHD and finally, drug intervention in ROS/RNS pathways, which could improve the clinical results after allogeneic HSCT.

Free Radicals' Toxicity in HSCT Patients

Superoxide (O_2•), nitric oxide (NO•), and their reaction product peroxynitrite (ONOO-) have been shown to exert toxic target molecule reactions when generated in excess, mainly during pathologic inflammatory situations [8, 9].

The HCST follows conditioning regimen using high doses of chemotherapy and/or radiation to effectively eliminate the blood forming elements of the bone marrow. Such regimen also serves to reduce the number of malignant cells in the body- since most HCST are performed in patients with leukemia. This conditioning protocol causes an increase in free radical formation, as well as depletion of tissue antioxidants [10, 11]. Free radical formation and depletion of tissue antioxidants as a result of chemotherapy and radiation was first demonstarated in the 1980's when Cyclophosphamide, frequently used in conditioning chemotherapy was found to deplete hepatic glutathione. In addition, lipid peroxidation has been suggested as one of the main causes of ionizing radiation damage and decreased essential antioxidants was found in the plasma of patients following high-dose radio/chemotherapy [10, 11, 13, 14]. Dürken et al. monitored the antioxidant status before and after HSCT finding a breakdown of plasma antioxidant defense and radical-vulnerable lipids, which was coupled with high circulating levels of iron [15, 16]. Similar results were obtained also in pediatric patients [17]. Evens et al. suggested that due to early saturation of transferrin and a rise in ferritin in HSCT patients, iron-generated ROS may lead to a pro-oxidant state and contribute to treatment-related morbidity and mortality following both autologous and allogeneic HSCT [18]. Recently, Sari et al. compared oxidative stress markers and antioxidant enzymes in the plasma of myeloablative and non- myeloablative conditioned patients failing to find any significant differences [19]. Their results indicate that the use of non-myeloablative conditioning regimen does not resolve the problem of oxidative stress. In murine models antioxidants treatment reduced oxidative stress and improved engraftment after allogeneic HSCT [20]. Hence, non-toxic, stable, antioxidants may be considered as a treatment for HSCT patients.

Although the cumulative data points out the contribution of conditioning regiments to imbalanced oxidative state in HSCT patients, the influence of this state on the clinical condition of the patients has to be further examined.

On the other hand, early in the 1990's, evidences started to accumulate on significant rise of NO• levels as a result of allogeneic activation [21, 22]. Increased serum NO• levels was demonstrated in GVHD animal model studies [12, 23]. Based on this data, Weiss et al. have performed follow-up measurements of the stable end-products of NO, nitrite/nitrate (NO2-/NO3-), in plasma of patients undergoing allogeneic and autologous bone marrow transplantation. They found, in a small number of GVHD patients, a significant rise in NO2-/NO3- levels [24]. Later on, Vora et al. confirmed the clinical results, but also demonstrated that nitrate and nitrite levels are raised in other serious post-transplant complications such as human marrow graft rejection and severe infections [25]. Choi et al., demonstrated that Plasma NO2-/NO3- in HSCT recipients is quantitatively associated with the acute GVHD symptoms presence, since the levels of NO2-/NO3- were significantly higher in patients with GVHD in grade higher than 2, compare to allogeneic HSCT patients with a lower GVHD severity, grade < 1 [26]. The correlation between plasma NO• and GVHD reported in these studies provides the basis for conducting further studies into the effects of NO• synthesis attenuation in GVHD, as a potential target of anti-GVHD prophylaxis and therapy, as will be further discussed.

The Role of RNS in the Patho-Etiology of GVHD

In mammals, NO is produced by one of three distinct isoforms of NOS: neuronal (nNOS), endothelial (eNOS) and inducible (iNOS). iNOS expression can be induced in a wide range of cells and tissues by cytokines and other agents. In healthy individuals, NO• is efficiently removed by reacting with oxyhemoglobin to form nitrate, which prevents NO• from directly reacting with oxygen to form significant amounts of ONOO-. However, pathological conditions can greatly increase the production of peroxynitrite. Even the generation of a moderate flux of peroxynitrite over long time periods will result in cell and tissue damage. The contribution of nitrosative stress to the pathophysiology of disease was described in inflammation, cardiovascular disease, neurodegeneration, diabetes, and other pathologies [8, 9].

A variety of murine and rat models were used in order to get better understanding of RNS involvement in allogenic activation in general, and particularly in GVHD. Early publications showed a significant rise of serum NO2-/NO3- levels in the allografted animals that preceded the clinical signs of rejection or GVHD in bone marrow/spleen cell, liver, heart or small bowl transplants [12, 27]. Treatment of recipients with immunosuppressive agents (FK 506, cyclosporine A), or with NO• synthesis inhibitors (L-NG-monomethyl arginine, aminoguanidine) reduced serum NO2-/NO3- levels as well as associated immunopathology, but not Interferon-gamma production [12]. Moreover, NO• synthesis in peritoneal macrophage and in other immune cell populations from allogeneic transplanted mice is enhanced [23, 28]. Recently, we reported up-regulation of iNOS gene expression in liver and colon of GVHD mice, but not in syngeneic transplanted mice [29].

Another outcome of the nitrosative stress in GVHD is immune dysfunction. Several studies have demonstrated that suppression of different immune cells function in mice with GVHD is mediated through the NO• pathway. For example, during GVHD, induction of the NO• pathway is an important mechanism which mediates B-cell hypo-responsiveness to LPS and that this pathway is induced by TNF-alpha [30]. T cell proliferation in response to activation, mainly the proliferation of the more sensitive CD8 cells, is also suppressed by NO• [31, 32]. Persistent suppression of the immune system exposes HSCT patients to high incidence of infectious complications and relapse.

Overall, this data indicates that pathologic elevation in NO• production, together with breakdown of plasma antioxidant defense and of radical-vulnerable lipids due to the conditioning regimen, leads to nitrosative stress in allogeneic HSCT patients. The nitrosative stress has a central role both in GVHD associated tissue damage and GVHD associated immune dysfunction (FIG 1). An ideal therapy would involve maintaining antioxidant defense with control of nitrosative stress.

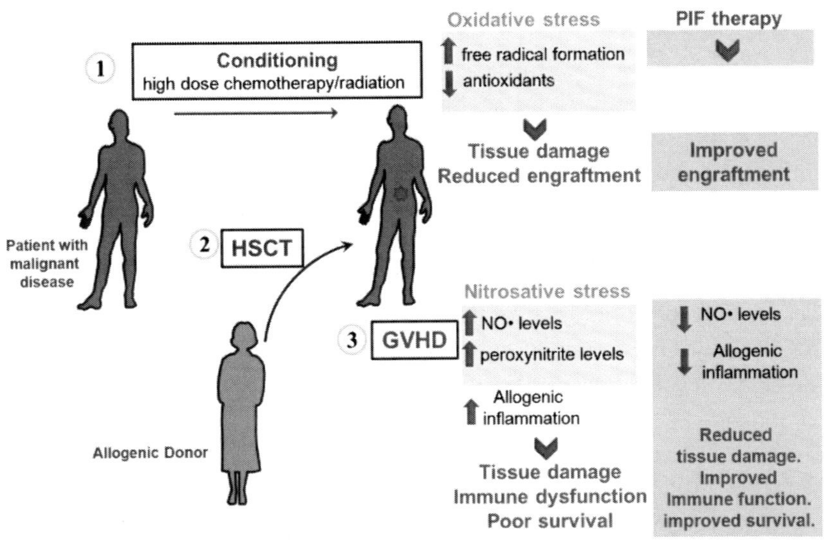

Figure 1. Oxidative and nirosative stress in allogenic HSCT patients. Stem cell transplantation proceeds with conditioning regimen of the recipient (1), which commonly includes high doses of chemotherapy / radiation. Oxidative stress is a byproduct of most conditioning protocols, due to increased free radicals formation and depletion of tissue antioxidants. This imbalance leads to reduced engraftment and tissue damage. Following HSCT from an allogenic donor (2), allogenic immune activation can cause the development of GVHD (3). Pathologic elevation in NO• production due to allogenic activation, coupled with high levels of oxygen free radicals lead to nitrosative stress in GVHD patients. Nitrosative stress has a central role in GVHD-associated tissue damage, immune dysfunction and mortality. PIF therapy lowers the conditioning regimen toxicity and therefore improves engraftment. Additionally, PIF enhances recovery and protects against development of acute GVHD by controlling both allogenic inflammation and NO• production.

Can Drug Intervention in RNS Pathway Improve the Clinical Results After HSCT?

The above results have encouraged scientists in the field to examine the effect of different ROS/RNS inhibitors on the clinical outcome in GVHD models. When the specific iNOS inhibitors L-NG-monomethyl arginine or aminoguanidine were used in organ transplantation models [33, 34] or in a GVHD model without bone marrow transplantation (BMT) [35, 36], the treatment prevented the increased NO• production, decreased mortality and attenuated pathogenesis. However, when these inhibitors where used in allogeneic BMT GVHD models [37, 38], the outcome was poor and mortality increased. The cause for these differences may be due to a critical role for small amounts of NO• in allo-engrafment and/or in T-cell regulation [38]. The over-efficient block of NO• production is therefore harmful for HSCT patients. A more effective approach would be a treatment that combines attenuation of NO• production with immunomodulation and does not reduce allo-engrafment.

We previously described PreImplantation Factor (PIF), an evolutionary conserved embryo-derived peptide (MVRIKPGSANKPSDD), expressed by the embryo/fetus and placenta and present in the maternal circulation of viable pregnancies [39-43]. We demonstrated that synthetic PIF modulates decidual immunity [44-46], orchestrates global anti-inflammatory effects in human peripheral blood mononuclear cells [47, 48] and has an immunomodulatory effect in murine models of autoimmune diseases [49, 50]. In allogeneic BMT GVHD models, PIF administration (short term, low dose) enhanced recovery and protected mice from the development of acute GVHD and the associated nitrosative stress. PIF protective effects were mediated mainly throgh the interaction with monocytes. In macrophages, PIF reduced LPS induced iNOS expression, thereby decreasing NO• secretion [29, 51]. In addition, PIF treatment can also lower the conditioning regimen toxicity, since when it was applied on acute radiation syndrome (ARS) mouse model, PIF improved hematologic recovery and reduced inflammation (Shainer at. al., in preparation). Based on these promising results we plan to use PIF in a clinical setting in the near future. Comprehensive toxicology studies demonstrated high safety for PIF administration, and clinical trial application is currently under FDA consideration.

Conclusion

The oxidative imbalance caused by conditioning regimens prior to HSCT and significant increase in NO• due to allogeneic activation lead to peroxynitrite formation and tissue damage in GVHD patients. Drug intervention in ROS/RNS pathways could improve clinical results post-allogeneic HSCT. Non-toxic, stable, antioxidants may be used to reduce oxidative stress due to conditioning regimen for both autologous and allogeneic HSCT patients. Specific iNOS inhibitors are not effective against nitrosative stress in allogeneic HSCT patients. The use of PIF, an immune-modulatory drug, will enable NO• reduction while preserving engraftment and immune defense.

Acknowledgment

PIF is a patented compound owned by BioIncept, LLC. Dr. Eytan R. Barnea is its (uncompensated) Chief Scientist. Dr. J.H. Barnea is its (uncompensated) President and CEO, and majority shareholder. Hadassah-Hebrew University Medical Center (O. Almogi-Hazan, R. Shainer, R. Or) received an unrestricted grant from BioIncept. All authors declare no conflict of interest.

References

[1] Jenq RR, van den Brink MRM. Allogeneic haematopoietic stem cell transplantation: individualized stem cell and immune therapy of cancer. *Nat Rev Cancer.* 2010;10:213-221.

[2] eggewiss R, Einsele H. Immune reconstitution after allogeneic transplantation and expanding options for immunomodulation: an update. *Blood.* 2010;115:3861-3868.

[3] Slavin S, Nagler A, Naparstek E, et al. Nonmyeloablative Stem Cell Transplantation and Cell Therapy as an Alternative to Conventional Bone Marrow Transplantation With Lethal Cytoreduction for the Treatment of Malignant and Nonmalignant Hematologic Diseases. *Blood.* 1998;91:756-763.

[4] Slavin S, Aker M, Shapira MY, Panigrahi S, Gabriel C, Or R. Non-myeloablative stem cell transplantation for the treatment of cancer and life-threatening non-malignant disorders; past accomplishments and future goals. *Transfusion and Apheresis Science.* 2002;27:159-166.

[5] Ferrara J, Levine J, Reddy P, Holler E. Graft-versus-host disease. *Lancet.* 2009;373:1550-1161.

[6] Blazar BR, Murphy WJ, Abedi M. Advances in graft-versus-host disease biology and therapy. *Nat Rev Immunol.* 2012;12:443-458.

[7] Miller M, Grisham M. Nitric oxide as a mediator of inflammation?-You had better believe it. *Mediators of I nflammation.* 1995;4:387-396.

[8] Valko M, Leibfritz D, Moncol J, Cronin MTD, Mazur M, Telser J. Free radicals and antioxidants in normal physiological functions and human disease. *The International Journal of Biochemistry & Cell Biology.* 2007;39:44-84.

[9] Pacher P, Beckman JS, Liaudet L. Nitric Oxide and Peroxynitrite in Health and Disease. *Physiological Reviews.* 2007;87:315-424.

[10] Clemens M, Ladner C, Schmidt H, et al. Decreased essential antioxidants and increased lipid hydroperoxides following high-dose radiochemotherapy. *Free Radic Res Commun.* 1989;7:227-232.

[11] Clemens M, Ladner C, Ehninger G, et al. Plasma vitamin E and beta-carotene concentrations during radiochemotherapy preceding bone marrow transplantation. *Am J Clin Nutr.* 1990;51:216-219.

[12] Langrehr JM, Murase N, Markus PM, et al. Nitric oxide production in host-versus-graft and graft-versus-host reactions in the rat. *The Journal of Clinical Investigation.* 1992;90:679-683.

[13] Gurtoo H, Hipkens J, Sharma S. Role of glutathione in the metabolism-dependent toxicity and chemotherapy of cyclophosphamide. *Cancer Res.* 1981;41:3584-3591.

[14] Purohit S, Bisby R, Cundall R. Structural modification of human erythrocyte membranes following gamma-irradiation. *Int J Radiat Biol Relat Stud Phys Chem Med.* 1980;38:147-158.

[15] Dürken M, Agbenu J, Finckh B, et al. Deteriorating free radical-trapping capacity and antioxidant status in plasma during bone marrow transplantation. *Bone Marrow Transplant.* 1995;15:757-762.

[16] Dürken M, Herrnring C, Finckh B, et al. Impaired plasma antioxidative defense and increased nontransferrin-bound iron during high-dose chemotherapy and radiochemotherapy preceding bone marrow transplantation. *Free Radical Biology and Medicine.* 2000;28:887-894.

[17] Evens AM, Mehta J, Gordon LI. Rust and corrosion in hematopoietic stem cell transplantation: the problem of iron and oxidative stress. *Bone Marrow Transplant.* 2004;34:561-571.

[18] Sabuncuoglu S, Kuskonmaz B, Uckun Cetinkaya D, Ozgunes H. Evaluation of oxidative and antioxidative parameters in pediatric hematopoietic SCT patients. *Bone Marrow Transplant.* 2012;47:651-656.

[19] Sari I, Cetin A, Kaynar L, et al. Disturbance of Pro-oxidative/Antioxidative Balance in Allogeneic Peripheral Blood Stem Cell Transplantation. *Annals of Clinical & Laboratory Science.* 2008;38:120-125.

[20] Amer J, Weiss L, Reich S, Shapira M, Slavin S, Fibach E. The oxidative status of blood cells in a murine model of graft-versus-host disease. *Annals of Hematology.* 2007;86:753-758.

[21] Hoffman R, Langrehr J, Billiar T, Curran R, Simmons R. *Alloantigen-induced activation of rat splenocytes is regulated by the oxidative metabolism of L-arginine.* 1990;145:2220-2226.

[22] Langrehr J, Hoffman R, Billiar T, Lee K, Schraut W, Simmons R. *Nitric oxide synthesis in the in vivo allograft response: a possible regulatory mechanism.* 1991;110:335-342.

[23] Hoffman R, Langrehr J, Wren S, et al. Characterization of the immunosuppressive effects of nitric oxide in graft vs host disease. *J Immunol.* 1993;151:1508-1518.

[24] Weiss G, Schwaighofer H, Herold M, et al. Nitric oxide formation as predictive parameter for acute graft-versus-host disease after human allogeneic bone marrow transplantation. *Transplantation.* 1995;60:1239-1244.

[25] Vora A, Monaghan J, Nuttall P, Crowther D. Cytokine-mediated nitric oxide release--a common cytotoxic pathway in host-versus-graft and graft-versus-host reactions? *Bone Marrow Transplant.* 1997;20:385-389.

[26] Choi I, Fung P, Leung A, Lie A, Liang R. Plasma nitric oxide is associated with the occurrence of moderate to severe acute graft-versus-host disease in haemopoietic stem cell transplant recipients. *Haematologica.* 2001;86:972-976.

[27] Kuo P, Alfrey E, Krieger N, et al. Differential localization of allograft nitric oxide synthesis: comparison of liver and heart transplantation in the rat model. *Immunology.* 1996;87:647-653.

[28] Nestel FP, Greene RN, Kichian K, Ponka P, Lapp WS. Activation of macrophage cytostatic effector mechanisms during acute graft-versus-

host disease: release of intracellular iron and nitric oxide–mediated cytostasis. *Blood.* 2000;96:1836-1843.
[29] Azar Y, Shainer R, Almogi-Hazan O, et al. PreImplantation Factor Reduces Graft-versus-Host Disease by Regulating Immune Response and Lowering Oxidative Stress (Murine Model). *Biology of Blood and Marrow Transplantation*. 2013;19:519-528.
[30] Falzarano G, Krenger W, Snyder K, Delmonte JJ, Karandikar M, Ferrara J. Suppression of B-cell proliferation to lipopolysaccharide is mediated through induction of the nitric oxide pathway by tumor necrosis factor-alpha in mice with acute graft-versus-host disease. *Blood.* 1996;87:2853-2860.
[31] Hoffman RA, Mahidhara RS, Wolf-Johnston AS, Lu L, Thomson AW, Simmons RL. Differential modulation of CD4 and CD8 T-cell roliferation by induction of nitric oxide synthesis in anigen presenting cells1. *Transplantation.* 2002;74:836-845.
[32] Krenger W, Falzarano G, Delmonte JJ, Snyder K, Byon J, Ferrara J. Interferon-gamma suppresses T-cell proliferation to mitogen via the nitric oxide pathway during experimental acute graft-versus-host disease. *Blood.* 1996;88:1113-1121.
[33] Langrehr JM, Machens C, Koch S, Zill E, Leder K, Neuhaus P. Hematologic parameters are improved by inhibition of NO synthesis during graft-versus-host disease after small bowel transplantation. *Transplantation Proceedings.* 2000;32:1288-1289.
[34] Worrall NK, Lazenby WD, Misko TP, et al. Modulation of in vivo alloreactivity by inhibition of inducible nitric oxide synthase. *The Journal of Experimental Medicine*. 1995;181:63-70.
[35] Ellison CA, Natuik SA, McIntosh AR, Scully SA, Danilenko DM, Gartner JG. The role of interferon-γ, nitric oxide and lipopolysaccharide in intestinal graft-versus-host disease developing in F1-hybrid mice. *Immunology*. 2003;109:440-449.
[36] Hoffman RA, Nüssler NC, Gleixner SL, et al. Attenuation of Lethal Graft-Versus-Host Disease By Inhibition of Nitric Oxide Synthase1. *Transplantation.* 1997;63:94-100.
[37] Drobyski W, Keever C, Hanson G, McAuliffe T, Griffith O. Inhibition of nitric oxide production is associated with enhanced weight loss, decreased survival, and impaired alloengraftment in mice undergoing graft-versus-host disease after bone marrow transplantation. *Blood.* 1994;84:2363-2373.

[38] Hongo D, Bryson JS, Kaplan AM, Cohen DA. Endogenous Nitric Oxide Protects against T Cell-Dependent Lethality during Graft-versus-Host Disease and Idiopathic Pneumonia Syndrome. *The Journal of Immunology.* 2004;173:1744-1756.

[39] Barnea E, Simon J, Levine S, Coulam C, Taliadouros G, Leavis P. Progress in characterization of pre-implantation factor in embryo cultures and in vivo. *Am J Reprod Immunol.* 1999;42:95-99.

[40] Barnea ER. Insight into Early Pregnancy Events: The Emerging Role of the Embryo*. *American Journal of Reproductive Immunology.* 2004;51:319-322.

[41] Stamatkin C, Roussev R, Stout M, et al. PreImplantation Factor (PIF) correlates with early mammalian embryo development-bovine and murine models. *Reproductive Biology and Endocrinology.* 2011;9:63.

[42] Stamatkin CW, Roussev RG, Stout M, et al. Preimplantation factor negates embryo toxicity and promotes embryo development in culture. *Reproductive BioMedicine Online.* 2011;23:517-524.

[43] Than NG, Paidas MJ, Mizutani S, Sharma S, Padbury J, Barnea ER. Embryo–Placento–Maternal Interaction and Biomarkers: From Diagnosis to Therapy – A Workshop Report. *Placenta.* 2007;28, Supplement:S107-S110.

[44] Barnea E, Kirk D, Paidas M. Preimplantation factor (PIF) promoting role in embryo implantation: increases endometrial integrin-$\alpha 2\beta 3$, amphiregulin and epiregulin while reducing betacellulin expression via MAPK in decidua. *Reprod Biol Endocrinol.* 2012;10:50.

[45] Duzyj CM, Barnea ER, Li M, Huang SJ, Krikun G, Paidas MJ. Preimplantation factor promotes first trimester trophoblast invasion. *American Journal of Obstetrics and Gynecology.* 2010;203:402.e401-402.e404.

[46] Paidas MJ, Krikun G, Huang SJ, et al. A genomic and proteomic investigation of the impact of preimplantation factor on human decidual cells. *American Journal of Obstetrics and Gynecology.* 2010;202:459.e451-459.e458.

[47] Barnea ER, Kirk D, Ramu S, Rivnay B, Roussev R, Paidas MJ. PreImplantation Factor (PIF) orchestrates systemic antiinflammatory response by immune cells: effect on peripheral blood mononuclear cells. *American Journal of Obstetrics and Gynecology.* 2012;207:313.e311-313.e311.

[48] Roussev RG, Dons'koi BV, Stamatkin C, et al. Preimplantation factor inhibits circulating natural killer cell cytotoxicity and reduces CD69

expression: implications for recurrent pregnancy loss therapy. *Reproductive BioMedicine Online.* 2013;26:79-87.

[49] Weiss L, Bernstein S, Jones R, et al. Preimplantation factor (PIF) analog prevents type I diabetes mellitus (TIDM) development by preserving pancreatic function in NOD mice. *Endocrine.* 2011;40:41-54.

[50] Weiss L, Or R, Jones RC, et al. Preimplantation Factor (PIF*) reverses neuroinflammation while promoting neural repair in EAE model. *Journal of the Neurological Sciences.* 2012;312:146-157.

[51] Shainer R, Azar Y, Almogi-Hazan O, et al. Immune Regulation and Oxidative Stress Reduction by Preimplantation Factor following Syngeneic or Allogeneic Bone Marrow Transplantation. *Conference Papers in Medicine.* 2013;2013.

In: Oxidative Stress
Editor: Cassidy Croft
ISBN: 978-1-63117-578-7

Chapter 8

Review of the Oxidative Stress Role in the Pathophysiology of Different Hearing Disorders: New Insight in the Role of Oxidative Stress in the Pathophysiology of Otosclerosis

*Milan Rudić**, *M.D., Ph.D.*
Research Associate, ENT Department
General Hospital Zadar, Croatia

Abstract

Inner ear hair cells are know to be highly energy demanding and oxygen consuming cells. The damage of the inner ear cells cell can occur as a results of local ROS (reactive oxygen species) production. The main source of these molecules within the cochlea appear to be the hair cells' mitochondria, or enzymes such as xanthine oxidase and NADPH oxidase. Once generated, ROS are responsible for direct cellular damage to lipids, proteins and DNA, triggering apoptosis or necrosis and may also diffuse among the inner ear scalae. In animal models, several conditions of ROS

* Tel: +385-23-505417; Mobile: +385-91-5695120; Email: milan.rudic@yahoo.com.

production related to cochlear damage have been reported, including exposure to noise and drugs (amynoglycosides and cisplatin). In humans, ROS appear to be involved in hairs cell damage in some cases of genetic hearing loss (i.e., Pendred syndrome, presbycusis and Meniere's syndrome). Several animal or in vitro models have been proposed for treatment against ROS-mediated damage (interruption of the lipid peroxidation process and preservation of the cell membrane integrity; prevention of noise induced inner ear damage by cochlear ischemia/ re-perfusion; and prevention of cell apoptosis).

In otosclerosis (localized bone dysplasia of the human otic capsule) the ROS could be produced in the otosclerotic foci and diffuse to the inner ear compartment through the cochlear endosteum, causing cochlear damage and sensorineural hearing loss. Indeed, recent studies for the first time confirmed the presence of ROS secondary messengers (4-hydroxynonenal) in the otosclerotic specimens. Different distribution pattern of HNE antibodies has been observed in otosclerotic specimens compared to the control ones, suggesting its potential role in the pathophysiology of the disease. However, further studies (both experimental and clinical ones) are needed in order to better understand and clarify the role of ROS in the pathophysiology of otosclerosis and different hearing disorders.

1. Oxidative Stress Overview

Oxidative stress takes place in tissues under the effect of toxic agents, inflammation, ischemia, or physical trauma. These situations may lead to an excessive formation of reactive oxygen species (ROS), and disequilibrium in the steady–state between formation and elimination of ROS [1]. This stress can cause various acute, as well as chronic diseases, such as cardiovascular, neurodegenerative diseases and malignant tumours [2,3,4]. Nowadays, there is growing evidence about the physiological generation of ROS that can occur as a byproduct of other biological reactions. NADPH oxidase is known to be the major source of ROS, but ROS generation also occurs with mitochondria, peroxisomes, cytochrome P-450, and other cellular elements [5]. Several growth factors and cytokines (e.g., TGF-β and PDGF) through binding to different types of cell membrane receptors can elicit a rise in intracellular ROS. Furthermore, it has been reported that ROS activate MAPK pathways in several systems, including extracellular signal regulated kinase (ERK) 1/2, Jun-NH2-terminal kinase and P38 MAPK cascades [6]. With an excessive amount of ROS in the cellular membrane environment, lipid peroxidation occurs and lipid cell constituents are damaged. Lipids are essential in cell membranes and among the first molecules susceptible to the damage caused by reactive oxygen species. Free radical reactions in tissues are accompanied by oxidative degradation of polyunsaturated fatty acids of membrane lipids [7]. This process results in the production of highly reactive aldehydes which are named "second messengers" as opposed to the primary free radicals that initiate lipid peroxidation [7]. Unlike reactive oxygen species (ROS), reactive aldehydes are relatively long-lived. Therefore, they might diffuse from the site of their production and attack distant intracellular or extracellular targets causing organ and tissular dysfunction involved in aging liver and kidney disease, neurological and cardiovascular systems, cancers, endocrine and metabolic disorders, diabetes and its complications and other oxidative stress-related pathologies [8]. Among many different aldehydes, most thoroughly studied are malondialdehyde, acrolein and the 4-hydroxyalkenal family, in particular 4-hydroxynonenal (HNE) [9].

2. Oxidative Stress and the Inner Ear Hair Cell Damage

Inner ear hair cells are known to be highly energy demanding and oxygen consuming cells. The damage of the inner ear cells cell can occur as a results of local ROS (reactive oxygen species) production. The main source of these molecules within the cochlea appear to be the hair cells' mitochondria, or enzymes such as xanthine oxidase and NADPH oxidase [10,11].

Once generated, ROS are responsible for direct cellular damage to lipids, proteins, and DNA, triggering apoptosis or necrosis and may also diffuse among the inner ear scalae [10,12,13]. In animal models, several conditions of increased ROS production related to cochlear damage have been described, including exposure to noise and to drugs (i.e., aminoglycosides and cisplatin) [10]. In humans, ROS appear to be involved in hair cell damage in some cases of genetic hearing loss (i.e., Pendred syndrome), presbycusis, and Menière's syndrome. Furthermore, the first evidence of the presence and production of a biologically relevant ROS, superoxide in the perilymph of patients affected by profound hearing loss and treated with cochlear implantation have been provided [10]. This molecule is produced by xanthine dehydrogenase/xanthine oxidase (XA/XO) enzyme system. High levels of ROS and related enzymes in human inner ear perilymph (above 25 mmoles per mg of protein) may be an expression of previous damage to the organ of Corti and to the inner ear [10]. In otosclerosis, (localized bone dysplasia of the human otic capsule) the ROS could be produced in the otosclerotic foci and diffuse to the inner ear compartment through the cochlear endosteum, causing cochlear damage and sensorineural hearing loss. [11, 14].

Several animal or in vitro models have been proposed for treatment against ROS-mediated damage [11]. In rats the increase of antioxidant supplies in the cochlea may effectively prevent hair cell damage and hearing loss [15]. Pharmacological interventions have been directed at: interrupting the lipid peroxidation process, thus preserving the integrity of cell membranes (i.e., by lazaroids), preventing noise-mediated inner ear damage by cochlear ischemia/reperfusion (i.e., by pentoxifylline and sarthran) and preventing cell apoptosis, by inhibitors of cell death pathways such as JNK inhibitors, D-JNK-1, riluzole or minocyclin [11,16].

2.1. Oxidative Stress and Drugs Induced Hearing Loss

2.1.1. Aminoglycoside and Cisplatin

The most common drugs associated with the hearing loss are amynoglycosides (antibacterial agents) and cisplatin (anticancer agent) [17]. They can be either “cochleotoxic” (affecting only the hearing organ, i.e., amikacin, neomycin and cisplatin) or “vestibulotoxic” (affecting the vestibular system, i.e., gentamicin). The severity of ototoxicity varies among the aminoglycosides: neomycin is considered highly toxic, gentamicin, kanamycin and tobramycin less, and amikacin and netilmicin are considered as the least toxic (mostly to the cochlea) [17]. Other drugs associated with different hearing disorders are: salicylate, diuretics like furosemide, ethacrynic acid, and bumetanide which in combination with aminoglycoside antibiotics can cause severe damage to the hearing. Recently, some phosphodiesterase inhibitors are reported to be associated with sudden hearing loss and/or vestibular disorders [17,18]. Other potentially ototoxic substances are organometals like organotins and mercury preparations, as well as solvents like toluene and styrene used in industry [17].

Cisplatin or aminoglycosides induced hearing loss is bilateral and begins at high frequencies, spreading to lower frequencies with prolonged treatment. Vestibulotoxicity of aminoglycosides can manifest as loss of balance with or without vertigo. Symptoms are usually delayed days or weeks after commencement of therapy and can continue to progress after treatment [17].

Certain risk factors are associated with the severe ototoxic side effects of these drugs (i.e., poor nutritional status, hypoalbuminemia, anemia, renal insufficiency, cranial radiation, pre-existing hearing loss, and co-treatment with other drugs) [17-18]

Both aminoglycosides and cisplatin are found to produce ROS. Current research suggest that the formation of the ROS is the main cause for the undesired side effects of the aminoglycosides and cisplatin [12,17]. Aminoglycosides, promote the formation of ROS by different mechanisms and signaling pathways (stimulation of NADPH, formation of redox-active complexes, via Rho-GTPases, mytochondrial mutation and dysfunction) [17,19]. Cisplatin also generates the formation of ROS by activation of NADPH and xanthine oxidase system. Aminoglycosids mostly cause cellular necrosis and apoptosis, while cisplatin primarily cause apoptosis of the outer hair cells, stria vascularis, spiral ligament and spiral ganglion cells [17,20,21].

The use of antioxidant therapy has been proposed as a potential treatment against drug associated hearing loss. Namely, administration of N-acetylcystein, and vitamin E. However there is a need for further research in finding new methods of delivery of these protective agents to the inner ear without interference against the desired therapeutic effects of the drugs used [17,22,23].

2.1.2. Mefloquine

Another drug associated with the hearing loss is mefloquine. Mefloquine is an antimalarial drug that is widely used for prophylactic and therapeutical treatment of malaria but with numerous side-effects like anxiety, panic attacks, nightmares, dizziness, headaches, balance disturbance and hearing loss [24]. In-vitro studies have shown that mefloquine damages cochlear and vestibular hair cells and spiral ganglion neurons through apoptosis [25,26]. Furthermore, mefloquine causes primary rat cortical neuron degeneration in embryonic rat neurons, and significant axonal degeneration [27]. The way in which mefloquine cause cytotoxic effect on hearing is through the generation of free heme, which than acts as s catalisator for the ROS formation [24,28]. Furthermore, recent study demonstrated that mefloquine treatment causes degeneration of cochlear hair cells and auditory nerves in a dose-dependent manner, and that it increases superoxide and protein carbonyl levels in the hair cells and spiral ganglion neurons in the cochleae suggesting that mefloquine-induced degeneration of the cochlear auditory nervous system is triggered by an increase in oxidative stress [24]. Results of the study confirmed that caspases-3-mediated apoptosis may be an important mechanism linking mefloquine, cochlear neuroaxonal and hair cell degeneration, and NAD+, and that NAD+ is a useful drug candidate in reducing or slowing the degeneration of cochlear axons and sensory hair cells caused by mefloquine treatment and oxidative stress damage to the cochlear cells [24].

2.2. Oxidative Stress and Presbyacusis

Age-related hearing loss (AHL), also referred to as presbyacusis, is the most common cause of hearing loss in aged people [29]. It occurs in 25–45% of people aged 65 years or older; 40% to 66% in people older than 75 years and more than 80% in people older than 85 years [29,30]. AHL is defined as progressive, bilateral, and symmetrical hearing impairment. It generally begins at high-frequency region and progresses toward the lower- frequency region. AHL is often associated with difficulty in speech discrimination and sound detection and localization. Eventually, it can affect the cognitive, emotional, and social function [29]. The pathophysiology of AHL is still unclear and needs to be clarified in order to develop new therapeutic strategies.

AHL is histologically characterized by structural changes in inner ear, such as degeneration of sensory cells, auditory neurons, and cells of the stria vascularis [29,30,31,32]. One of the causes of the age-related cochlear degeneration has been attributed to the accumulated effects of numerous insults, including exposure to intense noise and ototoxic drugs. However, age-related cochlear degeneration can occur in the absence of such insults. Reported that mammals reared in quiet environments without exposure to ototoxins showed progressive hearing loss with aging, suggesting the role of genetic and intrinsic factors in addition to environmental factors [29,33]. The free radical theory of aging has been suggested and for the AHL as well [29]. However, the role of free radical theory in the etiology of AHL is still controversial due to the lack of a strong and consistent evidence.

2.3. Oxidative Stress and Noise Induced Hearing Loss

The factors underlying noise-dependent damages have a complex nature and noise exposure is one of the most common causes of hearing loss, and oxidative stress and antioxidative protective mechanisms have been proposed as the most interesting issues in noise-related harmful effects [11, 34,35]. Although they are still under investigation, the exact mechanisms leading to hearing loss have not been fully understood so far. Noise exposure leads to a dramatic change in cochlear blood flow, including increased vascular permeability, capillary vasoconstriction and blood stagnation in strial capillaries [34]. This, in turn, causes an excessive ROS generation as an unwanted byproduct of high metabolic activity. Superoxide anion, hydroxyl radicals and reactive nitrogen species (RNS) as well as byproducts of lipid peroxidation and oxidative-induced DNA damage have been found to follow the intense noise exposure [34,36-38]. Acting on lipid molecules free radicals may lead to continuing cell damage after noise exposure and they can cause mitochondrial membrane injury, cytochrome C release, and ischemia/reperfusion damage in the inner ear [11,34-39]. Certain degrees of protections against NIHL were reported for antioxidant molecules such as glutathione, ebselen, alpha-tocopherol, acetyl-l-carnitine and *N*-acetylcysteine (NAC), Magnesium administration, Vitamin E and coenzyme Q10 [34,35,37-42]. d-methionine (oral antioxidant and a natural component of cheese and yogurt) has also been found to have otoprotective properties. Its ability to act as a free radical scavenger explains why it is protective against factors that can cause irreversible damage of the cochlea (e.g., cisplatin, aminoglycosides, noise) [34].

2.4. Oxidative Stress and Different Hearing Disorders

2.4.1. Oxidative STRESS and Otitis Media with Effusion and Chronic Otitis Media

Otitis media with effusion is one of the most frequent diseases in children. It can cause conductive hearing loss and have a negative impact on the speech development. Although OME is very common, its pathophysiology is still unclear. Recently the role of oxidative stress has been investigated in the pathophysiology of this disease [43-46]. Many various cellular element have been found in the middle ear fluid (inflammatory agents, neutrophils, macrophages, T and B lymphocytes). These inflammatory agents generate the production of superoxide radicals that have a potent bactericide activity, but during chronic inflammation this protective mechanism becomes damaging [44].

Several recent studies have investigated the role of oxidants and antioxidants in the chronic middle ear disease. The results suggest that indeed oxidative stress could have an important role in the development of the middle ear disease [43-46]. However, further analysis of these mechanisms could lead to the identification of the new treatment possibilities thus preventing severe possible complications.

2.4.2. Oxidative Stress and Pendred Syndrome

Pendred syndrome is an autosomal recessive disease that affects the inner ear and the thyroid and causes childhood deafness and postpuberty goiter. It is caused by loss-of-function mutations of the gene *SLC26A4*, which encodes the anion exchanger pendrin. Recently the studies suggested that the loss of pendredin leads to the free radical stress in stria vascularis thus causing the loss of Kcjn10 protein expression. The loss of Kcjn10 expression in stria vascularis causes the loss of endochondreal potential and the failure to develop hearing in the mouse model of Pendred syndrome [47].

2.4.3. Oxidative Stress and Ménière's Disease

Ménière's disease is characterized by the triad of symptoms (fluctuating hearing loss, episodic vertigo and tinnitus), and by endolymphatic hydrops found on post-mortem examination. Recent research studies suggest that oxidative stress could be involved in the development of endolymphatic hydrops and that cellular damage and apoptotic cell death causing sensorineural hearing loss found in later stages of the disease. Furthermore, it has been observed that patients with Ménière's disease are under systemic oxidative stress and that a key role in protection against protective oxidative stress, play vitagenes, that include heat shock proteins (Hsp70) as well as the thioredoxin/thioredoxin reductase system [48].

2.4.4. Oxidative Stress and Otosclerosis

Otosclerosis is a complex disease characterized by an abnormal bone turnover localised to the human otic capsule resulting in conductive hearing loss [49]. Its incidence in Western populations is 0.3%. In 80% of cases the disease has a bilateral form. It is more frequent in women than in men [50,51]. Several hypotheses have been proposed concerning the aetiology of otosclerosis including viral infection, and auto immunity, but the aetiology appears to be complex multi-factor and still unclear [52-55]. Recent research have been focused on the role of Angiotensin II and oxidative stress in the pathophysiology of otosclerosis. Angiotensin (Ang) II, a major effector peptide of the renin-angiotensin system is an important regulator of the cardiovascular system and body fluid homeostasis, and an important local cellular growth factor [56-58]. Ang II affects bone metabolism in a complex mechanism, still not revealed in details, either through receptors located in osteoblasts and osteoclasts or through regulation of the blood flow in marrow capillaries. Previous in vitro results have shown different effects of Ang II on bone cells. Ang II expressed stimulatory effect on the proliferation of osteoblast-rich cultured human bone cells, and stimulation of DNA synthesis, cell number and collagen synthesis in osteoblastic precursor cells. On the contrary, Ang II also caused deceleration of the differentiation and mineralization of osteoblastic cells. Furthermore, Ang II may exert stimulatory effect on osteoclastic bone resorption (promotion of the differentiation and activation of osteoclasts responsible for bone resorption via up-regulation of RANKL in osteoblasts) [59-64]. These observations suggested that Ang II could be considered as a new regulatory factor of bone metabolism and formation. Previously results have shown an existing association between otosclerosis and two genetic polymorphisms related to plasmatic Ang II concentrations, AGT M235T and ACE I/D [65,66].

Reactive oxygen species (ROS) have a major role in different signaling pathways of Ang II. Ang II stimulates the ROS formation via activation of NADPH oxidase and could therefore contribute to the onset of oxidative stress. Furthermore, several important physiological functions of Ang II (e.i. cell growth, hypertrophy, proliferation, apoptosis and cell migration) are directly mediated by ROS [67-71]. As highly reactive and unstable molecules ROS can react with bioactive macromolecules such as proteins, nucleic acids and lipids. Primary targets of ROS are polysaturated fatty acids in membrane phospholipids and in other lipid containing structures thus producing more stable reactive radicals in a process called lipid peroxidation. Lipid peroxidation products can cause lipid hydroperoxide-derived modifications of Ang II which can modulate its biological activity [67]. A major bioactive marker of lipid peroxidation, derived from ω-6 polyunsaturated fatty acids like arachidonic acid and linoleic acid, is 4-hydroxylnonenal (HNE), which is highly reactive aldehyde that acts as a second messenger of free radicals and a signaling molecule [7-9]. It is found in different human tissues and its physiological roles are not entirely understood. Previous studies revealed the involvement of HNE in differentiation, apoptosis and cell proliferation in various types of cells, including human osteoblast-like cells, in particular if present in physiological concentration. While its effects in various human diseases are intensively studied by continuously developing methods, recent studies have found HNE to be an important endogenous growth factor for osteoblasts grown *in vitro* on the surfaces of bioactive glass otherwise used in medicine for enhancement of osteogenesis [72-78].

Recent study have analysed the possible involvement of HNE in otosclerosis and its interactions with Ang II in growth regulation of cultured human osteoblast-like cells [79].

By analyzing the histologic samples of normal and otosclerotic stapes it was found that both samples expressed different positivity for HNE antibodies. While control samples showed clearly marked positivity in periosteal region, otosclerotic samples showed multifocal areas of HNE positivity mainly in the new bone or abnormal bone formation regions [79]. These observations suggest that HNE (secondary messenger of ROS) is indeed involved in the pathophysiological processes of the otosclerosis. Moreover, it was concluded that if the cells originate in periosteal region, HNE is involved in normal physiological process of cell growth but if the cells are forming new bone like in multifocal regions of otosclerotic bone, HNE is involved in pathophysiology of this disorder. So far it has been observed that several important physiological functions of Ang II are mediated through ROS (i.e., cellular growth, and inflammatory responses) [69]. Activating the NADPH oxidase enzyme system Ang II stimulates ROS generation mainly through its G protein-coupled Ang II type 1 (AT1) receptor [67]. In order to test the possible direct binding between the Ang II and HNE the Immunoblot analysis has been performed. The results showed that there could exist a possible interaction between the HNE and Ang II (histidin, serin, lisin and cistein amino-acids could be possible binding sites). In the performed experiment higher binding was observed for BSA and HNE then for BSA and Ang II (higher histidin concentration with the HNE). However, due to the experiment protocol (addition of HNE prior to Ang II) direct binding between them could not be confirmed. But, interaction is likely to exist in a tissue and intracellular level but mainly on the transmembrane proteins and receptors. HNE is mostly formed close to the cellular membrane and Ang II acts as a cytokine-like hormone and could react with the HNE. Indeed one of the signaling pathways of Ang II includes activation of mitogen-activated protein kinases (MAPK), including extracellular signal-regulated kinases (ERK 1 /2), c-junk N-terminal kinase (JNKs, also known as SAPKs), p38MAPKs and big MAPK-1. Previously it was observed that cells in respond to oxidative stress or HNE can also activate different mitogen activated proteins kinases (namely JNKs and ERK family MAP kinases) [80].

In studying the effect of Ang II and HNE on the cellular proliferation (HOS) the significant stimulation of cellular growth (DNA synthesis) was observed but in dose dependent concentrations. This might be due to the fact that HNE modulates the effect of Ang II or that Ang II adds to the already noted bifunctional-growth regulating effect of HNE on osteoblast-like cells.

To investigate the influence of Ang II and HNE on the cellular differentiation the alkaline phosphatase activity (ALP) was analyzed. In certain concentrations HNE (10μM) and Ang II (0.1 and 0.5nM) increased the activity of ALP while in concentrations of HNE (1μM or 2.5μM) and Ang II (0.1nM) no such effect was noted. These result are in contrast with previous results showing that HNE in concentration of 10μM caused decrease in cell differentiation [73].

The results of apoptosis induction showed that both HNE and And II expressed the concentration dependent results. While in certain concentrations the decrease of apoptotic cells was noted in others no such effect was observed. Results of the effect of the HNE on the apoptosis in concentrations of 10μM are in concordance with the previous observed HNE effect on osteoblast like cells (increased percentage of apoptotic cells)[73]. The observed bimodal effect of HNE on cellular growth is in concordance with previous reports suggesting that in cells exists a very narrow window of physiological levels of HNE. Alterations of those levels could strongly change the HNE effect on cell cycle. When intracellular HNE levels exceed its physiological range, programmed cell death (apoptosis) is triggered. On the contrary cellular proliferation is stimulated when HNE levels drop bellow the normal physiological range [81]. The mechanisms through HNE affects signaling processes in dose-dependent manner still need to be investigated. HNE is a strong electrophile and as such it reacts with nucleophilic groups of proteins, nucleic acid and lipids. It is possible that at low concentrations HNE selectively affects pathways in favor for cellular proliferation by interacting with nucleophilic groups having high affinity for HNE. At higher concentrations HNE could react with low affinity groups of cellular nucleophils thus triggering the cellular apoptosis [81]. Gluthatione S-transferases (GSTs) can modulate the intracellular concentrations of HNE by affecting its generation during lipid peroxidation by reducing hydroperoxides and also by converting it into gluthatione (GSH) conjugate (GS-HNE). Previously it was observed that otosclerotic cells produce bone matrix glyocosaminoglycans (GAG) with higher level of sulfatation [82]. Moreover otosclerotic cells express higher activity of the diastrophic dysplasia sulphate transporter (DTDST). This activity could be inhibited with the sodium-fluoride (NaF) and dexamethason [83].

Regarding the observed interaction between Ang II and HNE on the cellular proliferation, differentiation and apoptosis and with respect to the influence of both on the sulfatation of matrix proteins further studies are needed on possible interactions of HNE and Ang II and the role of GST in the regulation of these processes.

Further in vitro studies should be focused on investigating the presence of ROS in otosclerotic and control culture media. Furthermore the effect of antioxidants on proliferation, differentiation and apoptosis of otosclerotic cell cultures should be determined.

Clinical studies should be focused on evaluating the presence of ROS in stapedial samples (control and otosclerotic ones) as a possible prognostic factor for disease activity. Moreover measurement of the ROS presence in perilymph samples could be compared with the degree of hearing loss in otosclerosis.

Finally, like for other types of oxidative stress associated hearing loss future studies should be focused on developing new approaches for prevention and treatment (i.e., antioxidant therapy, interruption of the lipid peroxidation process, prevention of cochlear ischemia).

References

[1] Haliwell B, Gutteridge JMC. The chemistry of oxygen radicals and other oxygen-derived species. In : Halliwell B, Gutteridge JMC eds. Free radicals in biology and medicine, Oxford, Clanderon Press 1989;9:29-32.

[2] Ignarro LJ, Balestrieri ML, Napoli C: Nutrition, physical activity, and cardiovascular disease: An update. *Cardiovascular. Res.* 2007;73:326-340.

[3] Emerit J, Edeas M, Bricaire F. Neurdegenerative disease and oxidative stress. *Biomed. Pharma* 2004;58:39-46.

[4] Dreher D; Junod AF. Role of oxygen free radicals in cancer development. *Eur. J. Cancer* 1996;32B:30-38.

[5] Bedard K, Kruse KH. The NOX family of ROS-generating NADPH oxydases: physiology and pathophysiology. *Physiol. Rev. 2007*;87.245-313.

[6] Henrotin YE, Bruckner P. The role of reactive oxygen species in homeostasis and degradation of cartilage. *Osteoarthritis Cartilage* 2003;11:74-755.

[7] Esterbauer H, Schaur RJ, Zollner H. Chemistry and biochemistry of 4-hydroxynonenal, malonaldehyde and related aldehydes. *Free Radic. Biol. Med.* 1991;11:81-128.

[8] Negre-Salvayre, A.; Auge, N.; Ayala, V.; Basaga, H.; Boada, J.; Brenke, R.; Chapple, S.; Cohen, G.; Feher, J.; Grune, T.; Lengyel, G.; Mann, G.E.; Pamplona, R.; Poli, G.; Portero-Otin, M.; Riahi, Y.; Salvayre, R.; Sasson, S.; Serrano, J.; Shamni, O.; Siems, W.; Siow, R.C.; Wiswedel, I.; Zarkovic, K.; Zarkovic, N. Pathological aspects of lipid peroxidation. *Free Radic. Res.* 44:1125-1171; 2010.

[9] Zarkovic N. 4-Hydroxynonenal as a bioactive marker of pathophysiological processes. *Mol. Aspects Med.* 2003;24:281-291.

[10] Ciorba A, Gasparini P, Chicca M, Pinamonti S, Martini A. Reactive oxygen species in human inner ear perylimph. *Acta Otolaryngol.* 2010;130:240-246.

[11] Henderson D, Bielefeld EC. Harris KC, Hu BH. The role of oxidative stress in noise-induced hearing loss. *Ear Hear 2006*;27:1-19.

[12] Clerici WJ, Yang L. Direct effects of intraperylimphatic reactive oxygen species generation on cochlear function. *Hear Res.* 1996;101-14-22.

[13] Henderson D, McFadden SL, Liu CC, Hight N, Zheng XY. The role of antioxidants in protection form impulse noise. *Ann. NY Acad. Sci.,* 1999;884:368-80.

[14] Borovic S, Cipak A, Meinitzer A, Kejla Z, Perovic D, Waeg G, Zarkovic N. Differential sensitivity to 4-hydroxinonenal of normal and malignant mesenchymal cells. *Redox Rep.* 2007;12:50-54.

[15] Lorito G, Giordano P, Prosser S, Martini A, Hatzopoulos S. Noise induced hearing loss: a study on the pharmacological protection in the Sprague Dawely rat with N-acetyl-cysteine. *Acta Otolaryngol. Ital.* 2006;26:133-9.

[16] Corbacella E, Lanzoni I, Ding D, Previati M, Salvi R. Minocycline attenuates gentamicin induced hair cell loss in neonatal cochlear culture. *Hear Res.* 2004;197:11-18.

[17] Schacht J, Talaska AE, Rybak LP. Cisplatin and Aminoglycosides antibiotics: Hearing Loss and Its Prevention. *Anat. Rec.* 2012;295(11):1837-1850.

[18] Maddox PT, Saunders J, Chandrasekhar SS. Sudden hearing loss from PDE-5-inhibitors: A cellular stress etiology. *Laryngoscope.* 2009;119:1586-1589.

[19] Jiang H, Sha SH, Schacht J. Rac/Rho pathway regulates actin depolymerization induced by amynoglycoside antibiotics. *J. Neurosci. Res.* 2006b;83:1544-1551.

[20] Ylikoski J, Xing-Qun L, Virkkala J, Pirvola U. Blockade of c-Jun N-terminal kinase pathway gentamicin induced cochlear and vestibular hair cell death. *Har res.* 2002;163:71-81.

[21] Liang F, Schulte BA, Qu C, Hu W, Shen Z. Inhibition of the calcium- and voltage dependent conductance potassium channel ameliorates cisplatin-induced apoptosis in spiral ligament of the cochlea. *Neuroscience.* 2005;135:263-271.

[22] Feldman L, Efrati S, Eviatar E, Abramsohn R, Yarovoy I, Gersch E, Averbukh Z, Weissgart. Gentamicin-induced ototoxicity in hemodialysis patients is ameliorated by N-acetylcystein. *Kidney Int.* 2007;72:359-363.

[23] Kharkheli E, Kevanishvilli Z, Maglakelidze T, Davitshavili O, Schacht J. Does vitamin E prevent gentamicin-induced ototoxicity? *Georgian Med. News.* 2007:14-17.

[24] Ding D, Qi Weidong, Yu Dongzhen, Jiang H, Han C, Kim JM, Katsuno K, Hsieh YH, Miyakawa T, Salvi R, Tanokura M, Someya S. Addition of exogenous NAD+ prevents mefloquine-induced neuroaxonal and hair cell degeneration throuh reduction of caspase-3-mediated apoptosis in cochlear organotypic cultures. *PLos ONE.* 2013;8:e79817.

[25] Ding D, Qi W, Yu D, JIang H, Salvi R et al. Detection of apoptosis by RT-PCR array in mefloquine-induced cochlear damage. *J. of Otol.* 2011;6:1-9.

[26] Ding D, Someya S,Tanokura M, Jiang H, Salvi R. NAD attenuates mefloquine-induced cochlear damage from reactive oxygen species. *Abstr. Assoc. Res. Otolaryngol.* 2013.

[27] Dow GS, Hudson TH, Vahey M, Koenig ML. The acute neurotoxicity of mefloquine may be mediated through a disruption of calcium homeostasis and ER function in vitro. *Malar J.* 2003;2:14.

[28] Hood JE, Jenkins JW, Milatovic D, Rongzhu L, Aschner M. Mefloquine induces oxidative stress and neurodegeneration in primary rat cortical neurons. *Neurotoxicology.* 2010;31:518-523.

[29] Kinoshita M, Sakamoto T, Kashio A, Shimizu T, Yamasoba T. Age - related hearing loss in Mn-SOD knockout mice. *Oxi. Med. Cell Longev.* 2013;2013:1-12.

[30] Yueh B, Shapiro N, MacLean CH, Shekelle PG. Screening and management of adult hearing loss in primary care. *Scientific review Journal of the American Medical Association.* 2003;289:1976-1985.

[31] Schuknecht HF, Gacek MR. Cochlear pathology in presbycusis. *Annals of Otology, Rhinology and Laryngology*. 1993;102:1–16.

[32] Shimada A, Ebisu M, Morita T, Takeuchi T, Umemura T. Age-related changes in the cochlea and cochlear nuclei of dogs. *Journal of Veterinary Medical Science*.1998;60:41–48.

[33] Hellstrom Li, Schmiedt RA. Measures of tuning and suppression in single-fiber and whole-nerve responses in young and quiet-aged gerbils. *Journal of the Acoustical Society of America*. 1996;100:3275–3285.

[34] Rewerska A, Pawelczyk M, Rajkowska E, Politanski P, Sliwinska-Kowalska M. Evaluating D-methionine dose to attenuate oxidative stress-mediated hearing loss following overexposure to noise. *Eur. Arch. Otorhinolaryngol.* 2013;270:1513-1520.

[35] Fetoni AR, De Bartolo P, Eramo SLM, Rolesi R, Paciello F, Bergamini C, Fato R, Paludetti G, Petrosini L, Troiani D. Noise-induced hearing loss (NIHL) as a target of oxidative stress mediated damage: cochlear and cortical responses after an increase in antioxidant defensse. *J. Neurosci.* 2013;33:4011-4023.

[36] Chen YS, Tseng FY, Liu TC, Lin-Shiau SY, Hsu CJ. Involvement of nitric oxide generation in noise induced temporrary treshold shift in ginea pigs. *Hear Res.* 2005;203:94-100.

[37] Ohinata Y, Yamasoba T, Schacht J, Miller JM. Glutathione limits noise-induced hearing loss. *Hear Res.* 2000;146:28-34.

[38] Van Campen LE; Murphy WJ, Franks JR, Mathias PI, Toraason MA. Oxidative DNA damage is associated with intense noise exposure in the rat. *Hear Res*. 2002;164:29-38.

[39] Yamasoba T, Pourbakht A, Sakamoto T, Suzuki M. Ebselen prevents noise-induced excitotoxicity and temporary treshold shift. *Neurosci. Lett.* 2005;3:234-238.

[40] Hou F, Wang S, Zhai S, Hu Y, Yang W, He L. effects f alpha-tocopherol on noise induced hearing loss in guinea pigs. *Hear res.* 2003;2:1-8.

[41] Coleman JK, Kopke RD, Liu J, Ge X, Harper EA, Jones GA et al. Pharmacological rescue of noise-induced hearing loss using N-acetylcysteine and acetyl-L-carnitine. *Hear Res*. 2007;2:104-113.

[42] Fetoni AR, Ralli M, Sergi B, Parrilla C, Troiani D, Paludetti G. protective effects of N-acetylcysteine on noise-induced hearing loss in guinea pigs. *Acta Otorhinolaryngol. Ital.* 2009;29:70-75.

[43] Yilmaz T, Koccan EG, Besler HT, Yilmaz G, Gursel B. the role of oxidants and antioxidants in otitis media with effusion in children. *Otol. Laryngol. Head Neck Surg*. 2004;131:797803.

[44] Testa D, Guerra G, Marcuccio G, Landolfo PG, Motta G. Oxidative stress in chronic otitis media with effusion. *Acta Oto-Laryngologica.* 2012;132:834-837.

[45] Baysal E, Aksoy N, Kara F, Taysi S, Taskin A, Bilinc H, Cevik C, Celenk F, Kanhkama M. Oxidative stress in chronic otitis media. *Eur Arch. Otorhinolaryngol.* 2013;270:1203-1208.

[46] Cemek M, Dede S, Bayiroglu F, Caksen H, Cemek F, Yuca K. Oxidant and antioxidant levels in children with acute otitis media and tonsillitis: a comparative study. *Int. J. Ped. Otorhinolaryngol.* 2005;69:823-827.

[47] Singh R, Wangemann P. Free radical stress-mediated loss of Kcnj10 protein expresiion in stria vascularis contributes to deafness in Pendred syndrome mouse model. *Am. J. Physiol. Renal. Physiol.*2008;294:F139-F148.

[48] Calabrese V, Cornelius C, Maiolino L, Luca M, Chiaramonte R, Toscano MA, Serra A. Oxidative stress, redox homeostasis and cellular stress response in meniere's disease: role of vitagenes. *Neurochem. Res.* 2010;35:2208-2217.

[49] Donaldson JA. Snyder M. Otosclerosis. In: Cummings, CW, Frederickson JM, Harker LA, Krause, CJ, Schuller DE, eds. Otolaryngology-Head and Neck Surgery. St Louis, MI: Mosby-Year Book; 1993;2997-3016.

[50] Roland, PS. Samy, RN. Otosclerosis. In: Bailey J, Johnson J.T, Newlands S.D., eds. Head and Neck Surgery-Otolaryngology. Philadelphia, Lippincott Williams and Wilkins; 2006; 2126-2137.

[51] Menger, DJ, Tange, R. The etiology of otosclerosis: a review of the literature. *Clin. Otolaryngol.* 2008;28:112-120.

[52] Chole, R.A.; McKenna, M. Pathophysiology of otosclerosis. *Otol. Neurotol.* 2001;22:249-257.

[53] Thys M, Van Camp, G. Genetics of otosclerosis. *Otol. Neurotol.* 2009;30:1021-1032.

[54] Gordon MA. The genetics of otosclerosis: a review. *Am. J. Otol.* 1989;10:426-438.

[55] Topsakal V, Fransen E, Schmerber S, Declau F, Yung M, Gordts F, Van Camp G, Van de Heyning P. Audiometrics analyses confirm a cochlear component, disproportional to age, in stapedial otosclerosis. *Otol. Neurotol.* 2006;27:781-787.

[56] Gue RW, Yang LX, Li MQ, Liu B, Wang XM. Angiotensin II induces NF-κB activation in HUVEC via the p38MAPK pathway. *Peptides* 2006;27:3269-3275.

[57] Santos RAS, Campagnole-Santos MJ, Andrade SP. Angiotensin-(1-7): an update. *Regul. Pept.* 2000;91:45-62.

[58] De Gasparo, M, Catt KJ, Inagami T, Wright JW, Unger TH. International union of pharmacology. XXIII. The angiotensin II receptors. *Pharmacol. Rev.* 2000;52:415-472.

[59] Lamperter S, Kling L, Schrader M, Ziegler R, Pfeilschifter J. Effects of angiotensin II on bone cells in vitro. *J. Cell. Physiol.* 1998;175:89-98.

[60] Hiruma Y, Inoue A, Hirose S, Hagiwara H. Angiotensin II stimulates the proliferation of osteoblast-rich populations of cells from rat calvariae. *Biochem. Biophys. Res. Commun.* 1997; 230:176-178.

[61] Hagiwara H, Hiruma Y, Inoue A, Yamaguchi A, Hirose S. Deceleration by angiotensin II of the differentiation and bone formation of rat calvarial osteoblastic cells. *J. Endocrinol.* 1998;156:543-550.

[62] Hatton R, Stimpel M, Chambers TJ. Angiotensin II is generated from angiotensin I by bone cells and stimulates osteoclastic bone resorption in vitro. *J. Endocrinol.* 1997;152:5-10.

[63] Shimizu H, Nakagami H, Osako MK, Hanayama R, Kunugiza Y, Kizawa T, Tomita T, Yoshikawa H, Oihara T, Morishita R. Angiotensin II accelerates osteoporosis by activating osteoclasts. *FASEB J.* 2008;22:2465-2475.

[64] Asaba Y, Ito M, Fumoto T, Watanabe K, Fukuhara R, Takeshita S, Nimura Y, Ishida J, Fukamizu A, Ikeda K. Activation of renin-angiotensin system induces osteoporosis independently of hypertension. *J. Bone Miner. Res.* 2009;24:241-250.

[65] Imauchi Y, Jeunemaitre X, Boussion M, Ferrary, E, Sterkers O, Bozorg Grayeli A. Relation between renin-angiotensin-aldosterone system and otosclerosis: a genetic association and in vitro study. *Otol. Neurotol.* 2008;29:95-301.

[66] Rudić M, Nguyen C, Nguyen Y, Milković L, Zarković N, Sterkers O, Ferrary E, Bozorg Grayeli A. *Effect of angiotensin II on inflammation pathways in human primary bone cell cultures in otosclerosis. Audiol. Neurootol.* 2012;17:169-178.

[67] Lee SH, Goto T, Oe T. A novel 4-oxo-2(E)-nonenal-derived modification to angiotensin II: oxidative decarboxylation of N-terminal aspartic acid. *Chem. Res. Toxicol.* 2008;21: 2237-2244.

[68] Suzuki H, Frank GD, Utsunomiya H, Higuchi S, Eguchi S. Current understanding of the mechanism and role of ROS in angiotensin II signal transduction. *Curr. Pharm. Biotechnol.* 2006;7:81-86.

[69] Griendling KK, Ushio-Fukai M. Reactive oxygen species as mediators of angiotensin II signaling. *Regul. Pept.* 2000;91:21-27.

[70] Ohtsu H, Frank GD, Utsunomiya H, Eguchi S. Redox dependent protein kinase regulation by angiotensin II: mechanistic insights and its pathophysiology. *Antioxid. Redox. Signal.* 2005;7:1315-1326.

[71] Zhou C, Ziegler C, Birder LA, Stewart AFR, Levitan ES. Angiotensin II and stretch activate NADPH oxidase to destabilize cardiac Kv4.3 channel mRNA. *Cir. Res.* 2006;98:1040-1047.

[72] Borovic Sunjic S, Cipak A, Rabuzin F, Wildburger R, Zarkovic N. The influence of 4-hydroxy-2-nonenal on proliferation, differentiation and apoptosis of human osteosarcoma cells. *Biofactors.* 2005;24:141-148.

[73] Borovic S, Cipak A, Meinitzer A, Kejla Z, Perovic D, Waeg G, Zarkovic N. Differential sensitivity to 4-hydroxynonenal of normal and malignant mesenchymal cells. *Redox Rep.* 2007;12:50-54.

[74] Schaur RJ. Basic aspects of the biochemical reactivity of 4-hydroxynonenal. *Mol. Aspects Med.* 2003;24:149-159.

[75] Poli G, Schaur RJ. 4-hydroxynonenal in the pathomechanisms of oxidative stress. *IUBMB Life.* 2000; 50:315-321.

[76] Spickett CM, Wiswedel I, Siems W, Zarkovic K., Zarkovic N. Advances in methods for the determination of biologically relevant lipid peroxidation products. *Free. Radic. Res.* 2010; 44:1172-1202.

[77] Mrakovcic L, Wildburger R, Jaganjac M, Cindric M, Cipak A, Borovic-Sunjic S, Waeg G, Milankovic AM, Zarkovic N. Lipid peroxidation product 4-hydroxynonenal as factor of oxidative homeostasis supporting bone regeneration with bioactive glasses. *Acta Biochim. Pol.* 2010 ;57:173-178.

[78] Siems W, Grune T. Intracellular metabolism of 4-hydroxynonenal. *Mol. Aspects Med.* 2003;24:167-75.

[79] Rudić M, Milković L, Žarković K, Borović-Šunjić S, Sterkers O, Waeg G, Ferrary E, Bozorg Grayeli A, Žarković N. The effects of angiotensin II and the oxidative stress mediator 4-hydroxynonenal on human osteoblast-like cell growth: possible relevance to otosclerosis. *Free Radic. Biol. Med.* 2013;57:22-28.

[80] Uchida K. 4-hydroxy-2-nonenal: A product and mediator of oxidative stress. *Prog lip Res.* 2003;42:318-343.

[81] Awasthi S regulation of 4-hydroxynonenal mediated signaling by gluthatione S-transferases. *Methods Enzymol.* 2005;401:379-407.

[82] Bodo M, Carinci P, Venti G, Giammarioli M, donti E, Stabellini G, Paludetti G, Becchetti E, Glcosaminoglycan metabolism and cytokine

release in normal and otosclerotic human bone cells interleukin-1 treated. *Connect Tiss Res.* 1997;36:231-240.

[83] Grayeli AB, Escoubet B, Bichara M, Julien N, Silve C, Friedland G, Sterkers O, Ferrary E. Increased activity of the diastrophic dysplasia sulfate transporter in otosclerosis and its inhibition by sodium fluoride. *Otol. Neurotol.* 2003;24:854-862.

In: Oxidative Stress
Editor: Cassidy Croft
ISBN: 978-1-63117-578-7

Chapter 9

Oxidative Stress in Eales' Disease: An Update

R. Saravanan and K. N. Sulochana
R.S. Mehta Jain Department of Biochemistry and Cell Biology,
Vision Research Foundation, Sankara Nethralaya, Chennai, India

Abstract

Eales' Disease (ED) is an idiopathic, inflammatory, venous occlusive disease which primarily affects the peripheral retina of young adult males. The disease is more prevalent in the Indian subcontinent. ED was described by Henry Eales in 1880. Despite of the rigorous research effects, the etiopathogenesis of disease remains ambiguous. ED presents with inflammation, non-perfusion in peripheral veins, and retinal neovascularization. Loss of vision is due to repeated vitreous haemorrhage and its sequlae. Various research findings associate the disease with autoimmunity, oxidative stress and exposure to Mycobacterium *tuberculin* for the cause of the disease. There is no specific laboratory test available till date for its diagnosis. Therefore, the diagnosis of ED is arrived at by excluding other similar diseases. The scope of the present review is in highlighting the new findings on the strong association of oxidative stress with the disease.

There is strong evidence, for the involvement of oxidative stress and ED, both at the level of the local environment (i.e., vitreous humour and epiretinal membrane) and at systemic circulation. Elevated levels of thiobarbituric acid reactive substances (TBARS) were observed in serum, vitreous and monocytes samples of ED, as compared to controls. We have reported damage to DNA and proteins, from the accumulated 8-hydroxy-2'deoxyguanosine and 3-Nitrotyrosine in leucocytes respectively. Elevated levels of homocysteine (Hcy), and its metabolite thiolactone (HcyTL), are observed in the disease and are associated with the functional impairment of proteins due to homocysteinylation. Plasma Hcy and HcyTL levels are positively correlated with TBARS, while plasma glutathione (GSH) is negatively correlated with Hcy and HcyTL levels. Increased oxidative stress is also evidenced from the accumulation of advanced glycation and lipid oxidation end products in epiretinal membranes, observed in patients with ED who underwent vitrectomy. The antioxidant enzymes superoxide dismutase (SOD) and glutathione peroxidase (GPX) and GSH levels were found to be reduced in the vitreous and the erythrocytes of patients with ED. Most interestingly, significant increase in the levels of intra-cellular iron and copper in circulating monocytes was observed in the vitreous of patients afflicted with ED. A novel iron binding protein, 88 kDa in molecular weight and with a presumable antioxidant function has been characterized for its possible role in ED as a biomarker, and its involvement in its etiopathogenesis. Several iron binding proteins in circulation have been analyzed systematically and have been found to vary in ED, indicating a strong role for iron in the disease. A complete study into the significance of iron binding proteins in the mechanism of the disease is needed to decode their relevance in etiopathogenesis, and for subsequent application of this knowledge in therapeutics.

Keywords: Eales' Disease, TBARS, oxidative stress, homocysteine, iron, copper and 88 kDa protein

Introduction

Eales' Disease (ED) was first described by Henry Eales in 1880 and 1882 [1]. In current scenario ED is described as an inflammatory disease which primarily affects peripheral retina of the males in between second and fourth decades of life [2]. The prevalence is remains relatively higher in the Indian subcontinent although this disease is very rarely reported in the western countries [2]. In 50-90% of cases it affects both the eyes [3]. ED is presented with three hall mark clinical signs such as the inflammation in the peripheral retinal veins followed sheeting and sclerosis of the veins, non-perfusion in peripheral veins and retinal neovascularization. Recurrent vitreous haemorrhage from the neovascularized vessels is the major cause of tractional retinal detachment leading to loss of vision [4].

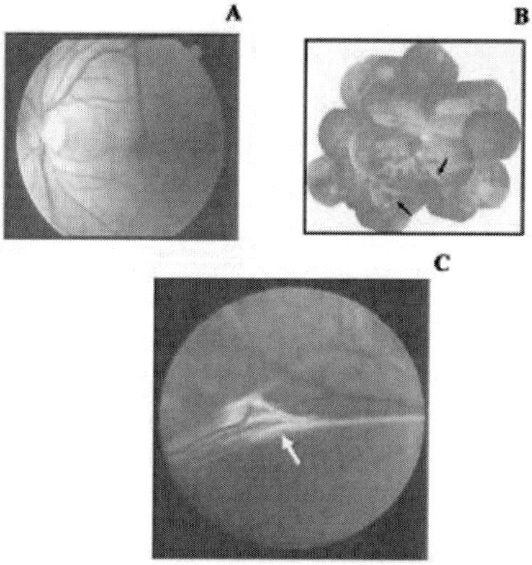

Figure 1. (A) Fundus picture of an healthy individual. (B) Montage fundus photograph of a patient with Eales' disease. Active inflammation of the retinal veins are denoted by arrow.(C) Fundus picture of a patients with ED in healed vasculitis stage, presenting with whitish fibrovascular sheahing.

Classification and assessment the severity of the disease is carried out as per new staging system described by Saxena et al. [5].

Table 1. New staging system for Eales's disease

Stage	Description
I	Periphlebitis of small (Ia) and large (Ib) caliber vessels with superficial retinal haemorrhages
IIa	Capillary nonperfusion
IIb	Revascularization elsewhere/of the disc
IIIa	Fibrovascular proliferation
IIIb	Vitreous haemorrhage
IVa	Traction/combined rhegmatogenous retinal detachment
IVb	Rubeosis iridis, neovascular glaucoma, complicated cataract, and optic atrophy

The natural course of the disease varies from remission to persistent progression to blindness [6]. Various research findings associated autoimmunity, oxidative stress and exposure to *Mycobacterium tuberculin* as the cause of the disease. Many investigators favoured association of tuberculosis with ED, owing to the presence of *Mycobacterium tuberculosis* gene in the surgically excised epiretinal membrane and in the vitreous from the patients with ED. There is no growth in culture *M. tuberculosis* from vitreous aspirates and it was considered as the hypersensitivity to MTB [7,8]. The association is debatable since prevalence disease in particular gender, age and geographical locations remains unexplained. In addition tubercular retinal perivasculitis, characterized with the presence of vitreous snowball opacities [9] which is not seen in ED. There is speculation on involvement of the auto immunity in ED. Majji et al. [10] reported presence of mast cells and eosinophils and Biswas et al. [11, 12] demonstrated infiltration of T lymphocytes in the epiretinal membrane. Hence immunological mechanism of Eales' retinopathy is not precisely understood and needs further studies.

Despite of the meticulous research in ascertaining disease etiopathogenesis, it remains elusive till date. The diagnosis of ED is made clinically by omitting various systemic and ocular diseases mimicking in the inflammatory and proliferative phases of the diseases. There is no specific laboratory test available till date for its diagnosis [13]. However clinical diagnosis the following tests listed in the table 2 were routinely carried out to exclude the other diseases mimicking ED.

The scope of the present review is in highlighting the findings on increased oxidative stress markers with decreased antioxidants levels and their strong association of with the disease.

Oxidative Stress

Cell efficiently and precisely maintains two major activities; first, energy level and second, redox status. Precise balance between the levels of free radicals and antioxidants are crucial, and any imbalance on either side is referred as oxidative or reductive stress. Reactive oxygen intermediates (ROI) are formed from consecutive one-electron reduction of oxygen (O_2).

Table 2. Investigations for Eales' Disease

To rule out the diseases mimic ED	Test
Leukemia and hematological diseases	Hemoglobin (Hb)
	Hemacrit(PCV)
	Total RBC count
	Total WBC count
	Differential WBC count
Sickle cell retinopathy	Sickle cell preparation
	Hemoglobin electrophoresis
Syphilis	Immunoglobin profile VDRL
	Treponema Pallidum Hemagglutination Test (TPHA)
Rheumatoid Arthritis	RA factor
SLE & other collagen diseases	Anti-nuclear antibody
Sarcoidosis	Serum angiotensin converting enzyme
	X-ray chest
Tuberculosis	Mantoux test
	Radiological tests
	X-ray chest
	PCR for *Mycobacterium tuberculosis*
	QuantiFERON - TB Gold IT test
Other tests:	Platelet count
	Erythrocyte sedimentation rate
	Reticulocyte count
	Plasma Glucose Fasting, Random and Postprandial
	Urea, creatinine
	Urine routine
	Basic coagulation test
	1. Bleeding time
	2. Clotting time
	3. Clot retraction
	4. Prothrombin time
	5. Partial Thromboplastin Time (PTT)
Tests to assess the oxidative status	
	TBARS
	Vitamins A, E,C
	Superoxide Dismutase, Glutathione peroxidase, Glutathione

ROI comprises of superoxide anion radical ($O_2^-/O_2^{\bullet-}$), hydrogen peroxide (H_2O_2), and hydroxyl radical ($OH^\bullet$). Reactive oxygen species (ROS) includes ROI, ozone (O_3) and singlet oxygen (1_2O). The reactive nitrogen intermediates (RNI) directly influence ROI levels are nitric oxide radical (NO or $NO^\bullet$), nitrogen dioxide radical ($^\bullet NO_2$), nitrite (NO_2^-), and peroxynitrite ($ONOO^-$) [14].

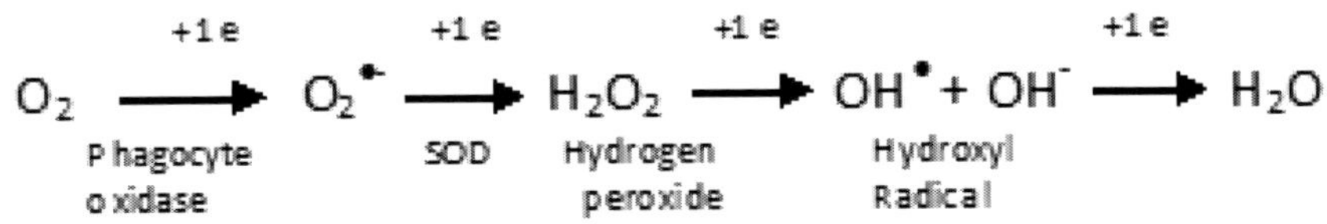

Figure 2. The step wise reduction of molecular oxygen via 1-electron transfers, producing ROS are shown in the above reaction.

NO and ROS acts as signalling molecules for various physiological functions. $O_2\cdot^-$ and NO$\cdot$ at a lower concentrations play important roles in the cellular signalling and regulation [15].

$O_2\cdot^-$ and H_2O_2 produced within mitochondria reacts beneficially to the cellular stresses induced by aging, such as mitochondrial dysfunction and DNA damage [16]. They also induce autophagy, inflammation and involved in the host defence and DNA base excision repair systems [17]. In higher levels these reactive molecules can cause lipid per-oxidation, DNA oxidation and glycoxidation. ROS/RNS are short-lived and their half-life ranges from nanoseconds to minutes (minute for stable oxidants) [18]. The concentrations of free radicals are maintained in narrow limits by harmonizing their production and removal rates by enzymatic antioxidants, such as glutathione peroxidase (GPx), catalase and superoxide dismutase (SOD), or nonenzymatic antioxidants like glutathione (GSH), urate, carotenoids, cysteine, bilirubin, and flavonoids and dietary vitamin C (Ascorbic acid) and vitamin E (α-Tocopherol).

The status oxidative stress can be analyzed by the biomarkers of oxidative or nitrosative stress/ damage isolated from tissues and biological fluids. Markers of oxidative/nitrosative stress either directly detected (electron spin resonance) or by measuring stable metabolites formed [19]. The bio-markers of protein oxidation includes a) carbonyl groups formation b) total protein thiol content c) oxidized aliphatic amino acid residues d) oxidized tryptophan and tyrosine residues, nitrated tyrosine residues [20]. Bio-markers of lipid peroxidation includes a) malondialdehyde (MDA) b) conjugated dienes c) lipofuscin d) lipid peroxides and e) isoprostanes. TBARS determination was used as most common biomarker in samples obtained from patients with ED [21].

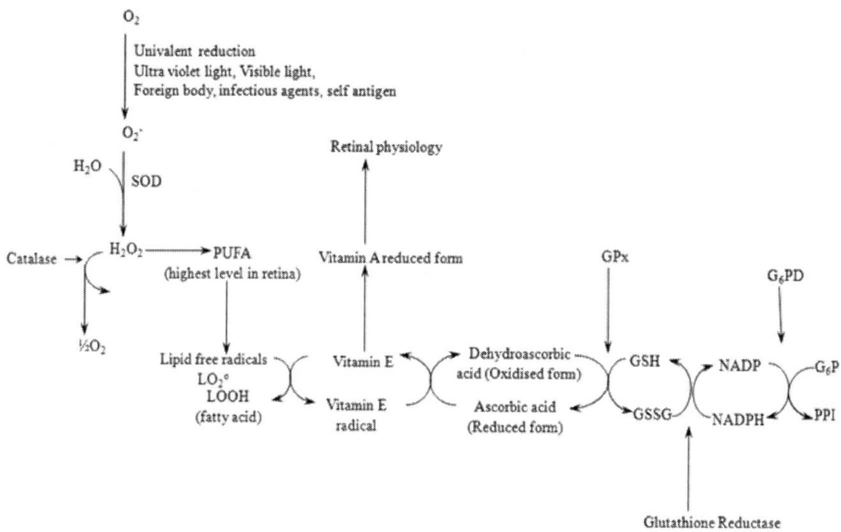

Figure 3. Schematic representation of antioxidant vitamins and GSH system in detoxification of ROS.

Free radical attack upon DNA generates a range of DNA lesions, including strand breaks and modified bases. $OH^{\bullet}$ attack on DNA leads to a large number of pyrimidine and purine derived base changes. 8-OHdG is considered to be the early biomarker to assess the intensity of free radical mediated DNA damage during inflammatory conditions [22].

Inflammation, angiogenesis and oxidative stress are shown to be interdependent in several human diseases [23]. ROS induced damage in ocular tissues reported in patients with uveitis [24]. In experimental autoimmune uveitis higher concentration peroxynitrite was noted in photoreceptors. It also correlated with the pathologic oxidation in photoreceptors [25]. Armstrong et al. proposed a mechanism wherein elevated lipid, induces the synthesis of cytokines and growth factors during neovascularization (NV) in retina [26]. The free radicals, induced stress and damage along with antioxidant levels in the ED are discussed in following headings.

Inflammation and Oxidative Stress in ED

During inflammation activated neutrophils and macrophages produces ROS and RNS [10,11]. The nitric oxide ($NO^{\bullet}$) and superoxide anion $O_2^{\bullet-}$ are produced in reactions catalyzed by the enzymes nitric oxide synthase and the NADPH oxidase respectively [27]. These $O_2^{\bullet-}$ and NO• radicals react to form peroxynitrite [28,29].·

$$O_2^{\bullet-} + NO\cdot \rightarrow ONO_2^-$$

ED is associated with raised levels of inflammatory marker C-reactive protein [30] and circulating interleukin (IL-6) [31] in the inflammatory stage. Monocytes and non classical inflammatory $CD16^+$ monocytes subset were found raised in ED. $CD16^+$ monocytes numbers correlated with the levels of serum proinflammatory cytokines such as TNF-α, IL-6, IFN-γ, and IL-1β [32,33]. CD 16^+ monocytes reported to be major source of secreted TNF-α in blood [34]. The $CD16^+$ monocytes can be crucial regulators with the secretion of proinflammatory cytokines that bring about the inflammatory process in the retina [32].

It was observed that disruption of blood retinal barrier, results in the migration of circulating phagocytes in to the retina of the patients with ED [35]. The inflammation may have resulted in ROI generation and oxidative stress in the retina of the ED patients.

Role of Iron in Oxidative and Nitrosative Stress in ED

A variety of oxidative stress bio-markers were assayed in serum, plasma, monocytes, epiretinal membrane and vitreous of patients with ED. $O_2^{\bullet-}$ can be metabolized to a lesser reactive hydrogen peroxide by two isoenzymes of Superoxide dismutases (SOD) namely CuZn-SOD and Mn-SOD [36]. Decreased SOD activity and GSH levels with increased TBARS were reported in the monocytes of ED patients [37].

H_2O_2 and O_2 are formed from dismutation $O_2\bullet^-$, catalyzed the SOD [29].

$$2\,O_2^{\bullet-} + 2H^+ \xrightarrow{\quad} \text{SOD} \quad H_2O_2 + O_2$$

H_2O_2 rapidly reacts with the other biomolecules is possible only when the reactions are catalyzed by metal-containing complexes or proteins [29]. Selvi et al. demonstrated raised serum Fe^{3+}/Fe^{2+} ratio in ED and it was found to be lowered after supplementation with antioxidant vitamins [38]. Fe^{3+} and • OH are formed when Fe^{2+} reacts with H_2O_2.

$$Fe^{2+} + H_2O_2 \xrightarrow{\text{Fenton reaction}} Fe^{3+} + {\bullet}OH + OH^-$$

The increased levels •OH free radicals were reported in the monocytes of patients with ED by using electron spin resonance spectrometry (ESR) [39].

•OH is a rapidly reacting molecule and a very strong oxidizing agent [40]. Its movement is diffusion limited [41] and it is able to react with all components of DNA bases as well as the deoxyribose backbone. DNA damage marker, 8-OHdG was found elevated by Gas chromatography-Mass spectrometry technique in the leucocytes patients with ED [37]. Treatment with iron chelator desferrioxamine, caused abrogation of •OH radical production, reduction in TBARS level, and increased SOD activity in monocytes from ED patients [39]. Desferrioxamine acts as powerful iron chelator, inhibits Fenton reaction and prevent the formation •OH. In oxidative stress or in induced inflammation, desferrioxamine treatment had ameliorated the complications of oxidative stress and mitigated the severity of inflammation [14]. From the above results we infer the •OH radical formed during an iron catalyzed reaction caused 8-OHdG and TBARS. Restoration of SOD activity after, vitamin supplement, desferrioxamine treatment suggests the exhaustion of antioxidants due to overproduction of free radicals.

In addition to the oxidative stress, nitrostative stress was also demonstrated in ED. In similar to ROS, RNS can also cause DNA damage, lipids and proteins. RNS can act as an oxidizing agent as well as nitrating agent [42]. Through the rapid reaction of NO• and $O_2^{\bullet -}$, peroxynitrite ($ONOO^-$) is formed which can result in oxidation, nitrosation (addition of $NO^{\cdot}$) or nitration (addition of NO_2). NO• is generated by three nitric oxide synthase (NOS) isoforms present in tissues: neuronal NOS (nNOS), endothelial NOS (eNOS), and inducible NOS (iNOS). For production of NO•, iron, O_2, and reducing equivalents, are required [43,44]. NO has high-affinity binding to heme and non-heme iron [45,46]. We found increased levels iron and copper by using atomic absorption spectrometry in monocytes of patients with ED compared to controls. TBARS levels were also reported to be higher along with increased iNOs protein expression and the 3 nitrotyrosine (NTYR) in the ED monocytes. NTYR is a stable product of tyrosine nitration, biomarker of protein damage induced by peroxynitrite and other reactive nitrogen species [47]. NO• is produced constitutively in nanomolar levels by eNOS and nNOS isoforms in the cells. iNOS expression in monocytes and macrophages is stimulated by inflammation and produces NO• in micromolar amounts [45]. After activation NO• can overwhelm Cu, Zn-SOD reaction and produce ONOO [45,48]. Peroxynitrite inactivates MnSOD by nitration of the critical tyrosine-34residue [49]. The presence of excess iron and copper in monocytes along with OH• radical, it is expected to damage biomolecules.

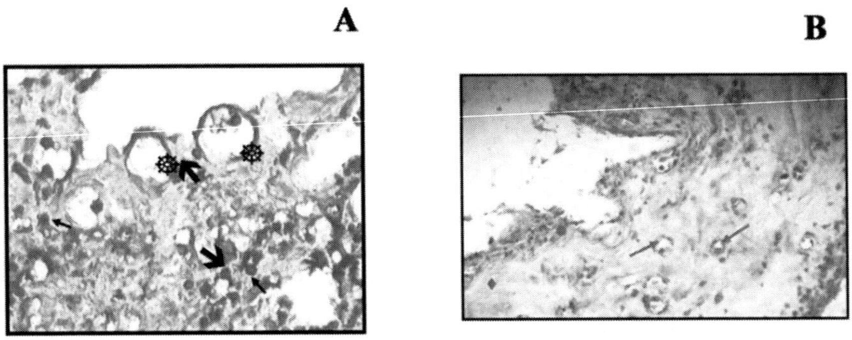

Figure 4. (A) iNOS immunolocalization in ERM. Strong expression could be noted in endothelium (arrow). (B) Immunolocalization of CML-AGE ERM-ED in the inflammatory cells is indicated by arrow (Mag. X 150).

Protein Damage in ED

Free radicals produced during oxidative stress can damage the peptide backbone, resulting in the generation of protein carbonyls. Accumulation of carbonyl groups on protein results in series of chemical modifications, which ultimately leads to the formation of advanced protein oxidation products (APO) or advanced glycation end products (AGE) [50]. AGE on binding with its receptor on retinal microvascular cells (endothelial cells or pericytes) or retinal pigment epithelial cells, has been shown to induce the expression of cytokines, growth factors and proteases, leads to retinal neovascularization [51]. Carbonyls compounds are generated by the oxidation of several amino acid side chains by the formation of schiff's base adducts between lysine, histidine, and cysteine residues and α,β-unsaturated aldehydes, forming advanced lipoxidation end products (ALEs). And by glycation / glycoxidation of Lys amino groups, forming advanced glycation end product [52]. Protein carbonyl group content reduced antioxidants correlates severity of ED [53]. The AGE accumulation in ED patients mainly in the form of CML [54] occurred in spite of their normo glycemic status. Since CML and pentosidine formation are closely linked to oxidative processes. CML may be formed from the lipid peroxidation (metal-catalyzed oxidation) as well as glycoxidation reactions [52].

Homocysteine Mediated Damage

Recently ED patients increased plasma homocysteine, homocysteine-thiolactone, TBARS, and decreased GSH levels [55]. Homocysteinemia may leads to production of reactive oxygen species such as H_2O_2, nitric oxide, the superoxide anion can form powerful oxidant peroxynitrite [56]. These sequence of events impairs the antioxidant defenses [57]. Homocysteine-thiolactone with reacts with proteins results in homocysteinylation of protein lysine residues [55]. This leads to protein damage, and is associated with the functional impairment of in ED. It could be one of the etiological factors for ED [58].

Serum Protein Marker 88 kDa in ED

The 88 kDa, protein was purified using HPLC, was characterized to be a glycoprotein, present in the vitreous, ERM and serum of ED patients. The protein was sequenced by in the N- terminal end and some of internal regions by automated Edman's degradation chemistry. The sequences obtained revealed no match in the protein and DNA database search. It shared common properties with haptoglobin including the electrophoretic mobility at α2 globulin region, positive acute phase protein, hemoglobin binding, and agglutination of RBC. The molecular weight of haptoglobin is 44 kDa. It has anti TBARS activity and 8% thiols by mass and oxidized ferrous ion to ferric ion and is a ferro oxidase [59, 60]. Further investigations are required to understand the role of the protein in the etiopathogensis of ED. Its identity interactive partners and its role in inflammation and angiogenesis are ongoing.

Increased ROS and Weakened Antioxidant Systems

Cytosol, the nuclear and mitochondrial matrices and extracellular fluids are protected by enzymatic and non-enzymatic antioxidant defence stratergies. Vitamin A, Tocopherols, carotenoids, and flavonoids in the lipid phase, While Ascorbate, glutathione, bilirubin, and thiols in the aqueous phase acts as antioxidant molecules effectively reinforcing the defense provided by the enzymes superoxide dismutase, catalase and glutathione peroxidases. Researchers had reported the increased level of the TBARS with reduced levels of the antioxidants in ED [62-66]. Bhooma *et al.* had reported elevated TBARS level in erythrocytes as well as the decreased levels of vitamin E, vitamin C, vitamin A in serum of both the active and in the healed perivasculitis stages of ED [62]. Other studies had shown supplementation with vitamin E and C had lowered the TBARS levels and Fe^{3+}/Fe^{2+} ratio; And also increased total antioxidant capacity (TAC) and vitamins levels in active vasculitis and healed vasculitis stages of ED [38]. Oral supplementation of vitamins E, C, and A, beta carotene; Cu; Zn; and Se for 3months, had significantly decreased the level of TBARS. It also increased the SOD activity, and GSH levels in the platelets from ED patients [63-65]. The clinical correlation or the benifical effects is not yet available.

Future Directions

Iron and copper are essential in the human body for the synthesis of variety of enzymes and other proteins that are involved in respiration, redox reactions and other metabolic pathways. Yet these two metals are potentially dangerous by their ability to participate in one-electron transfer reactions. This enables them to be powerful catalysts of autoxidation reactions. For instance, conversion of H_2O_2 to $OH^{\bullet}$ and decomposition of lipid peroxides to reactive peroxyl and alkoxyl radical. It is not only free metal ions that are catalytic. Haem and certain haem proteins can decompose lipid peroxides and interact with H_2O_2 to cause extensive structural and functional damage to the biomolecules. Therefore it is necessary to regulate the metabolism of these metal ions carefully, which are vital for physiological functions but are dangerous when their level exceeds the critical limit. The proteins which are involved directly or indirectly involved in regulation of iron metabolism are transferrin, haptoglobin (Hp) and Haemopexion (Hpx). The ferroprotein retains or exports ferric iron taken in dueodenum divalent metal transportor1 based on requirements. Ferric iron retained by the entrocytes in ferritin form. The exported iron is oxidized to the ferrous iron by hephastatin or ceruloplasmin and transported by transferrin. Ferroprotein is regulated by the hepicidin. Heme is transported by the heme-responsive gene 1 and oxidized by heme oxygenase 1 (HO-1) to produce ferrous iron.

Acknowledgment

We thank M Bharathselvi, for her support and help in editing and proof reading the manuscript.

References

[1] Eales H. Retinal hemorrhages associated with epistaxis and constipation. *Brim Med Rev* 1880;9:262-73.

[2] Das T, Biswas J, Kumar A, Nagpal PN, Namperumalsamy P, Patnaik B, et al. Eales' disease. *Indian J Ophthalmol* 1994;42(1):3-18.

[3] Biswas J, Ravi RK, Naryanasamy A, Kulandai LT, Madhavan HN. Eales' disease - current concepts in diagnosis and management. *J Ophthalmic Inflamm Infect*;3(1):11.

[4] Spitznas M, Meyer-Schwickerath G, Stephan B. The clinical picture of Eales' disease. *Albrecht Von Graefes Arch Klin Exp Ophthalmol* 1975;194(2):73-85.

[5] Saxena S, Kumar D. New classification system-based visual outcome in Eales' disease. *Indian J Ophthalmol* 2007;55(4):267-9.

[6] Kalsi R, Patnaik B. The developing features of phlebitis retinae (a vertical study). *Indian J Ophthalmol* 1979; 27: 87

[7] Therese KL, Deepa P, Therese J, Bagyalakshmi R, Biswas J, Madhavan HN. Association of mycobacteria with Eales' disease. *Indian J Med Res* 2007;126(1):56-62.

[8] Singh R, Toor P, Parchand S, Sharma K, Gupta V, Gupta A. Quantitative polymerase chain reaction for Mycobacterium tuberculosis in so-called Eales' disease. *Ocul Immunol Inflamm*;20(3):153-7.

[9] Gupta A, Gupta V, Arora S, Gupta A, Gupta V, Arora S, Dogra MR, Bambery P. PCR-positive tubercular retinal vasculitis Dogra MR, Bambery P. PCR-positive tubercular retinal vasculitis: clinical characteristics and management. *Retina* 2001;21(5):435-44.

[10] Forman HJ, Torres M. Redox signaling in macrophages. *Mol Aspects Med* 2001;22(4-5):189-216.

[11] Kobayashi SD, Voyich JM, Burlak C, DeLeo FR. Neutrophils in the innate immune response. *Arch Immunol Ther Exp (Warsz)* 2005;53(6):505-17.

[12] Majji AB, Vemuganti GK, Shah VA, Singh S, Das T, Jalali S. A comparative study of epiretinal membranes associated with Eales' disease: a clinicopathologic evaluation. *Eye (Lond)* 2006;20(1):46-54.

[13] Biswas J, Rao NA. Epiretinal membrane in Eales' disease and other vascular retinopathies. *Invest Ophllmlmol Vis Sci* 1990; **31**(Suppl): 369.

[14] Barry Halliwell JMCG, editor. *Free radicals in biology and medicine.* 4 ed. New York: Oxford University Press, 2007.

[15] Droge W. Free radicals in the physiological control of cell function. *Physiol Rev* 2002;82(1):47-95.

[16] Hekimi S, Lapointe J, Wen Y. Taking a "good" look at free radicals in the aging process. *Trends Cell Biol*;21(10):569-76.

[17] Scherz-Shouval R, Elazar Z. Regulation of autophagy by ROS: physiology and pathology. *Trends Biochem Sci*;36(1):30-8.

[18] Winkler BS, Boulton ME, Gottsch JD, Sternberg P. Oxidative damage and age-related macular degeneration. *Mol Vis* 1999;5:32.

[19] Valko M, Leibfritz D, Moncol J, Cronin MT, Mazur M, Telser J. Free radicals and antioxidants in normal physiological functions and human disease. *Int J Biochem Cell Biol* 2007;39(1):44-84.

[20] Dalle-Donne I, Rossi R, Colombo R, Giustarini D, Milzani A. Biomarkers of oxidative damage in human disease. *Clin Chem* 2006;52(4):601-23.

[21] Tsukahara H. Current status of redox markers in immunological and inflammatory diseases. *Rinsho Byori* 2005;53(8):759-67.

[22] Dizdaroglu M. Chemical determination of free radical-induced damage to DNA. *Free Radic Biol Med* 1991;10(3-4):225-42.

[23] Jackson JR, Seed MP, Kircher CH, Willoughby DA, Winkler JD. The codependence of angiogenesis and chronic inflammation. *Faseb J* 1997;11(6):457-65.

[24] Rao NA, Romero JL, Fernandez MA, Sevanian A, Marak GE, Jr. Role of free radicals in uveitis. *Surv Ophthalmol* 1987;32(3):209-13.

[25] Wu GS, Zhang J, Rao NA. Peroxynitrite and oxidative damage in experimental autoimmune uveitis. *Invest Ophthalmol Vis Sci* 1997;38(7):1333-9.

[26] Armstrong D, Ueda T, Ueda T, Aljada A, Browne R, Fukuda S, et al. Lipid hydroperoxide stimulates retinal neovascularization in rabbit retina through expression of tumor necrosis factor-alpha, vascular endothelial growth factor and platelet-derived growth factor. *Angiogenesis* 1998;2(1):93-104.

[27] Jarasch ED, Bruder G, Heid HW. Significance of xanthine oxidase in capillary endothelial cells. *Acta Physiol Scand Suppl* 1986;548:39-46.

[28] Kobayashi SD, Voyich JM, Burlak C, DeLeo FR. Neutrophils in the innate immune response. *Arch Immunol Ther Exp (Warsz)* 2005;53(6):505-17

[29] Bogdan C. Nitric oxide and the immune response. *Nat Immunol* 2001;2(10):907-16.

[30] Sandeep Saxena DK, Sangeeta Kapoor, Amita Jain. C-reactive protein in eales disease. *Annals of Ophthalmology* Winter 2002;34(4):179-180.

[31] Saxena S, Pant AB, Khanna VK, Agarwal AK, Singh K, Kumar D, et al. Interleukin-1 and tumor necrosis factor-alpha: novel targets for immunotherapy in Eales disease. *Ocul Immunol Inflamm* 2009;17(3):201-6.

[32] Sen A, Chowdhury IH, Mukhopadhyay D, Paine SK, Mukherjee A, Mondal LK, et al. Increased Toll-like receptor-2 expression on nonclassic CD16+ monocytes from patients with inflammatory stage of Eales' disease. *Invest Ophthalmol Vis Sci*; 2011; 52(9):6940-8.

[33] Gong Y, Wei SH, Zhang MN, Jin X, Hou BK, Wang D. Serum interferon-gamma/interleukin-4 imbalance in patients with Eales' disease. *Clin Exp Optom*; 2010;93(4):228-32.

[34] Belge KU, Dayyani F, Horelt A, Siedlar M, Frankenberger M, Frankenberger B, et al. The proinflammatory CD14+CD16+DR++ monocytes are a major source of TNF. *J Immunol* 2002;168(7):3536-42.

[35] Lightman S, Greenwood J. Effect of lymphocytic infiltration on the blood-retinal barrier in experimental autoimmune uveoretinitis. *Clin Exp Immunol* 1992;88(3):473-7.

[36] McCord JM, Fridovich I. Superoxide dismutase. An enzymic function for erythrocuprein (hemocuprein). *J Biol Chem* 1969;244(22):6049-55.

[37] Rajesh M, Ramesh A, Ravi PE, Balakrishnamurthy P, Coral K, Punitham R, et al. Accumulation of 8-hydroxydeoxyguanosine and its

relationship with antioxidant parameters in patients with Eales' disease: implications for antioxidant therapy. *Curr Eye Res* 2003;27(2):103-10

[38] Selvi R, Angayarkanni N, Bharathselvi M, Sivaramakrishna R, Anisha T, Jyotirmoy B, et al. Increase in Fe^{3+}/Fe^{2+} ratio and iron-induced oxidative stress in Eales disease and presence of ferrous iron in circulating transferrin. *Curr Eye Res* 2007;32(7-8):677-83.

[39] Rajesh M, Sulochana KN, Ramakrishnan S, Biswas J, Manoharan PT. Iron chelation abrogates excessive formation of hydroxyl radicals and lipid peroxidation products in monocytes of patients with Eales' disease: direct evidence using electron spin resonance spectroscopy. *Curr Eye Res* 2004;28(6):399-407.

[40] Koppenol WH, Stanbury DM, Bounds PL. Electrode potentials of partially reduced oxygen species, from dioxygen to water. *Free Radic Biol Med*;49(3):317-22.

[41] Buxton GV, Greenstock CL, Helman WP, Ross AB. Critical Review of Rate Constants for Reactions of Hydrated Electrons, Hydrogen Atoms and Hydroxyl Radicals (.OH/.O−) in Aqueous Solution. *Journal of Physical and Chemical Reference Data* 1988;17 513–886.

[42] Stamler JS. Redox signaling: nitrosylation and related target interactions of nitric oxide. *Cell* 1994;78(6):931-6.

[43] Werner ER, Gorren AC, Heller R, Werner-Felmayer G, Mayer B. Tetrahydrobiopterin and nitric oxide: mechanistic and pharmacological aspects. *Exp Biol Med (Maywood)* 2003;228(11):1291-302.

[44] Gorren AC, Mayer B. Nitric-oxide synthase: a cytochrome P450 family foster child. *Biochim Biophys Acta* 2007;1770(3):432-45.

[45] Toledo JC, Jr., Augusto O. Connecting the chemical and biological properties of nitric oxide. *Chem Res Toxicol*;25(5):975-89.

[46] Lancaster JR, Jr., Hibbs JB, Jr. EPR demonstration of iron-nitrosyl complex formation by cytotoxic activated macrophages. *Proc Natl Acad Sci U S A* 1990;87(3):1223-7.

[47] Rajesh M, Sulochana KN, Punitham R, Biswas J, Lakshmi S, Ramakrishnan S. Involvement of oxidative and nitrosative stress in promoting retinal vasculitis in patients with Eales' disease. *Clin Biochem* 2003;36(5):377-85.

[48] Beckman JS, Koppenol WH. Nitric oxide, superoxide, and peroxynitrite: the good, the bad, and ugly. *Am J Physiol* 1996;271(5 Pt 1):C1424-37

[49] Yamakura F, Taka H, Fujimura T, Murayama K. Inactivation of human manganese-superoxide dismutase by peroxynitrite is caused by exclusive

nitration of tyrosine 34 to 3-nitrotyrosine. *J Biol Chem* 1998;273(23):14085-9.

[50] Miyata T, Kurokawa K, Van Ypersele De Strihou C. Advanced glycation and lipoxidation end products: role of reactive carbonyl compounds generated during carbohydrate and lipid metabolism. *J Am Soc Nephrol* 2000;11(9):1744-52.

[51] Stitt AW. Advanced glycation: an important pathological event in diabetic and age related ocular disease. *Br J Ophthalmol* 2001;85(6):746-53.

[52] Fu S, Davies MJ, Stocker R, Dean RT. Evidence for roles of radicals in protein oxidation in advanced human atherosclerotic plaque. *Biochem J* 1998;333 (Pt 3):519-25.

[53] Rajesh M, Sulochana KN, Coral K, Punitham R, Biswas J, Babu K, et al. Determination of carbonyl group content in plasma proteins as a useful marker to assess impairment in antioxidant defense in patients with Eales' disease. *Indian J Ophthalmol* 2004;52(2):139-44.

[54] Swamy-Mruthinti S, Miriam KC, Kumar SK, Biswas J, Ramakrishnan S, Nagaraj RH, et al. Immunolocalization and quantification of advanced glycation end products in retinal neovascular membranes and serum: a possible role in ocular neovascularization. *Curr Eye Res* 2002;25(3):139-45.

[55] Bharathselvi M, Biswas J, Selvi R, Coral K, Narayanasamy A, Ramakrishnan S, et al. Increased homocysteine, homocysteine-thiolactone, protein homocysteinylation and oxidative stress in the circulation of patients with Eales' disease. *Ann Clin Biochem*;50(Pt 4):330-8.

[56] Loscalzo J. The oxidant stress of hyperhomocyst(e)inemia. *J Clin Invest* 1996;98(1):5-7.

[57] Nishio E, Watanabe Y. Homocysteine as a modulator of platelet-derived growth factor action in vascular smooth muscle cells: a possible role for hydrogen peroxide. *Br J Pharmacol* 1997;122(2):269-74.

[58] Jakubowski H. Pathophysiological consequences of homocysteine excess. *J Nutr* 2006;136(6 Suppl):1741S-1749S.

[59] Sulochana KN, Rajesh M, Ramakrishnan S. Purification and characterization of a novel 88 kDa protein from serum and vitreous of patients with Eales' disease. *Exp Eye Res* 2001;73(4):547-55.

[60] Rajesh M, Sulochana KN, Sundaram AL, Krishnakumar S, Biswas J, Ramakrishnan S. Presence of a 88 kDa Eales protein in uveitis,

tuberculosis, leprosy and rheumatoid arthritis. *Med Sci Monit* 2003;9(2):CR95-9.

[61] Dalle-Donne I, Rossi R, Colombo R, Giustarini D, Milzani A. Biomarkers of oxidative damage in human disease. *Clin Chem* 2006;52(4):601-23.

[62] Bhooma V, Sulochana KN, Biswas J, Ramakrishnan S. Eales' disease: accumulation of reactive oxygen intermediates and lipid peroxides and decrease of antioxidants causing inflammation, neovascularization and retinal damage. *Curr Eye Res* 1997;16(2):91-5.

[63] Srivastava P, Saxena S, Khanna VK, Kumar D, Nath R, Seth PK. Raised platelet thiobarbituric acid-reacting substances in proliferative Eales' disease. *Indian J Ophthalmol* 2000;48(4):307-9.

[64] Saxena S, Srivastava P, Khanna VK. Antioxidant supplementation improves platelet membrane fluidity in idiopathic retinal periphlebitis (Eales' disease). *J Ocul Pharmacol Ther*;26(6):623-6.

[65] Saxena S, Srivastava P, Kumar D, Khanna VK, Seth PK. Decreased platelet membrane fluidity in retinal periphlebitis in Eales' disease. *Ocul Immunol Inflamm* 2006;14(2):113-6.

Index

B

C

D

E

F

G

H

I

J

K

L

M

N

O

P

Q

R

S

T

U

V

W

X

Y

Z